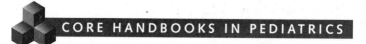
PEDIATRIC ENDOCRINOLOGY

W9-AEM-565

GRACE LIBRARY CARLOW COLLEGE
PITTSBURGH PA 15213

CORE HANDBOOKS IN PEDIATRICS

PEDIATRIC ENDOCRINOLOGY

Dennis M. Styne, M.D.

Rumsey Professor of Pediatric Endocrinology
University of California Davis
Chair Emeritus of Pediatrics
University of California Davis Medical Center
Sacramento, California

Ref.
RJ
418
S767
2004

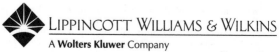

LIPPINCOTT WILLIAMS & WILKINS

A **Wolters Kluwer** Company

Philadelphia · Baltimore · New York · London
Buenos Aires · Hong Kong · Sydney · Tokyo

CATALOGUED

Acquisitions Editor: Timothy Y. Hiscock
Developmental Editor: Nicole T. Wagner
Production Editor: Emmeline A. Parker
Manufacturing Manager: Colin Warnock
Cover Designer: Jeane Norton
Compositor: Circle Graphics
Printer: R.R. Donnelley and Associates

© 2004 by **LIPPINCOTT WILLIAMS & WILKINS**
530 Walnut Street
Philadelphia, PA 19106 USA
LWW.com

All rights reserved. This book is protected by copyright. No part of
this book may be reproduced in any form or by any means, including
photocopying, or utilized by any information storage and retrieval system
without written permission from the copyright owner, except for brief
quotations embodied in critical articles and reviews. Materials appearing
in this book prepared by individuals as part of their official duties as U.S.
government employees are not covered by the above-mentioned copyright.

Printed in the USA

Library of Congress Cataloging-in-Publication Data

ISBN: 0-7817-3642-0

Care has been taken to confirm the accuracy of the information presented
and to describe generally accepted practices. However, the author and
publisher are not responsible for errors or omissions or for any consequences
from application of the information in this book and make no warranty,
expressed or implied, with respect to the currency, completeness, or accuracy
of the contents of the publication. Application of this information in a
particular situation remains the professional responsibility of the
practitioner.

The author and publisher have exerted every effort to ensure that drug
selection and dosage set forth in this text are in accordance with current
recommendations and practice at the time of publication. However, in view of
ongoing research, changes in government regulations, and the constant flow
of information relating to drug therapy and drug reactions, the reader is
urged to check the package insert for each drug for any change in indications
and dosage and for added warnings and precautions. This is particularly
important when the recommended agent is a new or infrequently employed
drug.

Some drugs and medical devices presented in this publication have Food
and Drug Administration (FDA) clearance for limited use in restricted
research settings. It is the responsibility of the health care provider to
ascertain the FDA status of each drug or device planned for use in their
clinical practice.

10 9 8 7 6 5 4 3 2 1

To my loving wife Donna, and to my children,
Rachel, Jonathan, Juliana, and Aaron.

♣ Contents

Preface ix

Acknowledgment xi

1. Introduction to Pediatric Endocrinology:
   The Endocrine System 1

2. The Evaluation of a Child or Adolescent with
   Possible Endocrine Disease 11

3. Disorders of the Hypothalamic–Pituitary Axis 17

4. Disorders of Vasopressin Metabolism 26

5. Abnormal Growth 44

6. Disorders of the Thyroid Gland 83

7. Disorders of Calcium Metabolism 110

8. Disorders of Sexual Differentiation 134

9. Disorders of Puberty 159

10. Disorders of the Adrenal Gland 196

11. Diabetes Mellitus 218

12. Obesity 248

13. Hypoglycemia 266

14. Endocrine Tumors of Childhood 287

15. Guide to Pediatric Endocrine Emergencies 295

16. Medications for Pediatric Endocrinology 306

17. Laboratory Values for Pediatric Endocrinology 314

Subject Index 359

♣ Preface

Thirteen years is quite a long gestation, but that is the period of time between the publication of the precursor to this book and its growth and development into its present incarnation. So much has happened in the rapidly advancing world of endocrinology that only a few basic concepts from the previous text have been retained. Over the years, many colleagues have inquired as to when an updated version might be published. I hope they find this handbook worth the wait!

Pediatric Endocrinology is in no way meant to replace the outstanding larger texts to which I refer the reader in the Suggested Reading section at the conclusion of each chapter. This book is for the practitioner puzzling over the approach to a child who has entered the examination room and seems to have an endocrine disorder, and for the student or house staff with a world of medicine to confront and not enough time to consult more comprehensive texts at that moment. This handbook is for anyone who wishes to have a consultation with a pediatric endocrinologist *in absentia*. I hope this book helps the reader to evaluate and treat the more straightforward issues in pediatric endocrinology, and possibly avoid an expensive and inconvenient consultation that, in fact, may not be indicated. Of course, there are complex issues within pediatric endocrinology that cannot be mastered without adequate experience; managing a baby with ambiguous genitalia is only one example of a subject that I have introduced in this text to allow the reader to understand the basics, but this handbook cannot possibly cover the complexities in their entirety. There is no claim that this book will give the reader the expertise of a pediatric endocrinologist; for that, a three-year fellowship is only the first step.

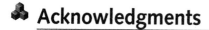 Acknowledgments

I am indebted to all my coworkers in the wide field of pediatric endocrinology, whose wisdom in print or in words I value and have tried to reflect in this handbook. This book grew out of my teaching and clinical experiences, and I am grateful to the uncounted students, house staff and postgraduate practitioners I have encountered in the last 25 years that I have pursued this field. I especially acknowledge the ever patient Tim Hiscock and Nicole Wagner of Lippincott Williams & Wilkins who took on this project and shepherded it through to the end. I am grateful to my first teachers of this field, Melvin M. Grumbach, Selna Kaplan, and Felix Conte at the University of California, San Francisco. They deserve much of the credit for any of my accomplishments, as they started me on my career.

1 ♣ Introduction to Pediatric Endocrinology: The Endocrine System

The endocrine system regulates reproduction, growth and development, homeostasis of the organism or maintenance of the internal environment, and the production, storage, and utilization of energy. The endocrine system originally was understood to regulate metabolism by biochemical messengers or hormones that were released from specialized organs (glands) into the general circulation so that they could act at a distance. Thus, hormones were classically defined as circulating messengers, with the location of their action far from the site of secretion. Hormone action also may be *paracrine* (acting on adjacent neighboring cells to the cell of origin of the hormone by diffusion) or *autocrine* (acting on the cell of origin of the hormone itself by diffusion); often agents acting in these ways are called factors rather than hormones. Indeed, these factors (e.g., growth factors) may be produced in most cells of the body rather than discrete glands (Fig. 1-1). The effects of hormones may be generally considered as directed toward the processes of cell differentiation, cell growth, and metabolism of the cell and the organism.

In the past, most of the endocrine glands appeared to be controlled by the pituitary gland, which was therefore considered to be "the master gland." The discovery of the hypophysiotropic hormones of the hypothalamus and their role in the control of pituitary secretion made it clear that a higher level of control of these functions exists. Now it is recognized that various regions of the brain regulate the hypothalamus and that many of the hormones of the pituitary-hypothalamic axis, or molecules that share much of their structure and function, also are found in the gastrointestinal tract and other tissues throughout the body, including the placenta. Overlap occurs between the control of the endocrine system and the nervous system; hormone secretion can be regulated by nerve cells, and endocrine agents can serve as neural messengers. Further, the endocrine system is regulated by factors important in the immune system (e.g., cytokines interact with the secretion of glucocorticoids, which then exert an influence on inflammation).

Hormones are often regulated in a feedback loop, so that the production of a hormone is controlled by its effect; for example, corticotropin-releasing factor (CRF) stimulates adrenocorticotropic hormone (ACTH) to produce cortisol, which in turn feeds back to suppress CRF and ACTH production so that equilibrium is reached and serum cortisol and ACTH remain in the normal range (Fig. 1-2). The set point of the equilibrium may change with development; in prepuberty, small amounts of sex steroids strongly suppress gonadotropin secretion, but during pubertal development, the sensitivity of this feedback loop decreases. Thus increased sex steroid production that causes the ensuing physical changes of puberty occurs without these sex steroids suppressing gonadotropin

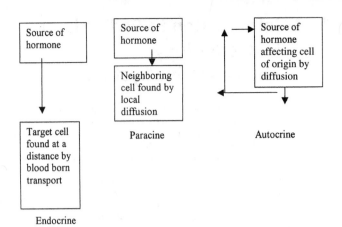

Fig. 1-1. Endocrine, paracrine, and autocrine effects.

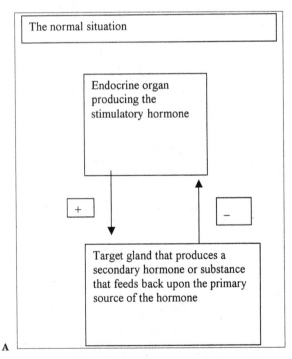

Fig. 1-2. Logic of evaluation of feedback loops. A: The normal situation.

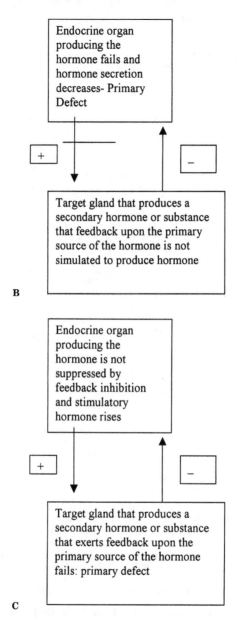

Fig. 1-2. (continued) B: Secondary or tertiary defect: stimulatory and target-hormone secretion decrease, and serum hormones decrease. C: Primary defect: stimulatory hormone increases, but target hormone secretion and serum concentrations decrease.

Table 1-1. The differential diagnosis of primary versus secondary or tertiary endocrine disease or autonomous function

Defects in hormone secretion		
Tropic hormone concentration (eg. ACTH)	Disorder	Target gland hormone concentration (eg. Cortisol)
High	Primary disorder of target gland (eg. Addison Disease)	Low
Normal	Normal function	Normal
Low	Secondary or tertiary disorder of origin of trophic hormones (eg. pituitary tumor decreasing ACTH secretion or hypothalamic tumor decreasing CRF secretion)	Low
Increase in hormone secretion		
Low	Autonomous function of the target gland hormone (eg. Autonomous Adrenal tumor)	High
High	Autonomous production of trophic hormone (eg. ACTH secreting pituitary tumor)	High

secretion, as would occur at a similar level of sex steroid secretion in the prepubertal state. A clinician may deduce the level of an endocrine defect in the system after measuring the serum concentrations of hormones at various steps of the process [e.g., a low serum cortisol and high adrenocortical-stimulating hormone (ACTH) indicates a primary defect at the level of the adrenal gland, whereas a low serum cortisol along with a low ACTH indicates a disorder of the pituitary gland or the hypothalamus (Table 1-1)].

ENDOCRINE DISORDERS GENERALLY MANIFEST IN ONE OF FOUR WAYS

1. By excess hormone effect [e.g., in Cushing syndrome, an excess of glucocorticoid is present; if the excess is secondary

to autonomous glucocorticoid secretion by a target organ (cortisol secretion by the adrenal gland), the trophic hormone ACTH will be suppressed].
2. By deficient hormone: in glucocorticoid deficiency, inadequate cortisol is present; if the deficiency is at the target organ (the adrenal gland), the trophic hormone (ACTH) will be elevated.
3. By an abnormal response of end organ to hormone: in pseudohypoparathyroidism, resistance is found to parathyroid hormone (PTH), and so PTH is elevated.
4. By gland enlargement that may cause effects as a result of size rather than function; with a large nonfunctioning pituitary adenoma, abnormal visual fields and other neurologic signs and symptoms will result, even though no hormone is produced by the tumor.

Tumors of endocrine organs (or even other organs such as the ectopic elaboration of ACTH from an oat cell carcinoma of the lung) may produce hormones. Endocrine disorders may be revealed by the response of various organs to an excess or deficiency of various hormones well before the size of the endocrine tumor makes it apparent.

Several classes of hormones and their respective receptors are found.

Peptide hormones are produced by various endocrine organs or in the cells of certain neoplasms. Peptide hormones act through specific cell-membrane receptors; the receptors consist of an extracellular domain, which directly interacts with the ligand hormone, a transmembrane domain that connects actions outside the cell with the actions destined to occur within the cell, and the intracellular domain that contains the cellular constituents that actually cause various biologic actions (Fig. 1-3). These internal cellular actions include phosphorylation of peptides or proteins and the generation of other molecules called second messengers that cause a cascade of events, ultimately leading to the metabolic action predicted by the presence of the hormone on the receptor (Fig. 1-4). G protein–coupled receptors [including ACTH, vasopressin, luteinizing hormone (LH), follicle-stimulating hormone (FSH), TSH, gonadotropin-releasing hormone (GnRH), thyroid-releasing factor (TRF), growth hormone–releasing factor (GHRH), CRF, somatotropin-releasing inhibiting factor (SRIF), glucagon, PTH receptors] have seven transmembrane domains and a G protein complex that regulates the second messengers such as calcium and cyclic adenosine monophosphate (AMP). Cytokine receptors for GH, prolactin, and leptin consist of an extracellular domain, transmembrane domain, and cytoplasmic domain (Fig. 1-5). The extra membrane domain may produce circulating binding proteins (e.g., the GHR bears the same amino acid sequence as a circulating growth hormone–binding protein (GHBP) with which GH circulates. The cytokine receptors must dimerize (two receptor molecules must join) to trigger a metabolic effect. The intracellular domain causes phosphorylation of tyrosine molecules (jak kinases), which then phosphorylate signal transducers, and activators of transcription (signal transducer and activator

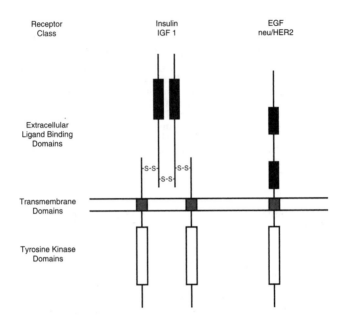

Fig. 1-3.   Schematic structure of cell-surface heterodimeric insulin/insulin-like growth factor 1 (IGF-1) receptor compared with single-chain receptor. The insulin receptor in a heterodimer is composed of two α and two β subunits. The type 1 IGF receptor has a similar structure. In contrast, growth hormone, epidermal growth factor, and other specific peptide hormones have single-chain receptors that may have to dimerize for a biologic action. (Reprinted from Kahn CR, Smith RJ, Chin WW. Mechanism of action of hormones that act at the cell surface. In: Wilson JD, Foster DW, Kroneberg HM. *Williams textbook of endocrinology,* **9th ed. Philadelphia: WB Saunders, 1998:95–144, with permission.)**

of transcription; STAT), which then travel to the nucleus to regulate deoxyribonucleic acid (DNA) action.

Peptide hormone–receptor number and avidity may be regulated by hormones; continuous rather than episodic exposure to GnRH downregulates GnRH-receptor number as well as receptor activity on pituitary gonadotropes. Mutations of receptors may cause disease by rendering the receptor inoperative, or alternatively, the receptor may work without the presence of the hormone, a situation called constitutive activation. The G protein complex may be abnormal in certain diseases (e.g., McCune-Albright syndrome is associated with constitutive activation of G stimulatory protein in affected cells). A constitutively active mutation in the seven-transmembrane domain may be present, as occurs in familial germ cell and Leydig cell maturation. Alternatively, dimerization may fail to occur in some cases of GH insensitivity.

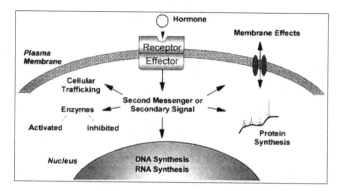

Fig. 1-4. The binding of a peptide hormone to its receptor, triggering second-messenger effects, once the peptide hormone attaches to the cell-surface receptor to elicit a response. This action triggers the production of a second-messenger production to bring about the change in cell function. (Reprinted from Kahn CR, Smith RJ, Chin WW. Mechanism of action of hormones that act at the cell surface. In: Wilson JD, Foster DW, Kroneberg HM, eds. *Williams textbook of endocrinology,* 9th ed. Philadelphia: WB Saunders, 1998:94–144, with permission.)

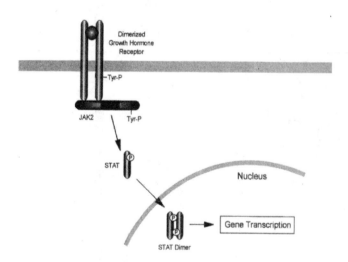

Fig. 1-5. The growth-hormone (*GH*) receptor, once bound to GH, dimerizes with another unoccupied receptor to stimulate tyrosine kinase, leading to cellular effects. The extramembrane portion of the GH receptor also may be cleaved and secreted into the circulation as GH-binding protein (*GHBP*). (Reprinted from Kahn CR, Smith RJ, Chin WW. Mechanism of action of hormones that act at the cell surface. In: Wilson JD, Foster DW, Kroneberg HM, eds. *Williams textbook of endocrinology,* 9th ed. Philadelphia: WB Saunders, 1998:94–144, with permission.)

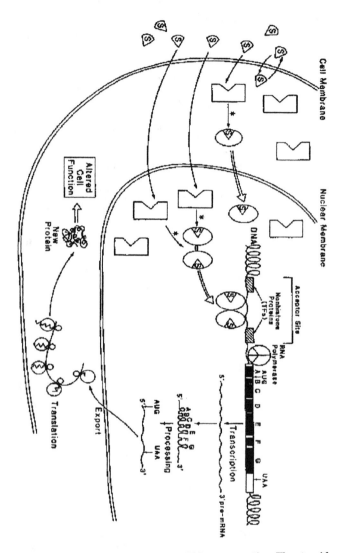

Fig. 1-6.   Molecular pathway of steroid hormone action. The steroid
circulates bound to protein, from which it dissociates to pass
through the cell membrane and reach the cytoplasm, where it binds
to a steroid receptor. Once bound to the steroid, the steroid receptor
is activated and changes conformation, allowing it to bind to the
steroid-response elements or receptor sites, causing the subsequent

The family of insulin receptors includes the insulin and insulin-like growth factor (IGF)-1 receptors (Fig. 1-3). These are hetero-dimeric, consisting of two α and two β chains. When the appropriate hormone binds to the extracellular domain, the conformation is altered, and phosphorylation of tyrosine occurs in the intracellular portion. Through a cascade of effects involving insulin-receptor substrates (IRSs), activation of mitogenesis and proliferation as well as effects on carbohydrate metabolism occur; insulin and IGF-1 have differing tendencies toward cell growth and metabolism, and each molecule has greater effect on its own specific receptor, although insulin can bind to the IGF-1 receptor, and IGF-1 can bind to the IR.

Steroid hormones circulate noncovalently bound to various binding proteins. Steroid hormones exert their effects by diffusion through the cell wall into the cytoplasm. Specific cytoplasmic steroid receptors bind to the steroid molecule and the hormone-receptor complex translocates to the nucleus (Fig. 1-6). The steroid receptor then binds at another location to DNA hormone-response elements to produce the synthesis of messenger RNA (mRNA) and ultimately the formation of proteins or peptides predicted by the hormone.

Thyroid hormone receptors are similar to steroid receptors in structure and function. The retinoid-X receptor (RXR) interacts with thyroid hormone receptors, vitamin D receptors, the peroxisome proliferator activating receptor-γ, as well as with retinoid receptors; RXR and the other receptor form heterodimers and exert effects through gene-response elements.

Because of the feedback loops, the interpretation of serum hormone levels must be related to their controlling factors; a given value of PTH may be normal in a eucalcemic patient, but the same value may be inadequate in a hypocalcemic patient with partial hypoparathyroidism, and this same value of parathyroid hormone may be excessive in a hypercalcemic patient who might have hyperparathyroidism.

A diurnal rhythm of hormone secretion often is found (e.g., serum ACTH increases in the early morning hours, followed by an increasing serum cortisol, followed by a decrease in the afternoon and evening). If the rhythm is disturbed, the amount of hormone present will vary from the normal pattern, and disease might occur; if the normal decrease of cortisol does not occur, Cushing syndrome might result, simply because the p.m. cortisol values match the a.m. values. Thus even though a great increase is not seen in serum cortisol values above normal a.m. values, a great increase in cortisol effect occurs.

Fig. 1-6. (continued) transcription of DNA into RNA and translation into proteins, which change cell function. The activated steroid receptor–steroid complex must dimerize in this example. (Reprinted from Tsai MJ, Clark JH, Schrader WT, O'Malley BW. Mechanism of action of hormones that act as transcription-regulatory factors. In: Wilson JD, Foster DW, Kroneberg HM, eds. *Williams textbook of endocrinology*, 9th ed. Philadelphia: WB Saunders, 1998:55–94, with permission.)

Knowing the basic functions of hormones and their interactions lends logic to the evaluation of patients with endocrine diseases. This volume attempts to emphasize such a systematic evaluation of endocrine disease. The chapters are based on organ systems and begin with a brief explanation of the basic physiology at work.

In each appropriate location, I have indicated the reference to the Online Mendelian Inheritance in Man web site, http://www.ncbi.nlm.nih.gov/Omim/. The format is as follows:

*, The gene location is reliably matched with the clinical situation.
#, Two or more genes can cause the phenotype.
Lack of either symbol, No mode of inheritance has been *proven*.

This source has frequently updated clinical and basic information on the subjects referenced. It is strongly recommended that the reader use this resource frequently.

SUGGESTED READINGS

Cohen P, Ballard PL. Mechanisms of hormone action. In: Rudolph CD, Rudolph AM, eds. *Rudolph's pediatrics*. New York: McGraw-Hill, 2002:2007–2011.

Chrousos GP. Organization and integration of the endocrine system. In: Sperling MA, ed. *Pediatric endocrinology*. Philadelphia: Saunders, 2002:1–14.

Menon RK, Trucco M. Molecular endocrinology. In: Sperling MA, ed. *Pediatric endocrinology*. Philadelphia: Saunders, 2002:15–32.

Rice AM, Rivkees SA. Receptor transduction of hormone action. In: Sperling MA, ed. *Pediatric endocrinology*. Philadelphia: Saunders, 2002:33–64.

Styne DM, Glaser NS. Endocrinology. In: Behrman RE, Kliegman RM, eds. *Nelson essentials of pediatrics*. Philadelphia: Saunders, 2002:711–766.

2 ♣ The Evaluation of a Child or Adolescent with Possible Endocrine Disease

As in most disciplines, the history and physical examination are crucial to determining a course of evaluation. A good pediatric history and physical examination will serve the evaluator well, but in a few areas, increased attention is worthwhile. The type of problem under consideration may change the direction of questioning and evaluation. The following general approach is discussed in more detail in the following chapters, but this outline is meant to direct the initial evaluation.

THE HISTORY AND PHYSICAL EXAMINATION

In many cases, the diagnosis is apparent from the medical history (Table 2-1). In general the parents will be the sources of information, but in many cases, it will be useful to obtain previous medical records, often from several sources because of the recent tendency for transferring care of a child if the child moves to new locations or has a mandatory change of insurance.

All aspects of pregnancy may be of importance. This includes medical complications, nutritional status, toxic or medication exposures (smoking, infections, medications), gestational age, complications or difficulties of delivery, and Apgar scores.

Medical history must include any possible chronic disorders that might have contributed to the disease under evaluation or complicate the treatment. Many chronic disorders may decrease growth rate. If no previous height measurements are available, a history of changes in shoe or clothing size can be of value to determine whether the child is growing adequately, although follow-up measurements over a period of at least 3 months (and longer if possible, as accuracy increases with the length of time of follow-up) are necessary for diagnosis. In older girls, or younger ones if the problem is appropriate, a menstrual history is necessary; age of menarche (onset), regularity, and amount of flow and discomfort are important. Are there abnormal patterns of urination or defecation?

Medication history must often be specific, as many do not consider vitamins as medicine, although excessive vitamins might be the very cause of a disorder (e.g., hypervitaminosis D). In addition, medications found around the house may be of importance; did the child get into the oral contraceptives or hormone-replacement therapy used by another member of the family? Diet and nutritional patterns are of general importance but also may contribute to the etiology of a condition [e.g., estrogen is not supposed to remain in beef bought in grocery stores (estrogen is often added to calves by subcutaneous implant, but it is supposed to dissipate by the time of slaughter), but might be found in a noncommercial source of beef].

Educational achievement, ability, and history are important. In addition, is the child manifesting psychological problems related to the condition (e.g., severe short stature)?

Table 2-1.   Generic history for pediatric endocrinology

Chief complaint
History of present illness
Birth history
  Gestational age
  Complications of pregnancy
  Toxic exposures
  Maternal accidents
  Medication intake including vitamins and "natural" treatments
  Substances used, including cigarettes
  Were ultrasounds obtained, and was the growth normal?
  Was fetal motion normal?
Newborn period
  Method of delivery
  Complications of delivery
  Apgar scores if known
  Birth weight
  Developmental assessment if known
  Use of oxygen or other types of support or treatment
  Hypoglycemia; documented by blood sugar value or inferred by
    activity or behavior?
Development
  Age of milestones: sitting, cruising, walking; speaking words,
    sentences. Perform a developmental test if problems are noted.
Family history
  Direct questions are often necessary, as family might not volun-
    teer information to general questions. Refer to chapters for
    associated conditions of importance.
  Note full siblings, half-siblings, stepparents, or biologic parent
    relationships.
  Construct a family tree if possible.
  Were there any miscarriages?
  Age and percentile of height and weight of siblings.
  Height and weight of parents; approximate weight, if obesity is
    noted, is important.
  Ethnicity of parents.
  Area where parents spent their childhood, especially if there is a
    possibility of famine, war, or refugee status in their history.
  Age of menarche in mother and sisters if old enough.
  Age father stopped growing or started to shave and the same
    information from brothers, if old enough.
  History of disease similar to patient or otherwise of importance in
    related individuals.
  Ask about early deaths due to heart disease or strokes specifically
    in all conditions under evaluation.
  Is there consanguinity?
  Social: who lives at home, what is their relationship, how do they
    interact, and are there adequate funds for the child's benefit?

Continued

Table 2-1. *Continued*

Diet: is there adequate food and of a healthful quality? Is there any aversion to eating, is there lack of satiety, or is there an unusual diet? In evaluation of obesity, much more detail of diet composition and even dietician consultation are important.

Surgical procedures

Allergies

Accidents, especially to the head

Medications taken, including vitamins or "natural substances." Direct questions are often necessary, as family might not volunteer information to general questions such as, "Does the child take any medications?"

School history: grade level, grades obtained, any changes, interrelationships with schoolmates, teasing or bullying interactions?

Educational achievement in patient and in siblings and parents.

Review of systems in general and directed specifically to the issues under consideration.

Areas of concern will vary with the disease under consideration, so check the appropriate chapters to determine specific symptoms and signs of importance.

In most situations today, ask about amount of television viewing per day, amount of activity, sports or other forms of exercise, and especially do so in obese children.

Family history is of great importance in the evaluation of most of the conditions in this book. The heights of parents and their age at puberty (menarche in mothers and age of physical changes of puberty or cessation of growth in fathers) will help determine if the child is following the appropriate pattern. Family history of chronic disease, including neurologic or endocrine conditions, is determined, and the construction of a family tree is helpful. In many cases, the questions must be direct, such as, "Has anyone in the family had thyroid disease?" rather than a general query. Did the parents immigrate from a developing country or live an underprivileged life to account for their own history or stature, if abnormal? Was the child adopted, or should another biologic parent who is no longer in the house be included in the history? Interfamilial interactions can be observed during the interview process to evaluate the possibility of psychosocial dwarfism or other psychosocial complications. If an autosomal recessive defect is suspected, determine whether consanguinity is present.

A history of surgery, allergies, and accidents to the central nervous system (CNS) or other important areas is pertinent.

Physical examination must be complete (Table 2-2). Accurate determination and plotting of height (in centimeters), weight (in kilograms), and body mass index (BMI) must accompany the

Table 2-2. Generic physical examination for pediatric endocrinology

All vital signs will vary with the age of the child, so refer to *Harriet Lane Manual* or other source for standards for age.

Pulse

Blood pressure (interpret in terms of blood pressure for height, and make sure there is an adequate-sized cuff).

Respiratory rate

(Temperature if pertinent to disease under consideration or intercurrent illness)

Infant length, measured as described in Chapter 5, performed by two adults

After age 2 years, measure height in centimeters on a stadiometer without shoes on; repeat 2 or 3 times if stature is main complaint, and make sure measurements are consistent and repeatable within 0.3 cm.

Weight in kilograms

Calculated BMI (kg/m^2)

Upper/Lower-segment ratio as necessary (especially in boys with disorders of puberty) (see Chapter 5)

Arm span as necessary (especially in chondrodystrophies or abnormalities of puberty) (see Chapter 5)

HEENT

　Look for midline defects, including cleft palate or lip.

　Observe for signs of syndromes.

　Cataracts or colobomas?

　Development and status of dentition for age. Single central maxillary incisor as a midline defect that might relate to hypopituitarism?

　Acne or comedones?

　Beard?

　Voice change?

Neck

　Motion

　Goiter? Measure width and height of thyroid lobes, and estimate thickness (e.g., 25% or 50% greater than normal) Nodules? Bruits?

　Acanthosis nigricans at back of neck?

Lungs: customary pediatric examination

Heart: customary pediatric examination

Abdomen: customary pediatric examination

Axillary hair or odor; enlarging axillary sweat glands?

Breast stage in girls (see Chapter 9)

Stage of pubic hair (see Chapter 9)

Stage of genital development in boys (see Chapter 9)

Continued

Table 2-2. *Continued*

Extremities: customary pediatric examination unless chondrodystrophy is suspected, and then note ratio of proximal to distal portions of extremities. Look for Madelung deformity in short stature
   (see Chapter 5). Note motion of joints and back. Evaluate upper-
   to lower-segment ratio. Observe for contractures or subtle signs of
   cerebral palsy.
Scoliosis evaluation
Skin
   Café-au-lait spots (number, type, shape, and size), subcutaneous
      calcifications, acanthosis nigricans
Neurologic: customary pediatric examination with special attention
   to the CNS in most cases
   Cranial nerves: signs of CNS disease, optic disk development,
      visual fields and, in delay of puberty, sense of smell
   Chvostek or Trousseau signs
   Tremor
   DTRs: customary pediatric examination

BMI, body mass index; HEENT, head, eyes, ears, nose, throat; CNS, central
nervous system; DTRs, deep tendon reflexes.

determination of vital signs (see Chapter 5 for details). An infant
should have weight and height interpreted in terms of gestational
age (by using intrauterine growth charts (see Chapter 5).

A patient who has stature below the third percentile for height
according to the new Centers for Disease Control (CDC) charts,
who is growing at a rate less than the fifth percentile for height
velocity for age, or is below the third percentile for corrected midparental height is worthy of evaluation; a combination of two or
more of these characteristics warrants increased concern. Determination of arm span and upper-to-lower ratio is useful in evaluation of short stature (e.g., to indicate hypochondroplasia or
achondroplasia or other abnormalities of proportionate growth)
or of delay in puberty (e.g., to look for the long arms and lower
upper- to lower-segment ratio of hypogonadism). The arm span
is measured with the patient standing with the back to the wall
with arms spread horizontally and is the distance from one
outstretched middle fingertip to the other. The lower segment
is measured from the top of the symphysis pubis to the floor,
whereas the upper segment is measured by subtracting the lower
segment from the height of the child. The upper- to lower-
segment ratio varies with age from 1.7 at birth to 1.4 at 2 years
to 1 at ~10 years, and values above 0.9 at adulthood (Fig. 5-7). An
increased upper-to-lower ratio is found in Klinefelter syndrome,
and a decreased ratio is found in untreated hypothyroidism,
among other possibilities.

If a problem of growth or pubertal progression is under evaluation, one must consider whether a low body weight is the source of the problem. If nutrition is suboptimal, usually the problem is not endocrine in origin, and other causes must be considered. Alternatively, if the child is starting puberty early or progressing too fast, is excess weight the cause? Weight-for-height curves are now superseded by Body Mass Index charts (found at www. CDC.com); low BMI for age might indicate malnutrition due to chronic disease, whereas elevated BMI for age might indicate rapid growth due to obesity.

The general appearance of the child may furnish a clue as to the chronicity of the problem and its emotional effects. Levels of energy and activity are important. Suspicion of a syndrome must be clarified by the examination. The head, eyes, ears, nose, and throat (HEENT) examination may point to a midline defect, syndrome, or neurologic condition. Is there a goiter or nodule of the thyroid gland? Cardiac, pulmonary, abdominal examinations must be thorough but do not differ appreciably from those in a general pediatric examination. Skin examination might reveal café-au-lait spots or subcutaneous calcifications. The extremities may appear to be curved or abnormal, as an indication of rickets; alternatively, an abnormality of gait may indicate one of these conditions. Neurologic examination is essential in most disorders considered in the book. Signs of dysfunction might suggest a neoplasm or a congenital defect associated with an endocrine condition.

In almost all conditions, it is important to determine the stage of pubertal development. This must be done with care and consideration, as the patient, especially in the teenage years, may be embarrassed; if the patient refuses and the caregiver cannot achieve acquiescence, this portion of the examination may have to be omitted on this visit, as it should not be done by force. Even with cooperation, in the modern social environment, a chaperone should be in the room during the examination. Determination of stage of breast and pubic hair growth is performed in girls, and genitalia and pubic hair (as well as beard), in boys, according to standard rating techniques (see Chapter 9). In addition, the development of axillary odor or hair, the presence of comedones or acne, and the maturation of facial features are noted in all. The appearance of abnormal distribution or amount of facial or body hair may be an indication of a problem.

3 ♣ Disorders of the Hypothalamic–Pituitary Axis

The reader will find more detailed discussion of specific hormones in the chapters related to their functions [e.g., growth hormone (GH) is presented in Chapter 5].

PHYSIOLOGY

The *hypothalamus* exerts endocrine effects either directly, in the production and release of vasopressin, or indirectly, through the release of hypothalamic peptides, which reach the anterior pituitary gland to cause the release of pituitary hormones. Higher regions of the central nervous system (CNS) control the hypothalamus. Thus, disorders of any of the regions, the CNS, the hypothalamus, or the pituitary gland, might cause endocrine disease, characteristically denoted as hypopituitarism. Hypothalamic releasing or inhibiting factors are small peptides produced in minute quantities and travel down the capillaries composing the pituitary portal system to regulate the pituitary hormones specific for the factor (Fig. 3-1). After secretion into the peripheral circulation, the pituitary hormones exert their effects on target glands and organs specific for that pituitary hormone. Target endocrine glands in most cases produce their own hormones that provide feedback to suppress their controlling hypothalamic and pituitary hormones in turn [e.g., insulin-like growth factor-1 (IGF-1), cortisol, sex steroids, and thyroxin all provide feedback to the hypothalamic–pituitary system to suppress the hypothalamic–pituitary hormones that stimulate them]. Prolactin is the only pituitary hormone that is mainly suppressed by a hypothalamic factor, prolactin inhibitory factor (dopamine), whereas all other pituitary hormones are mainly stimulated by hypothalamic factors (it is true that GH is suppressed by somatotropin release inhibiting factor [SRIF], but it also is mainly stimulated by growth hormone releasing factor [GRF]). Hypothalamic disease may lead to a decrease in secretion of most pituitary hormones and an increase in prolactin secretion, whereas a pituitary gland disorder may cause a decrease in prolactin secretion as well as a decrease in the other pituitary hormones. The hypothalamus contains the terminal of the axons of some vasopressin-secreting neurons while also serving as a location through which other vasopressin-secreting axons pass on their ways to their own terminal in the posterior pituitary gland. Thus hypothalamic damage may cause diabetes insipidus, whereas the result of pituitary stalk section is variable, depending on the level of lesion. If a pituitary stalk section or disorder is high on the pituitary stalk, all vasopressin-secreting neurons may be affected, and the result is diabetes insipidus, whereas if the pituitary stalk section is low, some vasopressin-secreting neurons may survive intact, and vasopressin secretion and action are still possible, so that diabetes insipidus may not develop.

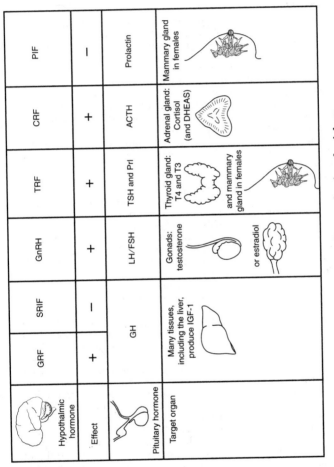

Hypothalmic hormone	GRF	SRIF	GnRH	TRF	CRF	PIF
Effect	+	–	+	+	+	–
Pituitary hormone	GH		LH/FSH	TSH and Prl	ACTH	Prolactin
Target organ	Many tissues, including the liver, produce IGF-1		Gonads: testosterone or estradiol	Thyroid gland: T4 and T3 and mammary gland in females	Adrenal gland: Cortisol (and DHEAS)	Mammary gland in females

Fig. 3-1.   Hypothalamic and pituitary endocrine physiology.

PATHOLOGY

Disorders of the hypothalamus or pituitary gland may logically be expected to affect endocrine function. However, disorders elsewhere in the CNS or radiation therapy to the CNS for other conditions may all cause significant endocrine effects. Although destructive lesions of the hypothalamic–pituitary axis usually decrease endocrine activity (e.g., hypogonadotropic hypogonadism), depending on location, disease of the hypothalamic–pituitary axis may instead cause increased function (e.g., precocious puberty). Alternatively, functioning lesions may cause endocrine effects because of secretions rather than because of destruction of tissue by their size or location [e.g., pinealomas secrete human chorionic gonadotropin (hCG) and cause precocious puberty in boys].

Specific terminology relates to the level of the endocrine lesion. A disorder of the target gland (e.g., thyroid, adrenal gland) is considered a primary disease. A lesion of the pituitary gland is considered a secondary defect, and a lesion of the hypothalamus is a tertiary condition.

CENTRAL NERVOUS SYSTEM DISORDERS

Tumors

Most CNS tumors will cause multiple pituitary defects. However, in hypothalamic disease, GH is usually affected, and GH deficiency is the most common outcome. GH deficiency may at first appear to be an isolated finding until more careful endocrine evaluation reveals other pituitary defects. A hypothalamic tumor may be indicated by the presence of galactorrhea, due to increased prolactin secretion in the absence of prolactin inhibitory factor, occurring along with deficiencies of other pituitary hormones.

Because tumors of this area are manifest after birth, late onset of hypothalamic–pituitary deficiencies without contributing history (e.g., surgery or trauma to the area) may very well indicate the development of a CNS tumor, especially if anterior and posterior deficiencies occur together. In contrast, congenital defects of hypothalamic–pituitary hormones appear at or soon after birth, so that early onset of combined posterior and anterior deficiencies may be significant but do not necessarily reflect the development of a tumor. Nonetheless, a magnetic resonance imaging (MRI) evaluation of a child with onset of hypopituitarism of any age is generally indicated to determine whether a definable anatomic defect is causing the condition.

Craniopharyngioma

A craniopharyngioma is rare but is the most common brain tumor associated with hypothalamic–pituitary dysfunction. This condition may be associated with a variety of abnormalities of puberty; lack onset of puberty is most common, although failure to progress through puberty once begun is possible, and even precocious puberty may occur, although less frequently. This tumor originates from epithelial rests along the pituitary stalk extending upward toward the hypothalamus. Craniopharyngiomas may be contained within the sella turcica extending outwards or extended upwards, or rarely, craniopharyngiomas may be found in the nasopharynx. The peak incidence of craniopharyngiomas is between ages 6 and 14 years.

Clinical presentation and history of craniopharyngiomas include headache, visual disturbances, short stature, symptoms of diabetes insipidus, and weakness of one or more limbs. CNS signs develop as the tumor encroaches on surrounding structures. Signs on physical examination include visual defects (including bilateral temporal field deficits due to impingement on the optic chiasm), optic atrophy, or papilledema. Signs may be noted of GH deficiency, abnormal puberty, and hypothyroidism. The patients do not always seek evaluation initially because of short stature, but many are below the mean in height and height velocity at the time of diagnosis. Laboratory evaluation may reveal deficiencies in one or more pituitary hormones, including gonadotropin, GH, thyrotropin (TSH), adrenocorticotropic hormone (ACTH), and vasopressin (AVP). The plasma concentration of prolactin (Prl) may be decreased, normal, or increased. The bone age is often delayed.

An abnormal sella turcica is found in 70% of patients with craniopharyngioma, and suprasellar or intrasellar calcification occurs in approximately 70% of patients. In contrast, such calcifications are found in fewer than 1% of normal individuals. Some asymptomatic patients come to diagnosis by the finding of calcification or abnormalities of the sella turcica on skull radiograph films taken for other indications (e.g., dental radiographs). Computed tomographic (CT) scans can reveal fine calcifications that are not apparent on routine roentgenograms, and CT or MRI scans with contrast (the latter being the diagnostic procedure of choice) can determine whether the tumor is cystic or solid and indicate the presence of hydrocephalus. However, MRI scans cannot reveal the presence of calcifications.

Transsphenoidal microsurgery is invoked to treat smaller craniopharyngiomas that are located mostly within the sella turcica. However, larger tumors that extend into the suprasellar area require craniotomy. Although it may appear that complete surgical removal is possible, a high recurrence rate is found if only surgery is invoked. Radiation therapy is often combined with more limited tumor removal (depending on the size and location of the tumor) to allow the likelihood of better neurologic, psychological, and endocrine results. Hypopituitarism with the need for replacement therapy with many or all of the pituitary hormones is a more likely outcome of radical attempts for removal of all craniopharyngioma tissue, but it is important to note that radiation therapy also will affect pituitary function and also may lead to the requirement for replacement therapy. Remarkable weight gain may occur, usually accompanied with hyperinsulinism, and even continued growth in the absence of GH is found after surgery for craniopharyngiomas.

A Rathke-cleft cyst can produce symptoms and signs similar to those of a craniopharyngioma, even though this is not a neoplasm.

The usual treatment is surgical drainage and excision of the cyst wall.

Other Extrasellar Tumors

Germinomas are extrasellar tumors most often found during the second decade of life; previously a variety of terms were used, including pinealomas, ectopic pinealomas, atypical teratomas, or dysgerminomas to describe germinomas. Germinomas are rare compared with all primary CNS tumors but can cause endocrine disease. Polydipsia and polyuria are among the most common symptoms, followed by visual difficulties and abnormalities of growth and puberty. The most common endocrine abnormalities caused by germinomas are deficiencies of vasopressin and GH, but other anterior pituitary hormone deficiencies (including gonadotropin deficiency) and elevated serum prolactin levels are frequent. Other germ cell tumors may arise in the suprasellar hypothalamic region, in the pineal region, or in another area of the CNS. Determination of the concentration of serum hCG (or a positive pregnancy test in the absence of pregnancy) and of α-fetoprotein are indicated, as these products are tumor markers for a germ cell tumor. The hCG secreted by germ cell tumors in boys interacts with the testicular luteinizing hormone (LH) receptor and may cause isosexual precocity by testosterone production. Girls do not develop precocious puberty, as hCG has no effect on ovarian function during prepubertal ages.

Isolated enlargement of the pituitary stalk on MRI is a suggestive finding that suggests the presence of a germinoma; sometimes the area must be observed with MRI for months before further enlargement of the area can be said to demonstrate the presence of the tumor. MRI scans with contrast enhancement are useful in the diagnosis of tumors more than 0.5 cm in diameter. Although the pituitary gland normally increases in size 100% between years 1 and 15, the size of the pineal gland does not normally change after age 1 year, so that enlargement of the pineal gland after infancy is suggestive of a mass lesion. Subependymal spread along the lining of the third ventricle all the way down to the lower spinal cord and cauda equina may occur in patients with germinomas. Germinomas are pure germ cell tumors and are radiosensitive; surgery is rarely required, except when needed for biopsy to establish a tissue diagnosis. However, a mixed germ cell tumor is treated with both radiation therapy and chemotherapy.

Hypothalamic and optic gliomas or astrocytomas, occurring either as part of neurofibromatosis (von Recklinghausen disease *162200 NEUROFIBROMATOSIS, TYPE I; NF1, due to mutations in the neurofibromin gene) or independently, also can cause various endocrine abnormalities.

Pituitary Tumors

Only 2% to 6% of pituitary adenomas occur in childhood and adolescence. Fifty percent of pituitary adenomas occurring before adulthood are prolactinomas, 20% are GH-secreting adenomas, and 30% are chromophobe adenomas. Hyperprolactinemia related to micro- or macroprolactinomas of the pituitary is uncommon in childhood and adolescence but may rarely cause a delay in puberty. Primary amenorrhea may be seen more often in these conditions. Galactorrhea may be absent by history, but it may be demonstrable by manual expression of the nipples; because serum prolactin will increase after manipulation of the nipples, serum samples must be obtained before examination or many hours later. Bromergocryptine is a dopamine agonist that can decrease serum prolactin concentrations and shrink the size of the tumors. The resulting reduction in serum prolactin levels usually allows pubertal progression as well as normal menstrual function. Alternatively, if medication is ineffective, microprolactinomas in children and adolescents may be treated with transsphenoidal resection.

Other pituitary adenomas may rarely cause pituitary gigantism because of excess GH secretion. Also rare are tumors secreting TSH or other pituitary hormones.

Langerhans Cell Histiocytosis

Langerhans cell histiocytosis (Hand-Schüller-Christian disease, or histiocytosis X) is characterized by the infiltration of the skin, viscera, and bone with lipid-laden histiocytic cells or foam cells. Diabetes insipidus, usually resulting from infiltration of the hypothalamus, the pituitary stalk, or both, is the most common endocrine manifestation, but GH deficiency and delayed puberty may occur. Other findings include cyst-like areas in flat bones of the skull, the ribs, the pelvis, and the scapula; in the long bones of the arms and legs; and in the dorsolumbar spine. Lesions of the mandible lead to the radiographic impression of "floating teeth" within rarefied bone and the clinical finding of absent or loose teeth. Infiltration of the orbit may lead to exophthalmos, and mastoid or temporal bone involvement may lead to chronic otitis media. The viscera also may be involved with this infiltration. Treatment of this condition is carried out with glucocorticoids, antineoplastic agents, and radiation, but more than half of patients have late sequelae or progression. Because a waxing and waning course of the disease is found, evaluation of efficacy of therapy is difficult. Letterer-Siwe disease (*246400) has similarities but may occur in an autosomal recessive pattern.

Postinfectious or Other Inflammatory Lesions of the Central Nervous System, Granulomatous Disease of the Area and Vascular Abnormalities, and Head Trauma

Postinfectious or other inflammatory lesions of the CNS, granulomatous disease of the area and vascular abnormalities, and head trauma may cause abnormal hypothalamic–pituitary function. Hydrocephalus may cause hypopituitarism, but precocious puberty also is a possible result, depending on the amount of pressure exerted on various locations. When hydrocephalus or subarachnoid cysts, which can cause similar effects, are decompressed, pituitary abnormalities may improve.

Radiation of the Head

Radiation of the head for treatment of CNS tumors, leukemia, or neoplasms of the head and the face, in which the radiation field involves the hypothalamus or pituitary field, may result in the gradual onset of hypothalamic–pituitary failure over a period of months to a few years. This etiology comprises an enlarging group of patients with hypopituitarism because of the increasing success in radiation treatment of such tumors. GH deficiency is the most common hormone disorder resulting from radiation of the CNS, but gonadotropin deficiency also occurs. Conversely, early or truly precocious puberty may occur after radiation therapy for CNS lesions. Newer radiation-treatment regimens with 18 Gy instead of 24 Gy may have less influence on the age of puberty. The combination of GH deficiency and precious puberty is a possible outcome and is difficult to detect clinically, as the growth rate of the child is greater than that found in patients with GH deficiency alone, because the sex steroid secretion increases growth rate during pubertal development. (see Chapters 5 and 9)

Developmental Defects

Idiopathic Hypopituitary Dwarfism

Congenital hypopituitarism usually is due to absence of hypothalamic-releasing factors; thus, ironically, the pituitary gland cannot release its hormones even though these hormones may be present in adequate supply in the pituitary gland. The pituitary gland can be usually be stimulated by exogenous hypothalamic-releasing factor administration (either once or in successive doses) in such cases of hypothalamic disease. Common to many patients with idiopathic congenital hypopituitary dwarfism is early onset of growth failure; late onset of diminished growth suggests the possible development of a CNS tumor, especially if posterior and anterior pituitary deficiencies are found. An association is seen between breech delivery, perinatal distress, and idiopathic hypopituitarism, especially in male patients. The familial forms of multiple pituitary hormone deficiencies with either autosomal recessive or X-linked inheritance are less common. The degree of hormone deficit and the age at onset of pituitary hormone deficiencies may vary within a single kindred, even if they have the same genetic defect.

Congenital defects of pituitary secretion also may result from anatomic malformations of the hypothalamus, from pituitary hypoplasia or aplasia, or from more subtle defects of hormone secretion. Congenital defects of the midline associated with hypopituitarism range from holoprosencephaly (cyclopia, cebocephaly, orbital hypotelorism) to single maxillary incisor and even to cleft palate (6% of cases of cleft palate are associated with GH deficiency, so that all growth failure in cleft palate should not be attributed to poor feeding or nutrition alone). The MRI findings of congenital hypopituitarism may include an ectopic posterior pituitary gland "hot spot" and the appearance of what appears to be a "pituitary stalk transection" and a small pituitary gland. In some patients, the neurohypophysis may appear absent because of a missing hot spot. Individuals with myelomeningocele (myelo-dysplasia) have an increased frequency of endocrine abnormalities, including hypothalamic hypothyroidism, hyperprolactinemia, and decreased gonadotropin concentrations, whereas some patients demonstrate true precocious puberty

Septooptic dysplasia (optic nerve hypoplasia, absent septum pellucidum, or variations of both caused by abnormal development of the prosencephalon) (septooptic dysplasia 182230 due to a mutation at 3p21.2-p21.1 at the HESX1 gene) may be associated with significant visual impairment, and pendular nystagmus results (to-and-fro nystagmus due to inability to focus on a target). Small, pale optic disks occur, but not the appearance of optic atrophy, which would suggest previous development of the optic nerves with subsequent deterioration due to acquired pathology. A midline hypothalamic defect may lead to the combination of GH deficiency and diabetes insipidus and may be associated with deficient ACTH, TSH, and gonadotropin secretion as well. Short stature and delayed puberty may be the most obvious results, although true precocious

Table 3-1. Genetic forms of multiple pituitary/hypothalamic hormone deficiencies

Defect	Hormones deficient	Inheritance	Other features
POU1F1	GH, Prl, TSH	Auto recessive and auto dominant	Severe impairment of postnatal growth
PROP1	GH, Prl, TSH, LH, FSH, and sometimes ACTH	Auto recessive and X-linked	
HEX1	Any or all, including vasopressin	Auto recessive	Septo optic dysplasia or hypoplasia
LHX3	GH, Prl, TSH, LH, FSH, but not ACTH		
LIM HOMEO BOX GENE 3;LIM3	Variable		Limited rotation of the head

GH, growth hormone; Prl, prolactin; TSH, thyroid-stimulating hormone; LH, luteinizing hormone; FSH, follicle-stimulating hormone; ACTH, adrenocorticotropic hormone.

puberty is an alternative outcome in rare cases of this midline defect. The septum pellucidum is absent in about 50% of cases of optic hypoplasia or dysplasia, and this defect is readily demonstrable by CNS imaging techniques, most frequently by MRI. The disorder may be related to a mutation of the HEXS1 gene.

Other developmental defects of the anterior pituitary gland associated with hypogonadotropic hypogonadism and other pituitary hormone deficiencies are caused by autosomal recessive mutations in homeobox genes encoding transcription factors involved in the early aspects of pituitary development (see Table 3.1). These include mutations in the LHX3 (*600577 LIM HOMEO BOX GENE 3; LHX39q34.3) associated with multiple pituitary hormone deficiencies including LH and FSH and severe restriction of head rotation) and PROP-1 genes (601538 PROPHET OF PIT1, PAIRED-LIKE HOMEODOMAIN TRANSCRIPTION FACTOR; PROP1 at 5q), which causes GH and TSH deficiency and more rarely ACTH deficiency; mutations of POU1F1 (PIT *173110 POU DOMAIN, CLASS 1, TRANSCRIPTION FACTOR 1; POU1F1 at 3p11) cause deficiency in GH, TSH, and prolactin (Table 3-1).

SUGGESTED READINGS

Kaplan SL. Neonatal hypopituitarism. In: Finberg L, Kleinman RE, eds. *Saunders manual of pediatric practice.* Philadelphia: WB Saunders, 2002:843–844.

Parks JS. Genetic forms of hypopituitarism. In: Finberg L, Kleinman RE, eds. *Saunders manual of pediatric practice.* Philadelphia: WB Saunders, 2002:840–843.

Pollock AN, Towbin RB, Charron MC, Meza MP. Imaging in pediatric endocrine disorders. In: Sperling MA, ed. *Pediatric endocrinology.* Philadelphia: WB Saunders, 2002:725–756.

4 ♣ Disorders of Vasopressin Metabolism

Disorders of vasopressin metabolism may cause increased or decreased urine formation and subsequent abnormalities in body water and serum sodium and other electrolytes. Although lack of antidiuretic hormone (ADH) is the main focus of the chapter, excessive urination also may be due to the desire for secondary gain in psychogenic polydipsia, to habitual excessive drinking, to urinary tract defects in concentrating ability, possibly due to urinary tract infections, as well as to osmotic diuresis. The most common etiology of a pathologic cause of polyuria is the glucosuria of diabetes mellitus (translated as "sweet urine") in contrast to the rarer condition of diuresis due to the lack of ADH that leads to central diabetes insipidus (DI; "weak urine").

NORMAL VASOPRESSIN PHYSIOLOGY

Arginine vasopressin is the human ADH (Fig. 4-1). It is produced in the magnocellular cells of the paraventricular and supraoptic nuclei of the hypothalamus in a large precursor molecule along with neurophysin II, to which vasopressin is bound in the circulation. The magnacellular neurons terminate, for the most part, in the posterior pituitary gland (the neurohypophysis), but some terminate in the third ventricle, and some terminate high in the pituitary stalk or in the median eminence of the hypothalamus. Vasopressin also is produced in the parvocellular cells of the paraventricular nuclei, as is corticotropin-releasing hormone (CRH), and both stimulate the secretion of adrenocorticotropic hormone (ACTH). An intracellular osmotic detector is located close to the supraoptic nuclei but separate from the nuclei containing ADH. This sensor detects changes in plasma osmolality as subtle as 1% to 2%, reaching a sensitivity that is better than many laboratory tests can accomplish. An increase in osmolality due to dehydration, or the infusion of a hypertonic solution such as concentrated saline, triggers the release of sufficient vasopressin to cause the kidney to retain water, thereby decreasing the serum osmolality to normal. When osmolality is less than 280 mOsm/kg, vasopressin is not released to any appreciable degree, but when it reaches 283 mOsm/kg or more, vasopressin is secreted in increasing amounts.

Stretch receptors in the right atrium and baroreceptors in the carotid sinus also regulate the release of vasopressin, so that a decrease in blood volume of 8% to 10% (equivalent to a major hemorrhage) will stimulate a large release in vasopressin, whereas smaller shifts may not cause any effects. Lung disease and respiratory support with ventilator therapy will trigger vasopressin secretion because of the increase in intrathoracic pressure, as detected by the stretch receptors of the atrium. During the daily routine of standing and walking, vasopressin concentrations change from moment to moment because of stimulation of the carotid baroreceptors. Other stimuli of vasopressin secretion

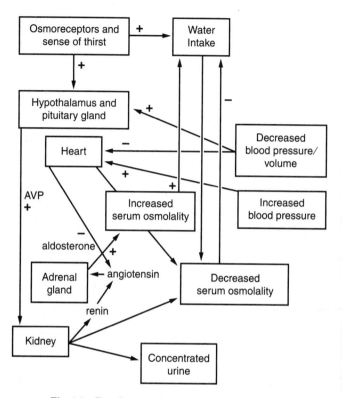

Fig. 4-1.   Regulation of serum sodium and water.

include nausea and certain drugs, such as chlorpromazine and antimetabolites, used in the treatment of cancer; the nausea of cancer treatment should therefore be an expected stimulus for vasopressin secretion and may cause the syndrome of inappropriate secretion of ADH (SIADH; see later). Nicotine exerts its effects through the precipitation of nausea, which stimulates the release of vasopressin.

Vasopressin exerts two major biologic effects: it increases permeability of the collecting duct of the nephron to water filtered in the urine, and, in large concentrations, ADH stimulates the contraction of arterial muscle, which increases blood pressure (BP; hence the name, vasopressin). The effects are mediated through G protein–coupled cell-membrane receptors. Of the three vasopressin receptors, the V_2 receptor located in the renal collecting duct mediates the actions of vasopressin on urine concentration. The medulla of the kidney normally maintains a high osmotic concentration of urea and sodium built up by the countercurrent exchange system. When vasopressin allows water filtered in the urine to pass through the walls of the collecting ducts, the water will, through the osmotic gradient, be drawn to the medulla, and the urine in the lumen of the collecting ducts will become more concentrated. The effects of vasopressin on salt balance are mediated through its effect on changes in water balance, as vasopressin itself has no direct effect on the transport of sodium or chloride. Thus if water is lost, serum sodium and osmolality increase, whereas if water is retained, serum sodium and osmolality decrease. If vasopressin cannot be released from the posterior pituitary, central DI develops. If the collecting duct cannot respond to the vasopressin, nephrogenic DI occurs. If a patient has been drinking large amounts of water for a prolonged period because of habit or psychogenic polydipsia, the medullary interstitial gradient becomes progressively more dilute ("washes out"), so that the maximal concentrating ability of the kidney is decreased, and polyuria results. Infection or various types of kidney disease also can decrease the concentrating ability of the kidney (causing functional nephrogenic DI).

The sensor responsible for the sense of thirst is located in the ventromedial nuclei of the hypothalamus. The sensation of thirst arises when serum osmolality increases to more than 293 mOsm/kg, which is 13 mOsm/kg higher than the limit for vasopressin secretion. Other sensors in the oral cavity interact with both the sense of thirst and vasopressin secretion, so that fluid ingestion is modulated quite closely, as appropriate fluid balance is essential for life.

Thus two basic mechanisms control serum osmolality: (a) vasopressin secretion exerting effects on the nephron, and (b) fluid dynamics mediated by fluid loss and the sense of thirst that affects fluid intake. Either mechanism can compensate for a defect in the other (once the infant stage of dependency on others to supply water is passed, a child who lacks vasopressin can drink enough to maintain fluid balance for a while), but if both mechanisms fail, and the individual has neither sense of thirst nor ability to concentrate urine, swings in osmolality may reach a life-threatening degree.

The consequences of hyperosmolality or hypoosmolality can be severe. The obvious impairment of renal function due to severe volume constriction and the pulmonary edema and heart failure that can be caused by volume excess are well appreciated. However, the effects of rapid fluid shifts on brain cells and brain function can be devastating and may be permanent, and these may occur because of DI or SIADH. A rapid increase in plasma osmolality can draw fluid from the brain and, especially in young infants, cause brain shrinkage and rupture of veins that bridge the distance from the rigid cranium to the more malleable brain substance. Although the brain is slower to correct osmolar balance than is the vascular compartment, during a more gradual increase in intravascular osmolality, the brain can produce "idiogenic osmols" that increase intracellular osmolality to balance an intravascular hyperosmolality. These osmolar-active molecules remain in the brain for hours and days after a decrease in intravascular osmolality occurs, leading to an imbalance of osmolar forces with the net shift of fluid toward the brain if serum osmolality decreases, resulting in cerebral edema that could cause cerebellar tonsillar herniation and death. Thus both hypoosmolality and hyperosmolality are damaging to the brain.

DIABETES INSIPIDUS

Central Diabetes Insipidus (*192340 ARGININE VASOPRESSIN; AVP at 20p13)

The inability to release adequate arginine vasopressin in the face of increased serum osmolality can be caused by central nervous system (CNS) tumor, trauma, infection, or granuloma as well as by a congenital defect of the brain structure (Table 4-1; Fig. 4-2). Some vasopressin secretion may remain in spite of DI, but the amount of vasopressin secreted is not commensurate with the need for water conservation, and excessive urination occurs. Depending on the nature of the defect, the sense of thirst may or may not remain intact, determined by whether the thirst center of the CNS is affected as well as the vasopressin neurons. If impairment of the sense of thirst occurs, maintenance of serum osmolality in the normal range becomes most difficult, as voluntary water intake must replace previously automatic functions, sensing thirst and drinking when thirsty.

Any hypothalamic–pituitary tumor can cause DI with or without other hypothalamic–pituitary disorders. Most commonly in the pediatric age group, a craniopharyngioma or germinoma is involved. Histiocytosis X or Hand-Schüller-Christian disease is an infiltrative lesion also associated with DI. The late onset of posterior pituitary disease manifest by DI, associated with any anterior pituitary deficiency or present in an isolated form, is an urgent reason for a full effort to diagnose a tumor or infiltrative lesion. Trauma, whether accidental, such as a fall off a horse or an automobile accident, or iatrogenic, such as surgery near the posterior pituitary for a craniopharyngioma, can lead to DI. Hydrocephalus or other types of increased intracranial pressure also can lead to vasopressin deficiency and DI.

Idiopathic, congenital DI without anatomic abnormalities can occur sporadically, in an autosomal dominantly inherited familial pattern (OMIM **125700 DIABETES INSIPIDUS, NEURO-HYPOPHYSEAL TYPE 20p13**) because of defects in the gene for vasopressin or can occur an X-linked pattern (**304900 DIABETES INSIPIDUS, NEUROHYPOPHYSEAL TYPE**). Congenital midline defects of the CNS also may lead to DI in addition to anterior pituitary deficiencies. Absence of the septum pellucidum may be associated with optic hypoplasia or dysplasia and is often associated

Table 4-1. Causes of disturbances of osmolality and serum sodium

Condition	Serum Na	Urine Na	Plasma Osm	Urine Osm	Serum AVP	PRA	Serum Aldo	Urine Aldo	Serum K	Plasma anti-natriuretic hormone
Central diabetes insipidus	High	Nl	High	Low	Low	Nl	Nl	Nl	Nl	
Nephrogenic diabetes insipidus	High	Nl	High	Low	High	Nl	Nl	Nl	Nl	
Psychogenic polydipsia	Low normal	Nl	Low normal	Low	Low	Nl	Nl	Nl	Nl	Nl
SIADH	Low	Nl-high	Low	High	High	Nl	Nl	Nl	Nl	High
Hyperaldosteronism	Nl with hypertension	Nl-low	Nl	Nl	Nl	Low	High	High	Low	High
Hypoaldosteronism	Low	High	Nl	Nl	Nl	High	Low	Low	High	
Hyporeninemic hypoaldosteronism	Nl	High	Nl	Nl	Nl	Nl-low	Low	Low	High	
Pseudohypoaldosteronism	Low	High	Nl	Nl	Nl	High	High	High	High	

Condition										
Cerebral salt wasting	Low	High	Low	High	Nl	High	High	High	Nl	High
Glucocorticoid insufficiency (dilutional hyponatremia)	Low	Low	Low	High	Nl (high in some studies)	Nl-high	Depends on cause of adrenal insufficiency	Depends on cause of adrenal insufficiency	Low-Nl	Low
Hypothyroidism (dilutional hyponatremia)	Low	Low	Low	High	Nl				Low	Low
Hyponatremia due to hyperglycemia	Low (1.6 mEq/mL decrease per 100 mg/dL elevation of glucose)	Osmotic diuresis	High	High	High					

From Quest Diagnostics/Nichols Institute and Majoub in Sperling textbook and Muglia, see Suggested Readings.
AVP, arginine vasopressin; PRA, plasma renin activity; Aldo, aldosterone; Nl, normal; SIADH, syndrome of inappropriate secretion of antidiuretic hormone.

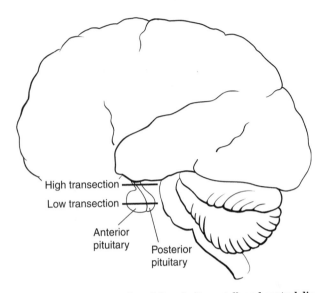

Fig. 4-2.   Level of transection of the pituitary stalk and central diabetes insipidus. If a transection of the pituitary stalk is high, the axons of all vasopressin-containing neurons are likely to be cut and to degenerate, leading to central diabetes insipidus. If the transection is low on the pituitary stalk, sufficient vasopressin-containing neurons are likely to remain to avoid central diabetes insipidus.

with hypothalamic abnormalities (OMIM **182230 SEPTOOPTIC DYSPLASIA at 3p21.2-p21.1**); initial clinical presentation may be a visual deficiency (with to-and-fro or pendular nystagmus due to the defect in the optic nerve) or an endocrine disorder, including DI. The Wolfram (OMIM 222300 WOLFRAM SYNDROME and *606201 WOLFRAM SYNDROME GENE 1; WFS1) or DIDMOAD (DI, diabetes mellitus, optic atrophy, and deafness syndrome) is caused by a mutation of a gene at 4p16.1. Although histiocytosis X and craniopharyngiomas usually occur at a later age, and the early onset of anterior and posterior pituitary disorders usually carries a more benign prognosis than does late onset, evaluation for a potential CNS tumor or anatomic abnormality should be carried out even in the youngest cases, unless a clear family pattern or gene diagnosis is made.

Nephrogenic Diabetes Insipidus

If the defect is in the nephron, ADH is produced in normal or increased amounts but is ineffective in stemming the production of urine. Originally nephrogenic DI was thought to be solely an

X-linked disorder, but numerous cases of sporadic occurrence or autosomal dominant inheritance have since been described. Congenital nephrogenic DI may be the result of

1. An X-linked mutation in the renal vasopressin receptor (V_2) at Xq28 (*304800 DIABETES INSIPIDUS, NEPHROGENIC, X-LINKED). A defect in the G protein of the adenyl cyclase system of the renal tubular cells.
2. An autosomal recessive mutation in the renal water channel aquaporin-1 at 12 q 13 (#222000 DIABETES INSIPIDUS, NEPHROGENIC, AUTOSOMAL RECESSIVE).
3. An autosomal dominant mutation in the aquaporin-2 at 12q13 (#125800 DIABETES INSIPIDUS, NEPHROGENIC, AUTOSOMAL DOMINANT).

Because the disorder classically is seen as a congenital condition, these babies are more prone to dehydration than are the majority of patients with central DI. Severe dehydration due to fluid loss may cause episodes of unexplained fevers, failure to thrive, and even lead to developmental delay; hypernatremia may be demonstrated during the episodes of dehydration. Usually, when the child reaches an age at which water can be obtained *ad lib,* the symptoms will decrease except at time of illnesses, when debilitation may cause a decrease in oral intake.

Acquired nephrogenic DI may be owing to drugs such as lithium chloride and demeclocycline or to electrolyte abnormalities such as hypercalcemia or hypokalemia.

Clinical Features of Diabetes Insipidus

Clinical features of DI of either the central or nephrogenic variety relate mostly to patterns of drinking and urinating. The patient will urinate large quantities throughout the day and night, awakening several times every night while constantly drinking (usually drinking cool water, as other fluids are less requested, at least not in the United States experience) because of continuous thirst. As noted, except for congenital defects, DI usually is first seen after infancy. If infants are affected, they will cry if deprived of their bottle and may drink their bath water or suck on their washcloths; these symptoms may be more common in those with nephrogenic DI than in those with the central form. Older children and adults will go to bed with gallons of water at their side for use throughout the night. At times of disability or when water cannot be obtained, the patient with DI will become severely dehydrated and could develop shock. Remarkable urine flow into the diaper of an infant or enuresis may be seen. Because of the massive flow of urine, the renal pelvises and ureters may show dilation on intravenous pyelogram as secondary complications. These features are in contradistinction to those found in the compulsive water drinker, who usually will get through the night without awakening, and the child drinking for secondary gain, who drinks small amounts frequently and who urinates frequently but in small quantities (psychogenic polydipsia).

Diagnosis of Diabetes Insipidus

Before proceeding with any evaluation for DI, it should be established that a patient who has polyuria and polydipsia without diabetes mellitus does not have chronic renal disease or urinary tract infection that explains the symptoms (Table 4-2; Fig. 4-3). For suggestion of a diagnosis of DI, a urine sample should be free of sugar and be dilute compared with plasma osmolality. The first question of importance is whether the patient really is urinating frequently in large quantities through the day and night or whether it is simply a pattern of frequent but small episodes of urination. The history should support a pattern suggestive of DI, and observation in the hospital or under the watch of reliable parents should be the first step to confirming increased urine volume output and

Table 4-2.   Water-deprivation test

Determine if patient is taking medications that can cause polyuria or has diabetes mellitus or other chronic disease that can cause decreased urine concentration (see text). Does patient have apparent psychological condition leading to psychogenic polydipsia? If not, proceed.

Normal overnight fast: if the patient does not normally drink overnight, fast, but if the patient does need to drink, allow this, but document time of intake and amount.

Determine first A.M. urine, serum osmolality, and hematocrit; if urine osmolality >600 (some have stated 450) mOsm, with serum osmolality ≤300 mOsm, vasopressin function is usually adequate.

If urine and serum do not match these guidelines, start observed fast (some suggest giving normal breakfast and then start observed fast, but if patient is stable, this may be omitted to shorten the test).

Check weight and urine osmolality hourly, and keep track of urine volume. Measure serum sodium and osmolality hourly, and measure serum vasopressin at 0 and the end of the test (certainly before any vasopressin is given) for future reference. All tests other than vasopressin should be ordered stat.

If urine osmolality >600 mOsm over a 1-hr period or more (some say 450) with serum osmolality ≤300 mOsm, or if urine osmolality >1,000 mOsm at any serum osmolality, function is normal.

If by 8 hr after beginning of observed fast, urine osmolality <600 (some say 450) mOsm, or at any time, if serum osmolality is >300 mOsm/L and urine osmolality stays below the guidelines, give 1 U/m^2 of aqueous vasopressin. If urine osmolality doubles the previous value over the next hour, the diagnosis is central DI. If no change occurs, the diagnosis is nephrogenic DI or some variant.

If blood pressure drops, pulse rises abnormally, or if weight drops >5%, consider stopping the test and obtaining last samples as listed. If the patient appears clinically stable, the test may be continued under careful scrutiny.

DI, diabetes insipidus.

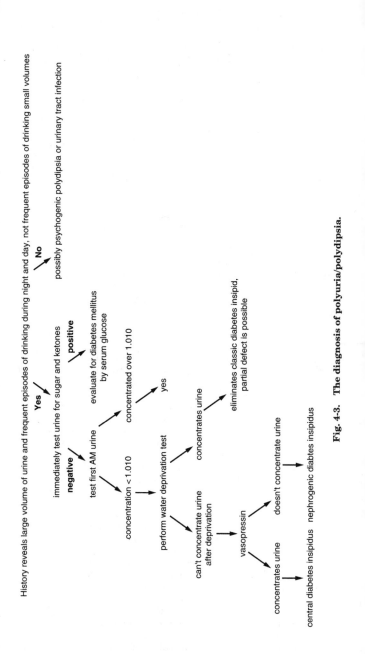

History reveals large volume of urine and frequent episodes of drinking during night and day, not frequent episodes of drinking small volumes

Yes → immediately test urine for sugar and ketones

No → possibly psychogenic polydipsia or urinary tract infection

positive → evaluate for diabetes mellitus by serum glucose

negative → test first AM urine

concentrated over 1.010 → yes

concentration < 1.010 → perform water deprivation test

concentrates urine → eliminates classic diabetes insipid, partial defect is possible

can't concentrate urine after deprivation → vasopressin

concentrates urine → central diabetes insipidus

doesn't concentrate urine → nephrogenic diabtes insipidus

Fig. 4-3. The diagnosis of polyuria/polydipsia.

fluid intake. The first voided urine sample in the morning is normally the most concentrated of the whole day, and a sample should be subjected to analysis of specific gravity and osmolality to see if this sample is concentrated more than 600 mOsm/L, which would eliminate the diagnosis in most cases (specific gravity may be increased fallaciously by contamination with nonosmotic substances, for example, stool, so measurement of osmolality is preferable). Serum osmolality and sodium should be determined; in DI, the values will be normal or slightly elevated if the patient has free access to water and a normal thirst mechanism, whereas in psychogenic polydipsia, the values will be normal or even low because of the dilutional effect of excessive water drinking. An ambulatory, conscious patient without a thirst mechanism will have a high osmolality and sodium because such patients do not have the normal drive to increase water intake as their serum sodium becomes increasingly concentrated; this condition has been called primary hypernatremia in some reports.

If the tests noted still suggest that the patient has DI, a careful water-deprivation test should be performed. These tests are difficult for the child and perhaps even more so for the family. The child must be expected to complain about lack of water whether DI or psychogenic polydipsia is involved, and the parents likewise might be uncomfortable over the procedure as the child cries for water. The most important consideration of such a test is to observe the child constantly for signs of dehydration that may be dangerous or for "cheating" when the child takes water surreptitiously, which will nullify the test results. The test should be done only with full staffing, and the later part of the thirst should not occur at night when the child might not be well observed.

The child should have a normal dinner, and the usual nighttime routine should continue. If the child stays at home for this night, whatever is the usual routine is followed (no fluid intake, if the child has been able to tolerate this schedule in the past, or fluid intake, if that is the norm). The next morning, the first voided urine should be analyzed for osmolality, the weight and BP should be determined, and serum sodium and a hematocrit should be determined. Assuming that the urine is not concentrated to 600 mOsm/L or greater and the serum osmolality is less than 300 mOsm/L, the test may commence. At that time, all oral intake should cease if it had not ceased during the night. Weight and BP should be taken hourly, serum osmolality and hematocrit determined every 2 hours, and all urine volume monitored and osmolality measured at every void. The test should cease if the BP decreases 10%, or the serum osmolality increases above 300 mOsm/L. If the urine osmolality increases above 600 mOsm/L but the serum osmolality is not above 300 mOsm/L, the test should stop, as there is no likelihood of DI. Otherwise, at the end of 8 hours or the time available with adequate staffing for the test, the serum and urine osmolality should be compared, and a serum vasopressin determination obtained to match with the osmolality determinations (the vasopressin value will not return for weeks from the laboratory but may prove useful if the diagnosis is still in doubt later).

As a patient becomes dehydrated, the urine osmolality will increase because of the delivery of increasingly concentrated filtrate to the kidney, but a patient with DI cannot concentrate the urine to more than 1.5 to 2 times the serum osmolality. If the serum osmolality increases to 300 mOsm/L or higher, the urine should normally be more than 450 mOsm/L and ideally more than 600 mOsm/L. In an intermediate situation in which a trend toward dehydration is developing, a continuation of the thirst may be necessary; this will be safe if careful observation of state of hydration, BP, and pulse is continued. Further, in partial DI, a patient may pass one test with just adequate urinary concentration, whereas, if the test is repeated the next day, the patient may be virtually unable to concentrate the urine because of the exhaustion of the patient's meager supply of vasopressin.

If the serum osmolality has increased without concentration of the urine and therefore no increase in urine osmolality, 0.05 to 0.15 mL of D-arginine-D-amino-vasopressin (DDAVP, see later for explanation of this medication) in a nostril (or, if DDAVP is unavailable or there is pathology of the nasal mucosa, a 1-U/m^2 subcutaneous dose of aqueous vasopressin) is administered, and the volume of urine and the urine concentration in the next 30 to 60 minutes is compared with the values obtained before the DDAVP or exogenous vasopressin was given. In central DI, at the end of the fast, the patient has secreted the maximal vasopressin that he or she is capable of secreting, but this diminished store of vasopressin is inadequate for the task of concentrating the urine. Thus, the exogenous vasopressin will further concentrate the urine significantly. A patient with nephrogenic DI will not be able to concentrate urine in spite of increasing serum osmolality, and the addition of exogenous vasopressin will not further increase urine osmolality or reduce urine volume, because the patient is resistant to vasopressin.

The diagnosis of psychogenic polydipsia may sometimes present problems. Because of excess water load before the onset of the test because of the patient's excessive drinking habits, the patient may have developed a dilute or "washed out" medullary gradient. The serum osmolality may not increase much above normal during the thirst, even if vasopressin is inadequate; if this owing to a long history of excess water intake, the patient may not reach full urinary concentration even if the fast is continued. However, the exogenous vasopressin will not cause further concentration of the urine because a patient with psychogenic polydipsia is perfectly able to release adequate endogenous vasopressin in the face of fasting, and exogenous vasopressin exerts no further effect than the endogenous vasopressin. Usually the psychological history in addition to the results of the water-deprivation test will lead to the correct diagnosis, as most children with psychogenic polydipsia will not have such urinary dilution after a fast as will those with nephrogenic DI.

Because central DI is likely owing to a congenital anatomic defect of the CNS or an acquired CNS tumor, an MRI is indicated. Loss of the T_1-weighted bright spot of the posterior pituitary gland during gadolinium MRI scan will result in central DI associated with the loss of vasopressin and neurophysin production that are responsible for the hot spot. However, in nephrogenic DI, a loss of the bright spot may be owing to continued and increased release of vasopressin. The CNS defect may be apparent on MRI, but in some cases, a thickening of the pituitary stalk is all that suggests a developing tumor; sequential follow-up MRI is indicated, as it may take years for the tumor to be truly discernible.

Treatment of Central Diabetes Insipidus

An untreated patient with DI, if old enough and able enough to take in sufficient water, will survive but will develop dilated ureters and renal pelvises because of the increased urinary flow and will be on the brink of severe dehydration if anything disturbs the balance achieved (see Chapter 15 for description of emergency treatment of hypernatremia due to DI). The appropriate therapy is vasopressin replacement in a convenient form. Native vasopressin has a short half-life and exerts hypertensive effects. DDAVP, an altered vasopressin molecule that has 140 times the urine-concentrating ability but almost none of the vasoactive effects of native arginine vasopressin, is the treatment of choice. A dose of DDAVP will usually last approximately 12 hours (or even 24 hours), whereas native vasopressin has a half-life of 20 minutes. The dose of oral DDAVP is titrated from 25 to 200 μg until adequate antidiuresis is achieved after a nighttime administration. A morning dose is given if significant polyuria still occurs during the day. Alternatively, DDAVP is administered in measured doses through inhalation by the nostrils, a method easier in older children than in infants. A syringe may be used to squirt DDAVP into the nostrils of the youngest children. A dose of 0.025 mL of a solution of 10 μg/0.1 mL (yielding 2.5 μg) is given with a plastic tube inserted into the nose and is repeated when the child complains of increasing thirst or an infant begins to increase urinary frequency again. A measured dispenser of nasal spray is an alternative treatment, with a dose of 10 μg per spray (0.1-mL volume). Oral vasopressin tablets are becoming more popular than the nasal route of therapy. Doses of 25 to 300 μg, 2 to 3 times per day, control most subjects. A patient must have a phase of urinary dilution or breakthrough urination before the next dose is given to ensure that water intoxication does not result. In the presence of an intact thirst mechanism, the patient should be able to maintain a normal sodium concentration with DDAVP treatment.

Lysine vasopressin or Lypressin is given as a nasal spray (50 U/mL or 2 U per spray) that lasts 2 to 8 hours, if a short action is desired (for example, in infants). This treatment is rarely used at present.

Intravenous (i.v.) management during surgery or recovery is given as 1.5 mU/kg/hr of vasopressin while carefully monitoring fluid intake to ensure appropriate fluid balance. Excessive fluid administration with i.v. vasopressin or any of the forms of vasopressin listed earlier will lead to an SIADH-like condition.

Patients with an absent thirst mechanism and diabetes insipidus are extremely difficult to treat. A set regimen is empirically determined under careful observation so that a given number of glasses of water or a volume of water per day sufficient to keep the serum sodium in the normal range is prescribed. An extra glass of water or more should be given for moderately increased activity or exposure to high temperature. Every week or two, the serum sodium should be measured, with determinations more often if stability has not been reached. The serious consequences of dehydration or overhydration should not be minimized in this complex condition that may lead to serious dehydration or death if not adequately treated.

Treatment of Nephrogenic Diabetes Insipidus

The goal of treatment of nephrogenic DI is to cause the kidney to retain water in the absence of any effects of vasopressin; the method may seem paradoxical, as a low-sodium diet and diuretic therapy is prescribed. With decreased serum solute due to the low sodium intake and the loss of sodium due to iatrogenic diuresis, the site of reabsorption of water shifts from the collecting duct where vasopressin exerts its effect to the proximal tubule where aldosterone, maximally stimulated by whole body sodium loss, will attempt to retain all available sodium and thereby carry water back into the vascular compartment along with the sodium, so that decreased urine flow results. Thus the treatment bypasses the tubule where vasopressin exerts no effect to an area where aldosterone can exert its effect. A thiazide diuretic with the addition of amiloride is suggested to counteract the hypokalemia caused by thiazide. Alternatively, thiazide diuretics and indomethacin are used, with a careful observation for nephrotoxicity.

THE SYNDROME OF INAPPROPRIATE SECRETION OF ANTIDIURETIC HORMONE

In the presence of vasopressin and excessive water intake, an expansion of intravascular volume will cause a decrease in serum sodium and serum osmolality as well as a sodium diuresis and some degree of concentration of the urine. This constellation seems paradoxical because the low serum sodium and osmolality could be corrected if the urine is maximally diluted and if maximal urinary sodium reabsorption is accomplished. Atrial natriuretic peptide may be responsible for the sodium diuresis, as it is elevated in times of volume overload. Vasopressin by itself exerts no effect on serum sodium, but the retention of water does in the presence of vasopressin. Because the combination of vasopressin secretion and water intake is responsible for SIADH, the syndrome is often iatrogenic; the patient already may be under a physician's care and may kept on the same regimen of fluid therapy after the vasopressin secretion begins after temporary DI or after vasopressin is administered as a medication. If fluid therapy in the treatment of conditions predisposing to SIADH were appropriately regulated, and if serum sodium concentrations were monitored routinely, the incidence of SIADH would decrease considerably. Patients with cancers that produce vasopressin in ectopic locations may be in the habit of drinking a set amount of fluid before the tumor developed; if the same fluid intake is continued after the ectopic vasopressin is present, SIADH may develop even before the cancer itself is diagnosed.

Any disorder of the lungs, including those requiring ventilator support, can cause the release of vasopressin, mediated by the volume or stretch receptors in the right atrium. Thus, the commonly prescribed increased fluids during episodes of pneumonia or other disorders of the lungs may precipitate an episode of SIADH. Infant botulism may lead to SIADH during ventilator support, and patients supported on ventilators for extended periods must have serum sodium regularly monitored. Most neurologic conditions, including meningitis, tumors, the postsurgical condition, and trauma, can increase vasopressin secretion; these potential complications are well recognized and account for the usual orders for reduced fluid administration in neurologic disease. After any surgery, increased vasopressin secretion occurs, and the patient is susceptible to SIADH; thus the orders to "push fluids" after surgery may precipitate an episode of SIADH. Any condition causing nausea and emesis, including carcinomatosis or the administration of chemotherapy, can increase vasopressin secretion. Further, drugs often used in cancer therapy, such as vancomycin, vincristine, and cyclophosphamide (Cytoxan), increase vasopressin secretion in addition to their tendency to cause nausea. Many types of cancers produce vasopressin in an ectopic hormone-secreting syndrome, so that a patient with cancer may be susceptible to SIADH from the cancer, from the nausea of the cancer therapy, and from the chemotherapeutic agent itself!

Another condition combining hyponatremia associated with various types of CNS disease is called cerebral salt wasting. In this condition, hyponatremia, excess urine sodium loss, but hypovolemia are demonstrated, in contrast to SIADH, in which intravascular volume is increased. In cerebral salt wasting, serum atrial natriuretic factor is increased and may be the primary defect, whereas serum aldosterone and vasopressin are normal or decreased. Treatment involves the replacement of sodium losses and volume.

Diagnosis of Syndrome of Inappropriate Secretion of Antidiuretic Hormone

Not all episodes of hyponatremia are owing to SIADH. The most frequent cause of hyponatremia in pediatrics is fluid overload with hypotonic fluids while receiving i.v. therapy under a physician's care. Congestive heart failure and the oliguric phase of acute renal failure may lead to hyponatremia. Other conditions lead to low sodium measured on laboratory instruments because of interfering or osmotically active substances in the serum, often called pseudohyponatremia; in hyperglycemia, hyperlipidemia, and hyperproteinemia (such as in multiple myelosis) serum sodium might fallaciously decrease. The effect of each elevation of blood glucose of 100 mg/dL is to depress serum sodium by 1.6 mEq/mL in the laboratory determination because of pseudo-hyponatremia. It is important to realize that an elevation of atrial natriuretic factor occurs in some cases of diabetic ketoacidosis, causing true hyponatremia requiring replacement rather than pseudohyponatremia due to hyperglycemia, which does not require sodium replacement. Pseudohyponatremia is asymptomatic and is not a physiologic problem, as the cells are actually exposed to normal amounts of sodium in spite of laboratory determinations. Thus in pseudohyponatremia, correction of the underlying condition is indicated, but sodium administration is rarely necessary.

The Treatment of Syndrome of Inappropriate Secretion of Antidiuretic Hormone

The treatment of SIADH is first and foremost prevention (see Chapter 15 for discussion of emergency treatment of hypernatremia due to SIADH). This is primarily an iatrogenic disease, and monitoring fluid therapy with frequent serum sodium concentrations will eliminate the possibility of severe shifts of sodium. Once SIADH develops, fluid restriction to the minimum possible but safe level is the correct approach. In many cases, maintaining i.v. fluids at a level just able to keep the i.v. line open is appropriate for a time as the attainment of fluid balance is indicated. With less severe hyponatremia, replacing urine output with an equal amount of i.v. fluid calculated every 2 to 4 hours is adequate fluid replacement. Because the urine flow is so low in SIADH, the tendency will be to fear that inadequate intravascular volume is the problem, and it may appear that the decision to administer boluses of fluid to increase urinary output is correct. If the oliguria is due to dehydration, the boluses are appropriate and will allow urination, but if SIADH has been diagnosed, the boluses will only intensify the SIADH, as the fluid will be retained. Careful review of the records, including an accounting of all fluids administered (a balance sheet of intake and output is essential), changes in body weight, and an estimation of intravascular volume or measurement of central venous pressure should clarify the diagnosis.

Other methods are available to break through the SIADH and allow urine flow so that intravascular volume decreases and the condition is modified. Lithium and democlocycline will interfere with ADH action on the kidney, but the inherent side effects limit their use in younger children. Replacement of the volume loss with 3% saline will help correct the hyponatremia without administering excessive fluid volume. If hyponatremia is severe and seizures have resulted, furosemide may be administered, as well as 3% saline, to bring about some degree of urination and volume depletion. This procedure of diuretic and hypertonic fluid administration can cause rapid fluid shifts, causing dilution and concentration at various times, and is potentially dangerous. Careful monitoring and maintaining a patent i.v. line to administer fluid volume if necessary are essential.

It should be emphasized that the sodium diuresis characteristic of SIADH is continuous during the active phase of the disorder, and sodium administered by any route will quickly be passed out in the urine and will not offer a long-term cure of hyponatremia. However, even if i.v. hypertonic saline increases serum sodium only temporarily, it may offer the only effective treatment for a hyponatremic seizure. If seizures are intractable, the combination of furosemide (Lasix) and hypertonic saline described earlier may be the only appropriate therapy. Whatever therapy is offered, constant observation must be given for severe fluid shifts.

THE TRIPHASIC RESPONSE AFTER SURGERY FOR CRANIOPHARYNGIOMA

A patient with a craniopharyngioma already may have DI before surgery is carried out for the tumor; if not, when the pituitary stalk is cut, DI may manifest immediately, possibly while the patient is in the operating suite (Fig. 4-4). After this, in a few days, often unrestrained release of vasopressin will occur as the cut nerve cells degenerate. If the high level of fluid replacement originally necessary for treatment of the DI is continued during this secondary phase of vasopressin secretion, full-blown SIADH will develop. During the following days, a third phase of permanent DI will occur in most patients. However, some patients who

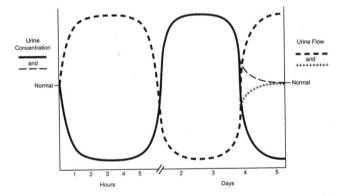

Fig. 4-4.   The triphasic pattern of urine concentration after pituitary surgery, usually for a craniopharyngioma. On the left Y axis is urine concentration relative to a conceptional normal, and on the right axis is urine flow relative to a conceptional normal state. If the transection is low on the pituitary stalk, normalization of urine flow (++++++) and urine concentration may occur (---), rather than diabetes insipidus in the third phase.

receive the surgical transection low on the pituitary stalk will resume close to normal vasopressin secretion, and the DI will cease. It is imperative that fluid output be monitored carefully after pituitary stalk surgery so that intake is matched to output, and fluid overloading does not occur during changing fluid dynamics, or that dehydration does not occur.

SUGGESTED READINGS

Albanese A, Hindmarsh P, Stanhope R. Management of hyponatremia in patients with acute cerebral insults. *Arch Dis Child* 2001;85:246–251.

Maghnie M, Cosi G, Genovese E, et al. Central diabetes insipidus in children and young adults. *N Engl J Med* 2000;343:998–1007.

Majzoub JA. Primary disturbances of water homeostasis. In: Rudolph CD, Rudolph AM, eds. *Rudolph's pediatrics.* New York: McGraw-Hill, 2002:2025–2028.

Muglia LJ, Majzoub JA. Disorders of the posterior pituitary. In: Sperling MA, ed. *Pediatric endocrinology.* Philadelphia: WB Saunders, 2002:289–322.

5 ♣ Abnormal Growth

Short stature is probably the most common complaint that brings a child to a pediatric endocrinologist, either by parental choice or by referral from the family's physician. Growth is a general indication of a child's health and can be considered a bioassay of the state of health of the child. Short stature, rather than indicating an endocrine abnormality, may herald the onset of nonendocrine systemic disease or a state of malnutrition. Whereas the goal of this chapter is the evaluation of endocrine disorders that affect growth, other chronic conditions should be ruled out before a sophisticated endocrine evaluation is started. Thus initial history and physical examination should determine whether a search for endocrine conditions is warranted. It is especially important to determine whether a nutritional condition has caused decreased growth rather than starting off on an endocrine evaluation.

HISTORY AND PHYSICAL EXAMINATION

In many cases, the diagnosis is apparent from the medical history. Query for abnormalities or toxic exposures of pregnancy, nutritional status during pregnancy, difficulties of delivery, degree of prematurity, if any, and even more important, evaluate weight for gestational age (Fig. 5-1) are important. Determination of age of puberty of parents (menarche in mothers and age of physical changes of puberty or cessation of growth in fathers) may suggest a tendency toward constitutional delay in growth or adolescence. Family history of chronic disease, including neurologic or endocrine conditions, and the child's history of symptoms of chronic disease of almost any organ can be of great importance, as most chronic diseases can decrease growth.

Physical examination must be complete to search for abnormalities of nutrition, chronic disease, and neurologic problems, especially of the central nervous system (CNS). If decreased nutrition appears to be the problem, most likely no endocrine condition is present, and other causes must be considered. Weight-for-height curves are now superseded by Body Mass Index charts (BMI charts found at www.CDC.com; see Chapter 12); low BMI for age might indicate malnutrition due to chronic disease, whereas elevated BMI for age might indicate rapid growth due to obesity.

MEASUREMENT OF GROWTH

Measurement of stature is the cheapest procedure available in the pediatric office and the one most often incorrectly performed if even performed at all! Failing to measure a child at a visit is a serious mistake that limits the assessment of the health of the child. Further, if a growth deficiency is developing as a consequence of the medical condition that precipitated the office visit, the most important measure of the defect in growth, the growth rate, cannot be assessed until another visit occurs, because two height measurements at least 3 months apart (and optimally 6 months apart) are needed to determine growth rate accurately. If previous height measurements from well-child visits were available, any change in growth rate would be noted earlier. Because many systemic diseases affect growth, a decrease in growth rate, which would serve as an early indication of the onset of such a disease, would be missed. Incorrect measurements are responsible for numerous inappropriate referrals for short stature. Further, incorrect measurement can obscure the effects of a medication meant to correct an abnormality of stature (e.g., the positive effects of growth hormone treatment can be evaluated only with accurate, sequential measurements).

An accurate measurement of infant length is extremely difficult and always requires two adults. The child must be laid on a flat surface with a device that has one plate horizontal to the plane of the top of the child's head and another plate horizontal to the first in the plane of the child's feet. The two plates should be at a 90-degree angle to a ruler on which the child's height is read. Several available devices range from inexpensive portable plastic caliper-like devices (e.g., infantometer) to scales with the measuring arms permanently attached (Fig. 5-2).

The worst method of measurement of infants is all too frequently in common use; a single observer makes a mark on the paper covering the examining table at the foot of the child and another mark at the head to measure the distance between the marks as an indication of the length of the child. It should be obvious that the paper is so flexible and so crumpled by the weight of the child as to make the distance between the head and feet quite variable, and that the movement of even a relatively quiet child will make such measurements useless. It may be glib to say so, but guessing the length of a term newborn as 21 inches is usually more accurate than using the paper technique described!

The measurement of a patient older than 2 years is done with the child standing. The switch from lying to standing measurements is responsible for a large number of inappropriate referrals because of the 1- to 2-cm decrease in height measurements that occurs when switching positions. It is important that the position of measurement be indicated on the chart next to the numeric measurement for children at this age of transition, so that unfounded worry about a declining growth rate does not develop. Regrettably, we must caution the observer to measure the child with the shoes off; if a child is measured in shoes one time and without them another time, a guaranteed 2- to 4-cm variation in height is found per visit, and this all too often happens during casual evaluations.

The device used to measure standing height must be a variation of a standard stadiometer (e.g., Harpenden stadiometer), which can measure to 0.1 cm. The child must have the back straight against the wall or to a hard, flat surface on which the stadiometer is attached. The child's back must be straight, and the heels and back must press posteriorly to the surface. The feet must be on a floor or hard surface rather than a soft carpet, as the bottoms of the feet are considered to be the beginning of the measurement. The top of the measurement must be a hard plate completely parallel to the plane of the feet, and the measurement

(text continues on page 48)

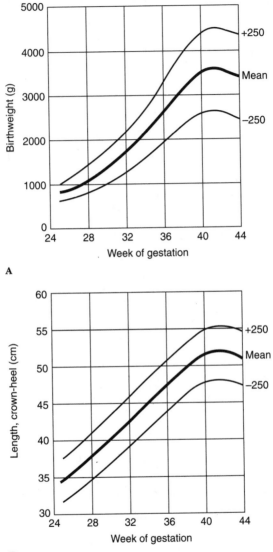

A

B

Fig. 5-1. Intrauterine growth charts showing the normal values of body weight, length, and head circumference for infants born at different gestational ages at sea level (Montreal). (From Usher R, McLean FM. Intrauterine growth of live-born caucasian infants at sea level: Standards obtained from measurements in 7 dimensions of infants born between 25 and 44 weeks of gestation. *J Pediatr* 1969;74:901, with permission.)

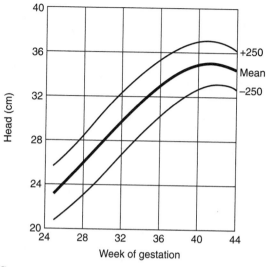

C

Fig. 5-1. (continued)

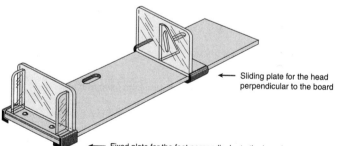

Fig. 5-2. A commercially available infantometer used for measuring lying length in infants. There is a ruler in centimeters fixed to the horizontal board.

must be read off a stationary ruler that is at right angles to the planes at the feet and head. A Harpenden stadiometer is the most accurate of such devices, as it indicates the height in millimeter increments, but inexpensive devices that follow these guidelines should give accurate measurements if correct measurement procedures are followed (Fig. 5-3). Unfortunately, the floppy-arm device attached to a pole rising above the common office scale is used in many offices; because the plate at the top of the pole is rarely parallel to the floor, there is no way to straighten the patient's back against a thin pole, and the child may slouch, the measurements are useless.

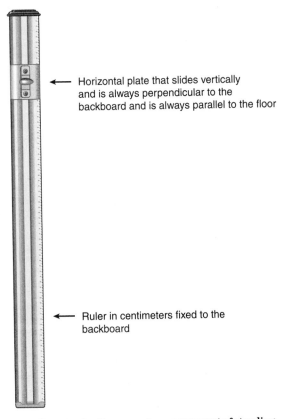

Horizontal plate that slides vertically and is always perpendicular to the backboard and is always parallel to the floor

Ruler in centimeters fixed to the backboard

Fig. 5-3.   A stadiometer for the accurate measurement of standing height to an accuracy of a few tenths of a centimeter. There is an indicator on the sliding plate that indicates the height. A standard bar of 2 meters is used to calibrate the measurement daily.

It is strongly recommended that all measurements be made by using the metric system. The tendency to round off numbers becomes problematic when an inch is the unit of measure; an inaccuracy of an inch or a half inch is a more serious error than a mistake of 1 or 0.5 cm; remember that a half-inch (1.25-cm) rounding error over a 6-month period can mean the difference between 4-cm/yr growth, which is abnormal, and 6.5 cm/yr, which is normal.

After the measurement is obtained, it must be displayed graphically on the growth chart. New charts of stature for age (as well as weight for age and BMI) from the National Center for Health Statistics are available at www.cdc.gov; they may be downloaded or printed (Fig. 5-4A and B). An abnormality of stature or growth rate is far more obvious on a graph than written as a number on the page. A decrease in growth rate in which a child "falls away from the curve" or "crosses percentiles of stature" becomes obvious on the graph. Growth-velocity charts (Fig. 5-5) demonstrate the rate of growth, are more sensitive to deviations from the normal growth velocity, and reveal abnormalities before they become apparent on the standard height-for-age charts found in Fig. 5-4 (see examples in Fig. 5-6).

Determination of arm span and upper-to-lower ratio is useful in evaluation of short stature (e.g., to indicate hypochondroplasia or achondroplasia) or of delay in puberty (e.g., to look for the long arms and decreased upper- to lower-segment ratio of hypogonadism). The arm span is measured with the patient standing with the back to the wall with arms spread horizontally and is the distance from one outstretched middle fingertip to the other. The arm-span measurement should be close to the measurement of the height; if it is shorter than the height, a chondrodystrophy may be limiting long-bone growth, whereas if it is longer than the height, an abnormality of the growth of the spine may be among other possibilities. The lower segment is measured from the top of the symphysis pubis to the floor, whereas the upper segment is measured by subtracting the lower segment from the height of the child. The upper- to lower-segment ratio varies with age from 1.7 at birth to 1.4 at 2 years to 1 at about 10 years, and values greater than 0.9 at adulthood (Fig. 5-7). An decreased upper-to-lower ratio is found in Klinefelter syndrome, and an increased ratio is found in hypothyroidism and chondrodystrophies.

Skeletal development, or bone age is more closely correlated with certain developmental landmarks than with chronologic age in conditions of delayed or advanced puberty. It is a reflection of the physiologic rather than the chronologic age of the child. A bone-age determination does not provide a diagnosis but may support a condition under consideration. The bone age is determined by a radiograph of the left hand and wrist as compared with the standards in the Greulich and Pyle atlas in most U.S. environments, although Europeans may prefer the Tanner Whitehouse (TW) method. The delay or advancement in bone age

(text continues on page 57)

CDC Growth Charts: United States

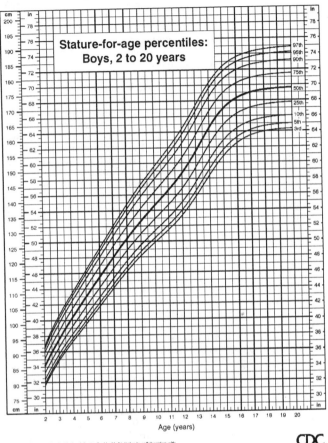

Stature-for-age percentiles:
Boys, 2 to 20 years

Age (years)

SOURCE: Developed by the National Center for Health Statistics in collaboration with the National Center for Chronic Disease Prevention and Health Promotion (2000).

CDC

Fig. 5-4.   A: Height for age percentiles in boys from 2 to 20 years (from Centers for Disease Control website, www.cdc.gov/growthcharts).

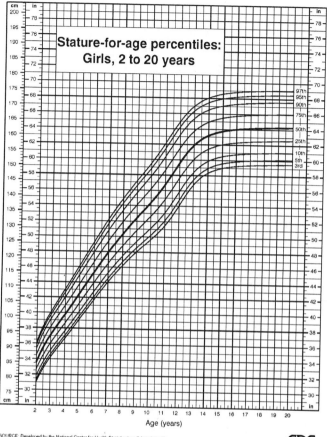

Fig. 5-4. (continued)   B: Height for age percentiles in girls from 2 to 20 years (from CDC website, www.cdc.gov/ growthcharts).

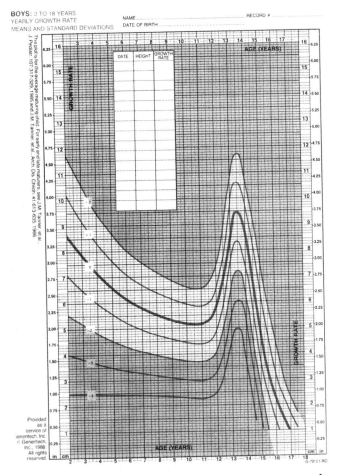

Fig. 5-5.   A: Growth-velocity chart. Yearly growth rate, means, and standard deviations for boys aged 2 to 18 years.

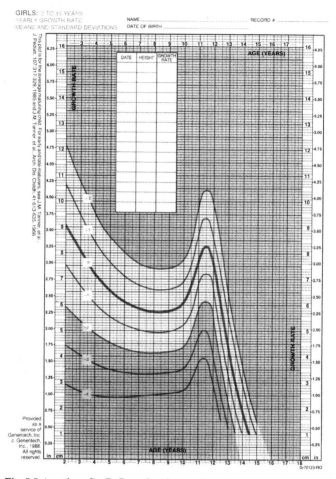

Provided as a service of Genentech, Inc. © Genentech, Inc. 1988 All rights reserved

Fig. 5-5. (continued)   B: Growth-velocity chart. Yearly growth rate, means, and standard deviations for girls aged 2 to 15 years.

CDC Growth Charts: United States

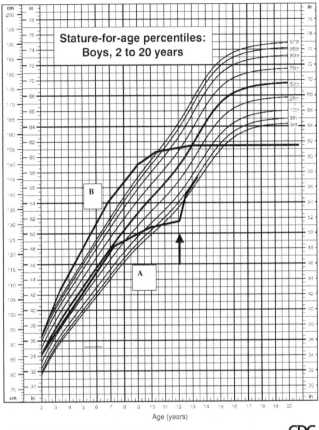

Stature-for-age percentiles:
Boys, 2 to 20 years

SOURCE: Developed by the National Center for Health Statistics in collaboration with
the National Center for Chronic Disease Prevention and Health Promotion (2000).

Fig. 5-6. Demonstration of the sensitivity of the growth-velocity charts compared to standard stature versus age charts.
A: A growth chart of two boys. Line A is a boy who decreases growth rate profoundly at age ~7 years. At age 12 years, some intervention occurs, and growth catches up at greater than average growth rate. This could be the institution of thyroxine in hypothyroidism, growth hormone (GH) in GH deficiency, or the removal of a glucocorticoid-secreting tumor. Line B represents a growth chart of a child growing faster than normal early in life, who slows to normal at 9 years and decreases thereafter, until ceasing to grow by age ~13 years; this is found in untreated precocious puberty.

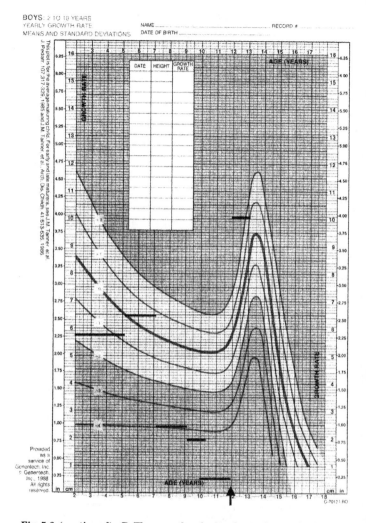

Fig. 5-6. (continued)   B: The growth-velocity chart of curve A, showing the more striking changes of growth rate at various ages. The growth rate between two ages is plotted as a horizontal bar, with the height of the bar demonstrating the annualized growth rate and the lateral limits spanning the ages under consideration.

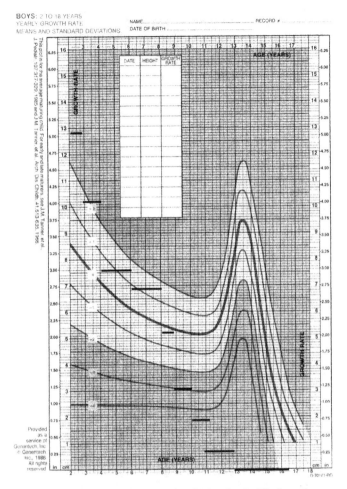

Fig. 5-6. (continued) C: The growth-velocity chart of the boy of
line B. The decrease in growth rate is more striking earlier than is
apparent on the statural growth chart. The growth rate between two
ages is plotted as a horizontal bar, with the height of the bar demonstrating the annualized growth rate and the lateral limits spanning
the ages under consideration.

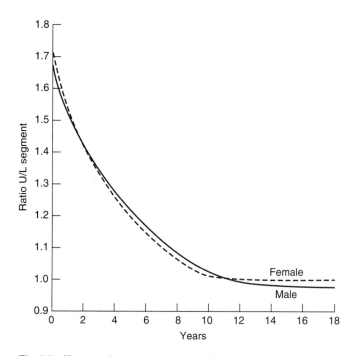

Fig. 5-7. **Upper- to lower-segment ratio. (From Engelback LW. The diagnosis and treatment of endocrine disorders in childhood and adolescence. Springfield, IL: Charles C Thomas Publishers, 1965, with permission.)**

is expressed in standard deviations from the average reading for chronologic age. Standard deviations vary with age; one standard deviation may be only 2 months during the first year to 1 year at 15 years. Increased accuracy in the technique is accomplished by radiologists with the most practice; unfortunately, most general radiologists who are not associated with a pediatric center do not read many bone ages, and their readings may not be quite correct. With a bone age over 6 years and an accurate determination of stature, final height can be predicted by the Bailey-Pinneau tables found at the end of the Greulich and Pyle atlas. The Roche Wainer Thissen (RWT) method allows prediction of eventual adult height in younger children. Other methods of height prediction are in use in Europe, and computerized methods of bone-age evaluation in development may increase accuracy in the future.

ENDOCRINE FACTORS IN POSTNATAL GROWTH

Growth hormone has a major effect on postnatal growth but has far less effect in prenatal growth, as growth hormone–deficient neonates are of normal or close to normal length. The release of growth hormone from its pituitary stores is stimulated by hypothalamic growth hormone (GH)-releasing factor and inhibited by somatostatin or GH-release inhibitory factor. GH has some direct effects (e.g., diabetogenic insulin-resistant effects), but most of the growth-promoting action of GH is mediated by insulin-like growth factor 1 (IGF-1). Serum GH concentrations are low throughout most of the day in normal patients but increase at intervals, and these peaks differentiate a GH-sufficient patient from a GH-deficient subject in most cases. Thus, random GH measurements do not reveal abnormalities of secretion unless the elevated levels found in GH resistance or pituitary gigantism are suspected; only sequential measurements through a 12- or 24-hour period (rarely performed because of expense) or measurements after the administration of a secretagogue are of interest. However, even secretory tests are suspect, as some children with normal GH secretion on testing can benefit from GH treatment, and others with low values on such a test are growing normally and need no GH.

Circulating GH is noncovalently bound to a GH-binding protein (GHBP). GH exerts a biologic effect by binding to a membrane-bound GH receptor. In the normal situation, a single GH molecule must bind to a GH receptor that dimerizes. The abundance of the membrane receptor for GH is reflected by the value of circulating GHBP, which itself has the amino acid sequence of the extra membrane portion of the GH receptor. In classic GH resistance (e.g., Laron dwarfism) the serum GHBP values are low, whereas serum GH is high. In other forms of GH resistance, the number of receptors and the measurement of GHBP are normal, but the function of the receptor is defective. In the absence of the gluconeogenic effects of GH, these patients tend to be hypoglycemic, as do GH-deficient patients themselves.

In GH deficiency, the bone-age development is delayed, whereas the upper- to lower-segment ratio is normal for bone age, in contrast to hypothyroidism, in which bone age is severely delayed, but the upper- to lower-segment ratio is quite increased because of lack of appropriate growth of the limbs. Patients with untreated GH deficiency have delay in the onset of puberty until the absent GH is replaced with treatment, and puberty progresses. It is thus difficult to determine which patient with untreated GH deficiency has delayed puberty because of this factor and which has gonadotropin deficiency in addition to the defect in GH secretion.

IGFs (previously called somatomedins), are produced in tissue throughout the body. IGF-1 is most closely associated with growth and has mitogenic effects in most dividing cells in the body. Plasma values of IGF-1 decrease in states of GH deficiency and increase in GH excess. IGF-1 is low in the neonate and increases slowly through childhood until a peak is reached during the pubertal period; normal values at puberty are in the range character-istic of acromegalic adults. Except for this increase that occurs near the time of the pubertal growth spurt, absolute plasma con-centrations of IGF-1 are not closely related to growth rate. The major problems with the interpretation of IGF-1 concentrations as a reflection of GH secretion are (a) the values in the first 3 years of postnatal life are close to or identical with those found in the hypopituitary state; (b) the values in constitutional delay in growth are appropriate for bone age rather than chronologic age and are often reported as abnormally low in constitutional delay in growth when, if corrected for bone age, the values would be normal; and (c) in states of poor nutrition, a condition that by itself can cause poor growth, IGF-1 values are as low as those in a GH-deficient subject. Thus the use of serum IGF-1 concentrations must be tem-pered with caution in the diagnosis of growth deficiency, and strict attention must be paid to nutritional status and physiologic state of development.

IGFs are associated with binding proteins in the circulation, and the binding proteins themselves might be indicative of GH status. IGFBP-3 is GH dependent, and low serum values in asso-ciation with low serum values of IGF-1 make the diagnosis of GH deficiency more likely than a decrease in serum IGF-1 by itself. Some suggest that the abandonment of secretory tests of GH and argue reliance on serum IGF-1 and IGFBP-3 is sufficient for diagnosis of GH deficiency. Not all insurance companies or state agencies agree to pay for GH treatment without a GH secretory test, so we cannot yet completely abandon this testing procedure.

Concentrations of IGF-2 are decreased in GH deficiency but not increased in GH excess. Levels also may be increased in patients with osteosarcoma. Although plasma IGF-1 concentrations alone may not be reliable in the diagnosis of GH deficiency, the finding of both low values of IGF-1 and IGF-2 has been stated to be quite reliable in pointing to the diagnosis. In general, however, IGF-2 measurements are not used clinically.

Thyroid hormone is essential for postnatal growth but has lit-tle effect on fetal longitudinal growth, as congenital hypothy-roidism is associated with normal or even slightly greater than normal birth length. Thyroid hormone also is necessary for the normal secretion of GH, as hypothyroid patients may not respond to GH-stimulation tests with GH secretion, thereby confusing the diagnosis of hypothyroidism with GH deficiency. Hypothyroid patients who have accompanying GH deficiency cannot respond to GH therapy unless they are rendered euthyroid. In the absence of adequate thyroid hormone, a patient has reduced limb growth, leading to a delayed or higher upper- to lower-segment ratio. Bone-age development also is retarded in hypothyroidism, and when the epiphyses do appear, they are often irregular and abnormal, with multiple epiphyses (epiphyseal dysgenesis). Usually puberty is delayed if thyroid hormone is decreased, but with profound hypothyroidism, some aspects of puberty may occur prematurely, particularly in girls (see Chapter 9).

Sex steroids advance growth, skeletal age, and pubertal development in the postnatal state. Gonadal steroids are essential for the pubertal growth spurt and are responsible for approximately half of the growth achieved during puberty. If excessive sex steroid concentrations are maintained for a long period (e.g., virilizing congenital adrenal hyperplasia), the epiphyses will fuse prematurely, and the previously tall child will become a short adult; epiphyseal fusion is owing to the action of estrogen, which may be secreted directly or result from the aromatization of testosterone. Absence of gonadal steroids will delay skeletal maturation and decrease the pubertal growth spurt, but in some cases, hypogonadism will allow prolonged growth that leads to taller-than-predicted adult stature.

Glucocorticoids are the most effective growth suppressors when present in excess; thus, Cushing syndrome due to endogenous (e.g., an adrenal adenoma) or exogenous (e.g., for rheumatoid arthritis or renal disease) glucocorticoids can cause the cessation of growth and result in short stature. Inhaled glucocorticoids for asthma therapy may have measurable but smaller effects on growth than do oral glucocorticoids. If glucocorticoids for treatment of a chronic disease can be minimized by the use of decreased dosage, alternate-day treatment, or even alternative therapy, growth will usually benefit. Decreased glucocorticoids will not affect growth as long as the patient is not disabled or anorexic from the condition.

Insulin in excess will increase growth rate in the fetus (e.g., infant of a diabetic mother) and after birth (e.g., patients with insulinomas or islet cell hypertrophy). Insulin deficiency will decrease growth if replacement is inadequate because of the many serious effects of diabetes. Further, in the absence of insulin receptors, as in Donohue's "leprechaun" syndrome (246200 LEPRECHAUNISM at 19p13-2), an autosomal recessive condition, fetal and postnatal growth will be poor.

Genetic factors are of obvious importance in growth. The correlation between midparental height and children's height can be used to adjust the position of a child on a growth chart. Therefore, a child at the fifth percentile of the standing growth chart who has short parents may be closer to a conceptual tenth percentile for the family when adjusted for midparental height. The average difference in adult stature of 5 inches between men and women in the United States is used for the process; thus 5 inches is subtracted from a father's height to allow plotting his adjusted height appropriately on a daughter's chart (as shown on figure 5-8) and 5 inches is added to a mother's height to allow plotting her adjusted height on a son's chart (plotted at 18 to 20 years, an age when growth normally ceases and is effectively adult height). Then the father's height and adjusted mother's height is averaged, and the midparental height that results (the adjusted midparental height) is plotted on the far right of the son's growth chart (e.g., at 18 years, or adult stature) or the mother's height and the adjusted father's height are averaged, and the resulting midparental height plotted on the far right of the daughter's

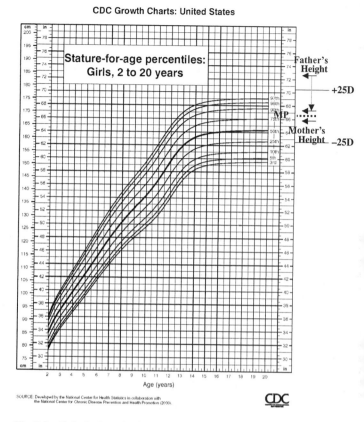

CDC Growth Charts: United States

Stature-for-age percentiles:
Girls, 2 to 20 years

Father's Height

+25D

MP

Mother's Height   −25D

97th
95th
90th
75th
50th
25th
10th
5th
3rd

Age (years)

SOURCE: Developed by the National Center for Health Statistics in collaboration with
the National Center for Chronic Disease Prevention and Health Promotion (2000).

**Fig. 5-8. Calculation of target height for children by using the
stature-for-age percentiles for girls aged 2 to 20 years growth chart
(from CDC website, www.cdc.gov/growthcharts). The mother's height
is plotted on the right directly, while the father's height must be
reduced by 5 inches on a girl's chart. The mid-parental height (MPH)
is the average of the mother's height and the corrected father's
height. The limit of 2 standard abbreviations (SD) are approximately
4 inches above and below the MPH.**

growth chart (Fig. 5-8). The limits of 2 standard deviations (in the
United States, a standard deviation is 2 inches for adult height,
so 2 SD is 4 inches) or 4 inches are noted above and below the midparental height. This then is the target height of the child. One
can conceptually adjust the growth chart for the family by interpreting the midparental height as the 50th percentile for this particular family and interpreting the height of the child by the
resulting new percentiles on the conceptual chart. Thus a boy who
plots at the 3rd percentile for the United States who has short
parents might plot well within the target height (or on the con-

ceptually reinterpreted chart at the 10th percentile for the family; Fig. 5-8A and B).

Nutrition is one of the most essential factors for growth and reproductive development. In the evaluation of children immigrating to the United States from developing countries or from countries torn by war or famine, it may be inappropriate to consider the parents' heights in the evaluation of the child; the parents may have been subject to malnutrition during their growing years and may be inappropriately short, whereas the child may benefit from better nutrition in their new home and have the opportunity to be taller than the parents. Voluntary decrease in nutrients (excessive dieting or even anorexia nervosa) or chronic disease can exert the same effect as economic malnutrition on decreasing growth. Thus, socioeconomic and psychosocial factors are important considerations in the interpretation of growth rate.

Chronic disease may decrease growth apart from effects on decreasing nutritional intake. For example, the decrease in stature in children with juvenile rheumatoid arthritis is not completely nutritional in origin.

Psychological problems can affect growth either from a nutritional standpoint or through an endocrine effect. Psychosocial dwarfism is a temporary condition of hypopituitarism precipitated by abnormal parent-child interaction; it may be improved by moving the child out of the home.

ABNORMALITIES OF GROWTH

Short Stature

Nonendocrine Causes of Short Stature

Constitutional delay in growth and adolescence (constitutional delay) is best considered a variation of normal development (Table 5-1). After a normal birth length and weight, growth rate subtly decreases during the first 2 years so that stature becomes considerably shorter than average for age by age 2 to 3 years, but the child then follows the channel of growth on the chart just reached [i.e., growth rate then normalizes (Fig. 5-9)]. In addition, bone age is delayed at least two SDs by the definition of constitutional delay. Thus the condition is a variation in the normal tempo of development rather than a disease. The child is usually thin, often male, and the growth rate is appropriate for the skeletal development but not for the chronologic age (Fig. 5-9). Thus the growth rate must be interpreted in terms of bone age rather than chronologic age. If the patient has genetic short stature in addition to constitutional delay in growth, the degree of short stature may be so obvious that the patient will seek advice sooner; if constitutional delay occurs in a child without genetic short stature, the degree of short stature may not stimulate a medical evaluation until a delay in puberty is noted. Often one parent or a sibling has a history of constitutional delay (e.g., mother did not begin menstruating until 15 to 16 years, or father did not stop growing until well after high school).

Table 5-1.   Etiologies of short stature

Variations of normal
Constitutional in growth and development with delayed bone age
Genetic short stature with short familial heights

Endocrine disorders
GH deficiency
  Congenital
    Isolated GH deficiency
    With other pituitary hormone deficiencies
    With midline defects
    Pituitary agenesis
    With gene deficiency
  Acquired
    Hypothalamic/pituitary tumors
    Histiocytosis X (Langerhans cell histiocytosis)
    CNS infections and granulomas
    Head trauma (birth and later)
    Hypothalamic/pituitary radiation
    CNS vascular accidents
    Hydrocephalus
    Empty sella syndrome
    Autoimmune hypophysitis
  Functional GH deficiency
    Psychosocial dwarfism
GH resistance
  Laron dwarfism (increased GH and decreased IGF-I)
  Pygmies (normal GH and IGF-II but decreased IGF-I)
Hypothyroidism
Glucocorticoid excess
  Endogenous
  Exogenous
Diabetes mellitus under poor control
Diabetes insipidus (untreated)
Hypophosphatemic vitamin D–resistant rickets
Virilizing congenital adrenal hyperplasia (tall child, short adult)
  $P-450_{c21}$, $P-450_{c11}$ deficiencies

Skeletal dysplasias
Osteogenesis imperfecta
Osteochondroplasias

Lysosomal storage diseases
Mucopolysaccharidoses
Mucolipidoses

Syndromes of short stature
Turner syndrome (syndrome of gonadal dysgenesis)
SHOX deficiency
Noonan syndrome (pseudo-Turner syndrome)
Autosomal trisomy 13, 18, 21
Prader-Willi syndrome

Continued

Table 5-1. *Continued*

Laurence-Moon or Bardet-Biedl syndromes
Autosomal abnormalities
Dysmorphic syndromes (Russell-Silver, Cornelia de Lange)
Pseudohypoparathyroidism

Chronic Disease
Cardiac disorders
  Left-to-right shunt
  Congestive heart failure
Pulmonary disorders
  Cystic fibrosis
  Asthma
GI disorders
  Malabsorption (e.g., celiac disease)
  Disorders of swallowing
  Inflammatory bowel disease
Hepatic disorders
Hematologic disorders
  Sickle cell anemia
  Thalassemia
Renal disorders
  Renal tubular acidosis
  Chronic uremia
Immunologic disorders
  Connective tissue disease
Juvenile rheumatoid arthritis
Chronic infection
  AIDS
  Hereditary fructose intolerance

Malnutrition
Fad diets and anorexia nervosa
Kwashiorkor, marasmus
Iron deficiency
Zinc deficiency
Anorexia due to chemotherapy for neoplasms
Amphetamine treatment for hyperactivity with decreased caloric
  intake

Modified from Styne DM. Growth disorder. In: Fitzgerald PA, ed. *Handbook of clinical endocrinology.* Norwalk, CT: Appleton & Lange, 1986: 73–99, with permission.
AIDS, acquired immunodeficiency syndrome; CNS, central nervous system; GI, gastrointestinal; IGF, insulin-like growth factor; GH, growth hormone.

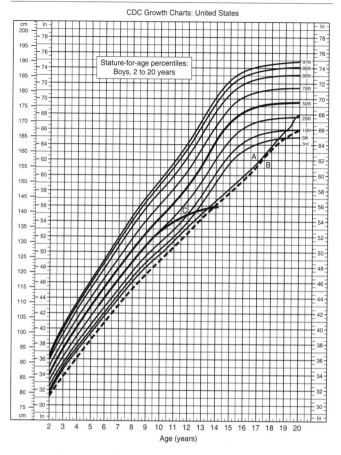

CDC Growth Charts: United States

Stature-for-age percentiles:
Boys, 2 to 20 years

**Fig. 5-9. Growth chart demonstrating the various patterns of
growth. A: A boy with genetic short stature who parallels the normal
curve just below the 3rd percentile and who has no delay in bone age.
He reaches a height at a percentile similar to the percentile at which
he grew during childhood. B: A boy with constitutional delay in
growth, who parallels the normal growth curve but has a delayed
bone age, and so continues to grow after the average boys have
stopped. He will reach a final height in the normal range above the
percentile he followed during childhood. C: Growth of a boy with a
serious disease, which could be a brain tumor that interferes with
growth hormone secretion, glucocorticoid-induced growth failure,
or a host of serious chronic diseases. His growth decreases remarkably
at age 10 years, which is the age at onset of his disorder. Note that this
child reaches a height at age 14 years comparable to those in curves A
and B but does so in quite a different pattern. He surely should have
been diagnosed with a problem soon after the change in growth velocity (drawn on chart from CDC website, www.cdc.gov/growthcharts).**

Patients with constitutional delay will enter puberty at a later age than their peers (by definition, older than 13 years in girls and 14 years in boys) but at an age appropriate for their bone age. Although considerable variation exists, as a rule of thumb, boys will enter puberty when their bone age is 12 years, and girls, when their bone age is 11 years. The predicted height of boys with significant delay in bone age calculated by the use of the Bayley Pinnea tables in the Greulich and Pyle atlas may overestimate adult height; thus their adult height, although within the normal range, might be lower than expected.

Genetic short stature refers to the child of shorter than average parents (Fig. 5-9). These children are expected to reach a reduced final height, as their short stature is not accompanied by a delay in bone age.

Small for gestational age (SGA) infants are born with weights below the tenth percentile for their gestational age; for a term baby, this translates into a weight less than 2,500 g. Standards are available (e.g., figure 5-1) for weight according to gestational age to interpret the birth weight of premature infants. Intrauterine growth retarded or restricted (IUGR) babies are usually considered to have poor intrauterine growth monitored by ultrasound and usually are born SGA. However, they may increase their growth rate before birth and even be born larger than the SGA guidelines; the terminology is often confused in various texts, but we adhere to the definition of SGA based on birth weight compared with gestational age and IUGR based on fetal growth rate here. Symmetrical SGA indicates that a decreased head circumference accompanies the decreased length, whereas asymmetrical SGA indicates that the head circumference is spared and is normal for age; symmetrical SGA may simply indicate a more severe condition, whereas asymmetrical SGA is less severe. Most, approximately 75%, of affected SGA children will catch up to the normal growth percentiles, but a minority remain small for their entire growing period and attain short adult heights; the symmetrical SGA subjects are those most likely to continue to have retarded growth. SGA patients are characteristically thin, have bone age appropriate for chronologic age, and therefore have a normal age at onset of puberty and usually have a rate of growth within the normal range.

Many syndromes encompass SGA in their features. A complete list of such conditions is beyond the compass of this volume, so the reader is referred to a more complete source such as *Smith's Recognizable Patterns of Human Malformation*. Common examples include fetal alcohol syndrome (also associated with microcephaly, short palpebral fissure, epicanthal folds, small jaws and short philtrum of the lip, cardiac defects, and some delay in mental development), maternal smoking, and maternal abuse of various other substances. Russell-Silver dwarfism syndrome (180860 RUSSELL-SILVER SYNDROME; RSS at 7p12-p11.2) in addition to SGA is characterized by hemihypertrophy, lateral asymmetry, asymmetry of arms and/or legs, fifth finger clinodactyly, syndactyly of toes, craniofacial disproportion, delayed fontanel closure, tri-angular facies, turned-down corners of the mouth, and sometimes cryptorchidism. On radiograph, vertebral abnormalities including absent sacrum and absent coccyx may be seen. It is usually spo-radic but is rarely described with maternal uniparental disomy (UPD).

Numerous syndromes, including abnormal karyotypes, will have short stature as one of their characteristics. Turner syn-drome has absence or abnormalities of the X chromosome (see Chapters 8 and 9). The autosomal dominantly inherited Noonan syndrome (*163950 NOONAN SYNDROME 1; NS1 at 12q24) includes many features that resemble those of Turner syndrome and others that do not, but does not include SGA. Some charac-teristics are short stature (of prenatal onset); failure to thrive in infancy; triangular, low-set posteriorly rotated ears; nerve deaf-ness; ptosis; hypertelorism; down-slanting palpebral fissures; epi-canthal folds; myopia; blue-green irides; deeply grooved philtrum; high peaks of upper lip vermilion border; high-arched palate; micrognathia; dental malocclusion; low posterior hairline; webbed neck; cystic hygroma; congenital heart defect (usually of the right side) including pulmonic stenosis, septal defects, patent ductus arteriosus; shield chest; pectus carinatum superiorly and pectus excavatum inferiorly; hypogonadism and cryptorchidism; verte-bral abnormalities; cubitus valgus; clinodactyly; brachydactyly; blunt fingertips; lymphedema; wooly-like consistency of hair; articulation difficulties; and, in 25%, mental retardation.

Other syndromes combine short stature and obesity, a combi-nation that should awaken concern over an organic etiology for short stature, as patients with otherwise uncomplicated obesity are usually tall for age. The Prader-Willi syndrome (#176270 PRADER-WILLI SYNDROME; PWS—Due to deletion or mater-nal uniparental disomy of 15q11.2-q12) has poor weight gain in infancy and early childhood because of poor neonatal feeding caused by diminished swallowing and sucking reflexes. This con-dition is followed by insatiable polyphagia and rapid weight gain occurring after 1 year, leading to obesity. Other features include narrow bitemporal head dimension, almond-shaped eyes, stra-bismus, myopia, thin upper lip, down-turned corners of mouth, viscous saliva, hypoventilation and hypoxia, hypogonadotropic hypogonadism, cryptorchidism, small penis and scrotum, hypo-plastic labia, amenorrhea, and limb and skeletal abnormalities including scoliosis, kyphosis, osteopenia, small hands and feet (acromicria), and narrow hands with a straight ulnar border. CNS abnormalities include fetal and neonatal hypotonia (such poor fetal motion leads to the assumption of fetal death in some cases), men-tal retardation, behavioral problems, sleep disturbances, hypore-flexia, articulation difficulty, skin and scab picking, and high pain threshold. This and the Laurence-Moon and Bardet-Biedl syn-dromes, other causes of short stature, are described in Chapter 9.

Other conditions discussed elsewhere in the volume include pseudohypoparathyroidism as well as Cushing syndrome, hypothyroidism, and growth hormone deficiency, which lead to short stature and obesity.

Chronic disease of any organ system can cause growth retardation, and any pediatrics textbook will have numerous etiologies on virtually every page. Indeed, the onset of a chronic disease may be indicated by a decrease in the growth rate noted on the child's growth chart.

Malnutrition, a frequent cause of short stature, may be due to maternal neglect, poverty and lack of available food, neurologic impairment that decreases interest in food or causes inability to swallow it, malabsorption, or even voluntary lack of food intake. Serum IGF-1 may be decreased with any of these, and the unwary investigator may incorrectly consider that GH deficiency is at fault; in states of malnutrition, GH is often elevated, whereas IGF-1 is decreased, and GH administration will do no good.

"Failure to thrive" includes a wide variety of conditions in which an infant is not growing well. Usually, the weight is affected before and to a greater degree than the length or height; this is in contrast to the effects of hypothyroidism and GH deficiency where weight for height is maintained or increased, but growth slows, leading to a chubby appearance. These infants may have as an etiology, reflux, parents inexperienced in feeding infants, aberrant intrafamilial dynamics, and many other chronic conditions alluded to earlier and found in general pediatrics texts. Decreased BMI according to standard charts is usually an indication of a nutritional disease rather than an endocrine problem, although some endocrine conditions (e.g., hyperthyroidism or the diencephalic syndrome can indeed have decreased weight for height).

Endocrine Causes of Short Stature

Growth Hormone Deficiency

Classic GH deficiency has been reported as frequently as 1 in 4,000 children; even if this report is not generally applicable to all populations, GH deficiency qualifies as a more common disease rather than a "zebra." When acquired GH deficiency (such as that caused by head and neck irradiation used to treat children with cancer) is added to the equation, the condition is even more common. GH deficiency must always be considered as a possible etiology in a patient with growth failure and no other identified cause.

Idiopathic GH deficiency is usually owing to decreased hypothalamic GHRH. Rarely patients have no pituitary glands or somatotrophs, and gene defects can cause GH deficiency (see later). Most patients are less strikingly affected, and the dividing line between GH deficiency and normal GH secretion is becoming increasingly blurred. Our classic tests have proven less effective than previously thought.

Congenital GH deficiency does not affect fetal growth, as the child has a near normal birth length, although a minor decrease may occur, according to some studies. Soon after birth, however,

careful observation will indicate an abnormally low growth rate
on careful measurements, and plotting an accurate growth chart
will demonstrate this finding. The patient will be obviously short
for age by age 2 to 4 years, and the diagnosis often will be suggested at this point, if not earlier. Classic GH-deficient patients
will have a cherubic appearance because of their chubbiness.
They will manifest a high-pitched voice caused by their small
larynx but have adequate intellectual and vocal ability to speak
appropriately for chronologic age. They appear precocious because
their appearance suggests a younger age, but their speech and
abilities suggest an older one. Male children may have microphallus (stretched penis length less than 2 cm, which is 2.5 standard deviations below the mean), especially if there is associated
gonadotropin deficiency. Hypoglycemia may occur because of the
absence of the gluconeogenic effects of GH, which also acts as
an antiinsulin factor and would increase serum glucose by two
means in a normal individual. If adrenocorticotropic hormone
(ACTH) also is absent, more profound hypoglycemia is possible
(cortisol also stimulates gluconeogenesis and opposes insulin
action), and in either situation, hypoglycemic seizures may occur.
The combination of hypoglycemic seizures and normal birth
length without complications of the birth process should alert
the observer of the possibility of neonatal hypopituitarism; if the
patient is a boy with microphallus, the diagnosis is even more
likely. Midline defects ranging from cleft palate to encephalocele
are associated with congenital hypopituitarism. Optic hypoplasia
with any degree of visual impairment, usually associated with
pendular (to and fro without any predominant direction) nystagmus, is a frequent indication of associated hypopituitarism.
Absence of the septum pellucidum is found in about 50% of
patients with optic hypoplasia and pituitary impairment. Thus if
there is diminished vision due to optic hypoplasia with or without
absence of the septum pellucidum (septooptic dysplasia; see Chapter 9) in association with hypoglycemia and, in a boy, microphallus, the diagnosis of hypopituitarism must be ruled out before
most other conditions are considered. If hypoglycemia is apparent and not adequately treated, developmental delay may be the
outcome instead of the usually normal intellect found in children
with GH deficiency. Hypoglycemia in the newborn period due to
GH or cortisol deficiency requires a lower glucose infusion rate
(usually less than 10 mg/kg/min) than states of insulin excess
(often more than 12 to 15 mg/kg/min) require to maintain blood
sugar (see Chapter 13).

Breech delivery occurs in greater prevalence in patients with
congenital hypopituitarism, especially in boys. Any type of birth
trauma may increase the risk of congenital hypopituitarism.

Familial GH deficiency may occur in autosomal recessive or
dominant patterns or in an X-linked pattern due to mutations in
the gene for GH or for pituitary development. GH deficiency 1B
(#262400 PITUITARY DWARFISM I) is autosomal GH deficiency
due to mutation in the GH gene; with treatment with GH and

therefore exposure to GH for the first time, GH antibodies may develop and eliminate the effects of GH on growth. Hypopituitarism due to a defect in the LHX1 gene (#262600 PITUITARY DWARFISM III at 9q34.3) leads to hypopituitarism and loss of prolactin (Prl), luteinizing hormone (LH) and follicle-stimulating (FSH), GH, and thyroid-stimulating hormone (TSH) in an autosomal recessive pattern associated with severe restriction of head rotation. Mutation of PROP-1 (*601538 PROPHET OF PIT1, PAIRED-LIKE HOMEODOMAIN TRANSCRIPTION FACTOR; PROP1 at 5q) causes GH and TSH deficiency, and more rarely, ACTH deficiency. Mutations of POU1F1 (PIT *173110 POU DOMAIN, CLASS 1, TRANSCRIPTION FACTOR 1; POU1F1 at 3p11) cause deficiency in GH, TSH, and Prl.

GH resistance is indicated by elevated GH with decreased serum IGF-1. The first described form of hereditary GH insensitivity, Laron dwarfism (#262500 pituitary dwarfism II at 5p13-p12), is due to an absence of receptors for GH, and serum GHBP is low. The pattern is autosomal recessive. Other forms of GH resistance have postreceptor defects, so that serum GHBP is normal. Affected patients cannot respond to GH administration with increased growth or increased IGF-1 concentrations; patients do respond to IGF-1 administration in clinical trials with increased growth, and this is the only modality that will be effective. In this syndrome, puberty is delayed, the forehead is prominent, sclerae are blue, and dentition is delayed. This is an autosomal recessive condition; the GHR gene is mapped to 5p13-p12 *600946 GROWTH HORMONE RECEPTOR; GHR.

Pygmies (#265850 PYGMY) have normal GH concentrations and normal IGF-1 but very low IGF-2 concentrations. They are of normal height until puberty but lack a pubertal growth spurt. Because the population is described with nutritional deficiencies as well as the genetic defect, multiple causes of short stature may exist.

Biologically inactive GH (#262650 PITUITARY DWARFISM IV) has been postulated as a cause of growth failure with normal serum GH concentrations as measured by radioimmunoassay but poor growth; growth rate increases with administration of exogenous GH administration, even though the endogenous GH appears ineffective. The prevalence of affected patients is unknown; autosomal recessive inheritance is suggested. Partial GH deficiency appears to be a more common explanation for this condition and is represented by subjects who have adequate GH secretion on testing but respond to GH administration with increased growth.

Diagnosis of Growth Hormone Deficiency

The diagnosis of GH deficiency has become more complex with increased knowledge of GH physiology. Some patients respond to GH treatment without demonstrated classic GH deficiency; most of these more subtle indications are beyond the range of this chapter and are best investigated and diagnosed by a pediatric endocrinologist.

Classic GH deficiency is defined by the inability to increase GH concentration above an accepted limit generally 10 ng/mL in most laboratories (although certain assays are more sensitive, and lower cutoff of normal levels are used) after two stimulatory tests. This limit is somewhat arbitrary and is higher than values used in previous decades. Further, prepubertal children may not respond as well as pubertal children to GH stimulatory tests, so that different standards may be useful at different ages (according to published studies), but are such standards are not available from commercial laboratories. To standardize the responses before and after puberty, some investigators suggest priming the prepubertal child with a dose of estrogen or propranolol (propranolol can precipitate hypoglycemia and should not be used if hypoglycemia is already present). As mentioned, the measurement of a single sample for basal GH concentrations is useless in the diagnosis of GH deficiency.

Secretagogues invoked in the testing for GH deficiency are given early in the morning after an overnight fast (hypoglycemic patients should not be forced to fast unobserved so the test must be modified!). Two tests are usually performed because any normal child can fail to increase GH concentration after one test; two tests yield a false positive (failure of a normal child to reach the normal limit of serum GH) more than 10% of the time.

Several pharmacologic tests are commonly invoked as secretagogues. L-Dopa is used in doses of 125 mg for body weight up to 15 kg, 250 mg for weight up to 35 kg, and 500 mg for body weight over 35 kg is given; samples are taken at 0, 30, 60, and 90 minutes. Nausea and vomiting are possible side effects for a few hours after administration, so it might be used as the second of two tests. Clonidine in a dose of 0.1 to 0.15 mg/m^2 can be given and samples obtained at the same time sequence; side effects are possible hypotension and lethargy for several hours, so we prefer the lower range of dosage. Intravenous arginine infusion of 0.5 g/kg body weight up to 20 g over a 20-minute period can be given with samples taken at the same time periods as mentioned earlier; no side effects are likely, but the test is considered to be less effective than others. Growth hormone–releasing factor (GHRH) is commercially available for testing but offers little improvement in testing over the other regimens. When it is administered in a dose of 5 to 10 g/kg, serum GH concentrations will promptly increase in normal individuals. GH-deficient patients demonstrate either no increase in GH or a blunted increase. Those with a pituitary defect have no response, whereas those with a hypothalamic defect may respond. Insulin-induced hypoglycemia (0.075 to 0.1 units/kg body weight of insulin given i.v.) is an effective but extremely dangerous test; the patient must be shown to have a normal fasting blood sugar just before the test, must not have a known tendency toward hypoglycemia, a patent i.v. line must be available to infuse dextrose should a hypoglycemic seizure occur, and the patient must be watched carefully by a physician during the test. Glucose and GH should be measured at

0, 15, 20, 30, 60, and 90 minutes and cortisol at 60 and 90 minutes if this test is performed to test ACTH reserve as well as GH secretion. If severe hypoglycemia occurs, dextrose must be administered immediately; no greater than 25% dextrose at 1 mL/kg should be infused so that blood sugar will increase but so no severe change in osmolality will occur.

Nonpharmacologic tests are available in addition to the stimulatory tests. After 10 minutes of vigorous exercise, normal children will increase their GH in 80% of trials. Sequential serum samples may be taken at night in the hope that the peak that customarily occurs 90 minutes after the onset of sleep may be captured, but this method is expensive and inconvenient. Sampling for GH levels every 10 to 15 minutes for 24 or 12 hours has been suggested as a way to determine whether a normal circadian rhythm of GH secretion is present; the facilities for such a study are generally unavailable.

Plasma IGF-1 concentrations can be used to assist in the diagnosis of GH deficiency but must be interpreted with caution. Low values may mean malnutrition as well as GH deficiency; in malnutrition, GH values usually increase, and IGF-1 values decrease. In delayed puberty, values are more appropriate for bone age than for chronologic age and may be incorrectly interpreted as abnormally low in such a situation; thus a 14-year-old with an 11-year-old bone age who has an IGF-1 value inappropriate for a 14-year-old but appropriate for an 11-year-old is normal. The measurement of IGF-BP3 in addition to IGF-1 may add accuracy to the diagnosis of GH deficiency.

Treatment of Growth Hormone Deficiency

The treatment of GH deficiency is accomplished by the use of biosynthetic recombinant DNA–derived GH. Previously, cadaver-donated pituitary-derived GH was administered, but the recognition that some batches were contaminated with the prions of Jakob-Creutzfeldt disease led to the discontinuation of such therapy. Biosynthetic GH is available with the 191–amino acid sequence of the natural GH molecule from several companies. Daily subcutaneous injections are administered in dose starting at about 0.18 to 0.3 mg/kg/week given 6 or 7 days per week up to about twice this dose in puberty. Dosage is titrated to the growth response. Experimental protocols are under way to determine whether titrating the GH dose to achieve a normal serum IGF-1 value allows increased effect.

Numerous methods of administration of GH are used, with more in development. Thus, standard syringe-and-needle administration of either premixed solutions of GH or lyophilized preparations that must be reconstituted have been joined by the use of mechanical pens that use cartridges of premixed GH, and even needleless devices are available. A long-acting preparation of GH may be given every 2 to 4 weeks, albeit with a larger needle and larger volume of injection.

GH is presently indicated for GH-deficient patients, Turner syndrome (see Chapters 8 and 9), growth failure of renal insufficiency, Prader-Willi syndrome, and IUGR (evaluated as SGA). GH has just been approved for use in otherwise normal boys predicted to be shorter than 5'3", or girls predicted to be shorter than 4'11" as adults. GH has been used in critically injured patients with mixed or even harmful results, so it is not presently recommended for such situations. It also is said to be used illicitly by athletes and weight lifters to increase muscle strength, but no benefit has been proven in these conditions. GH treatment of adults with GH deficiency is indicated to maintain bone density and improve skin and muscle condition. The use of GH in frailty of aging is under investigation.

Complications of GH treatment include a tendency toward slipped capital femoral epiphyses (this side effect is presently under review, so it is not clearly related to treatment), and patients must be asked about hip and leg pain or the development of a waddling gait; the treatment is surgical. Pseudotumor cerebri may cause a severe headache along with papilledema: although it should be reversible, if it is allowed to continue, impairment or loss of vision may result. Hypothyroidism may develop during GH therapy and a free T_4 value should be obtained annually or if growth rate decreases. Development of antibodies to GH is less a problem with the use of human sequence GH but should be considered if a patient ceases to grow as expected while receiving therapy with GH.

Controversy exists over the negative psychological effects of short stature. This lack of agreement of studies is partially because it is the patients who are brought to evaluation who are studied rather than the children in the community with short stature who do not come to medical attention. Nonetheless, psychological support must be considered for a short child whether or not medical therapy is offered. Parents should be counseled against thinking that the fact that their child is shorter than average is a tragedy and that therapy is required at all costs. In view of the constant bombardment by the media that leadership, friendship, and indeed the company of the opposite sex requires tall stature, some boys (and some girls) may become depressed and possibly suicidal; the most severe of these tendencies are rare, but the physician must be sensitive to such a possibility. If the child's parents are shorter than average and unhappy about it, they may tend to read into the child's future the unpleasant experiences they had, which may not, after all, directly reflect on their height. Children should be counseled toward sports that will realistically allow success and foster self-confidence; for example, soccer is far more appropriate than basketball, and martial arts classes can lead to greater self-confidence in an insecure shorter child. The ultimate psychological outlook of a short child may result, in large part, from the manner in which the child was approached by family, teachers, peers and physicians during the early years after the diagnosis.

Other Endocrine Disorders

Psychosocial dwarfism may occur in one child among several other normal siblings. Abnormal parent-child interaction leads to functional hypopituitarism with GH deficiency on provocative testing; GH secretion will revert to normal within days after removal from the offending situation. Affected children have a pot-bellied, immature appearance. They may exhibit aberrant behavior such as drinking from toilet bowls, begging for food from neighbors, and foraging for food in garbage cans, in spite of apparently normal caloric intake at home. These patients may have had psychological abuse but rarely have signs of physical abuse. When removed from their homes, such children may exhibit catch-up growth in foster homes or in the hospital, environments where one would not expect a child to thrive. Even if psychotherapy is administered for prolonged periods, the outcome is uncertain.

Maternal deprivation (perhaps a sexist term, but as the mother usually is responsible for feeding the child, an often-used term) is the diagnosis applied to infants with poor growth rates due to parental neglect. These children may have actual caloric deprivation in addition to psychological neglect. The term also is applied to situations in which the mother is inexperienced in child-feeding, practices in which education can provide marked improvement.

Hypothyroidism will decrease the growth rate and retard skeletal development. Most children with congenital hypothyroidism will be diagnosed with neonatal screening procedures, but acquired hypothyroidism is still a frequent occurrence in later childhood and adolescence (see Chapter 6).

Cushing syndrome refers to excess glucocorticoid exposure from endogenous or exogenous sources. Topical and even inhaled preparations of glucocorticoid can retard growth and must be considered a potential cause of decreased growth (see Chapter 10).

Pseudohypoparathyroidism is first seen as a chubby appearance, short stature, short fourth metacarpals, round facies, and mental retardation. Hypocalcemia and hyperphosphatemia can be treated with medical therapy, but the poor growth cannot be improved with this method (see Chapter 7).

Diagnosis of Short Stature

A patient who has stature below the third percentile for height according to the new CDC charts, who is growing at a rate less than the fifth percentile for height velocity for age, or is below the third percentile for corrected midparental height, is worthy of evaluation; a combination of two or more of these characteristics warrant increased concern (Fig. 5-10; Table 5-2). A full history and physical examination are essential for the evaluation of short stature to reveal familial influences, nutrition, or systemic diseases. Interfamilial interactions can be observed during the interview process to evaluate the possibility of psychosocial dwarfism. If no previous height measurements are available, a history of changes in shoe or clothing size can be of value to determine whether the child is growing adequately, although follow-up measurements over at least 3 months (and longer if possible) are necessary for diagnosis.

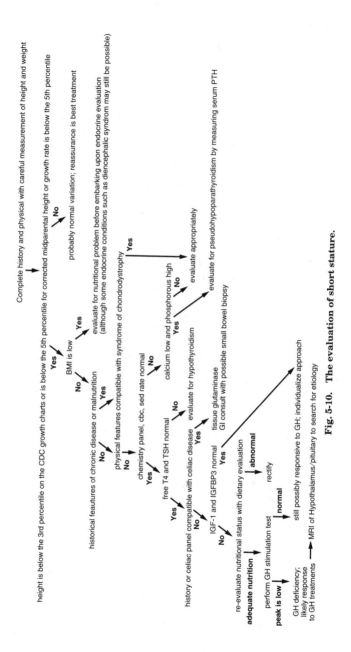

Fig 5-10. The evaluation of short stature.

Table 5-2.   The evaluation of short stature

Test	Rationale
CBC	*Anemia:* nutritional, chronic disease, malignancy *Leukocytosis:* inflammation, infection *Leukopenia:* bone marrow failure syndromes *Thrombocytopenia:* malignancy, infection
ESR, CRP	Inflammation of infection, inflammatory diseases, malignancy (electrolytes, liver enzymes, BUN).
Chemistry panel	Signs of acute or chronic hepatic, renal, adrenal dysfunction; hydration and acid-base status
Carotene, folate, tissue trans-glutaminase antibody, or celiac panel	Assess malabsorption; detect celiac disease
Urinalysis	Signs of renal dysfunction, hydration; renal tubular acidosis
Karyotype	Evaluate for genetic syndromes
Cranial MRI imaging	Assesses hypothalamic-pituitary tumors (craniopharyngioma, glioma, germinoma) or congenital midline defects
Bone age	Determine physiologic maturation, and evaluate height potential
IGF-I, IGF BP3	Reflects growth hormone status or nutrition
Free thyroxine and TSH	Detects hypothyroidism
Prolactin	Elevated in hypothalamic dysfunction or destruction, suppressed in pituitary disease

BUN, blood urea nitrogen; CBC, complete blood count; CRP, C-reactive protein; ESR, erythrocyte sedimentation rate; IGF BP3, insulin-like growth factor–binding protein 3; MRI, magnetic resonance imaging; TSH, thyroid-stimulating hormone.
Modified from Styne DM, Glaser NS. Growth disorder. In: Behrman RE, Kliegman RM, eds. *Essentials in Pediatrics.* Philadelphia: WB Saunders Company, after Sperling, with permission.

Physical examination begins with the accurate measurement of height, weight, head circumference, arm span, upper-to-lower ratio, and vital signs. Height and height velocity are plotted on appropriate charts (see Fig. 5-5). BMI is determined by using CDC charts to evaluate nutritional status. Signs of disease or syndromes are evaluated.

If no diagnosis is obvious from history or physical examination, a laboratory evaluation is performed. A screening chemistry panel for liver and kidney function, a bicarbonate and electrolyte determination to evaluate the possibility of renal tubular acidosis or a metabolic acidosis syndrome, evaluation of carotene or folate for determination of fat absorption, a complete blood count with differential, and a urinalysis including microscopic examination may indicate a problem not obvious from the physical examination. A free thyroxine determination and TSH also are obtained to determine whether hypothyroidism is present. An IGF-1 concentration may be falsely low because of factors listed earlier, but if the IGF-1 and IGF-BP 3 are normal, classic GH deficiency is not likely. A urinary free cortisol determination is obtained, possibly with dexamethasone suppression (see Chapter 10) if obesity complicates short stature and Cushing syndrome is under consideration. An elevated serum Prl concentration will suggest hypothalamic deficiency; if it is low, it will suggest pituitary disease. A celiac panel will determine if unexpected celiac disease is the etiology of the problem. A bone-age determination will not lead to a diagnosis (although it may support several potential diagnoses), but will indicate the amount of remaining growth. If neurologic symptoms are noted or if a CNS tumor is in the differential diagnosis, an MRI evaluation with contrast of the pituitary–hypothalamic area is in order; in the past, a lateral radiograph of the skull was performed, but a more detailed evaluation is appropriate if the concern is raised. It is essential that thin cuts be ordered and taken through the hypothalamic–pituitary area on the MRI so that a small tumor or congenital abnormality is not missed.

GH testing is usually performed if no other diagnosis is apparent from the evaluation. As mentioned earlier, the diagnosis of classic GH deficiency is relatively straightforward, but the emergence of other, more subtle conditions for which GH treatment may be helpful has confused the situation.

Tall Stature

Nonendocrine Causes of Tall Stature

Constitutional tall stature is the other side of the coin from constitutional short stature, although it is far more rarely reported or even evaluated (Table 5-3). Patients are taller than average, have a moderately advanced bone age but a height velocity appropriate for bone age, and have no sign of the disorders described later. Puberty will be early in children with constitutional tall stature, so that final height will not be out of normal range, although height during childhood was greater than normal. Obesity will advance bone age and physiologic development and, except for the weight, simulates constitutional tall stature.

Genetic tall stature occurs in a family with one or, more often, two parents taller than the normal adult range. The child may be born at a normal length and weight but, because of a higher range of normal growth rate, will reach a taller than average height as an adult. The adjusted midparental height will help in the evaluation of genetic tall stature.

Girls more often will be concerned about being taller than average than will boys; often fears are intensified by parental concerns about tall stature and effects on social development. However,

Table 5-3.   Etiologies of tall stature

Variations of normal
    Constitutional
    Genetic
    Exogenous obesity

Endocrine disorders
    Pituitary gigantism
    Sexual precocity
    Thyrotoxicosis
    Beckwith-Wiedemann syndrome

Nonendocrine disorders
    Marfan syndrome
    Klinefelter syndrome
    XYY syndrome
    Cerebral gigantism (Sotos syndrome)
    Homocystinuria
    Weaver-Smith syndrome

Modified from Styne DM. Growth disorder. In Greenspan FS, Gardner DG, eds. *Basic and clinical endocrinology.* New York: Lange, 2001: 163–200.

such fears have decreased in view of the success of tall fashion models, actresses, and athletes. Thus treatment is rarely invoked today because of ethical issues, but high-dose estrogens can effectively slow longitudinal growth while advancing puberty, causing a rapid increase in bone age and thereby limiting adult height in girls. Because of theoretic risks of high-dose estrogen therapy, such as thrombotic effects, the development of ovarian cysts, and future menstrual disorders, therapy, if considered, is not to be undertaken without a careful description of the possible side effects. Further, the child must be included in discussions concerning her adult height. In rare circumstances, a girl with a predicted height of more than 6 feet, who is age 10 to 12 years with a bone age no older than 10 to 11 years, may hope to realize a decrease in her final height of up to 2 inches with the use of estrogen therapy. Again, this therapy is not recommended by this author but is presented for completeness.

Boys concerned about too great an adult height are rare, but testosterone therapy can be used to precipitate pubertal development and limit final height. Such therapy is not recommended either.

Cerebral gigantism (*117550 CEREBRAL GIGANTISM at 5q35) or Soto syndrome is recognized by the prominent forehead and sharp chin, with prognathism, high-arched palate, down-slanting palpebral fissures, hypertelorism, strabismus, and nystagmus. Developmental delay, behavioral problems with expressive difficulties, and possibly seizures are often found. No evidence if found of GH excess, but bone age is advanced, and hands and feet are large, with genu valgum. Rapid growth is most characteristic of infancy, and height velocity decreases by mid-childhood or adolescence, leading in many cases to normal adult stature.

The Weaver syndrome (#277590 WEAVER SYNDROME) is associated with prenatal as well as postnatal increased stature and advanced bone age but no acceleration of growth velocity, as seen in Soto syndrome. It is usually sporadic. Facial features include macrocephaly, large bifrontal diameter, flattened occiput, long philtrum, round face in infancy, retrognathia, prominent chin with central dimple, large ears, strabismus, hypertelorism, epicanthal folds, down-slanting palpebral fissures, and depressed nasal bridge. Numerous skeletal abnormalities include scoliosis, kyphosis, coxa valga, limited elbow extension, limited knee extension, flared metaphyses (especially distal femora and humeri), camptodactyly, broad thumbs, prominent fingertip pads, large hands, clinodactyly, talipes equinovarus, calcaneovalgus, metatarsus adductus, short fourth metatarsals, prominent toe pads, pes cavus, and overriding toes. Behavior and learning disorders, seizures and hypotonia, and abnormalities of CNS anatomy occur in some.

Marfan syndrome (#154700 MARFAN SYNDROME; MFS at 15q21.1) includes disproportionate tall stature with long-bone overgrowth (dolichostenomelia), arm span exceeding height, and a very low upper- to lower-segment ratio, arachnodactyly (or long, thin fingers and toes), and hyperextensibility of the joints, as well as joint contractures. Other skeletal anomalies include scoliosis, kyphoscoliosis, thoracic lordosis, spondylolisthesis, lumbosacral dural ectasia, pectus excavatum, pectus carinatum, and pectus asymmetric deformity. Optic anomalies include subluxation of the lens (ectopia lentis) with myopia, corneal flatness, retinal detachment, iris hypoplasia, early glaucoma, early cataracts, and down-slanting palpebral fissures. In addition, the face is long and narrow face, with dolichocephaly, high-arched narrow palate, micrognathia, retrognathia, and crowded teeth. Respiratory findings include pneumothorax, pulmonary blebs, and in the worst cases, emphysema. Cardiac abnormalities include aortic root dilatation, aortic regurgitation, ascending aortic aneurysm, aortic dissection, mitral regurgitation, mitral valve prolapse, congestive heart failure, pulmonary artery dilatation, tricuspid valve prolapse, and premature calcification of mitral annulus. The skin reveals striae distensae. The disorder results from a mutation in the fibrillin gene.

Homocystinuria (*236200 HOMOCYSTINURIA at 21q22.3) is an autosomal dominant condition with a phenotype somewhat similar to that of Marfan syndrome; one point of difference is the usual upward dislocation of the lens in Marfan syndrome and usual downward dislocation in homocystinuria (ectopia lentis). The disorder is owing to mutations in cystathionine β-synthase, which leads to the laboratory findings of homocystinuria and methioninuria. Myocardial infarction, mitral valve prolapse, pectus excavatum or carinatum, osteoporosis, biconcave "codfish" vertebrae, kyphoscoliosis, dolichostenomelia, arachnodactyly, and limited joint mobility may occur.

Mental retardation, psychiatric disorders, and seizures are all characteristic of homocystinuria. Treatment involves a low-methionine, cystine-supplemented diet for pyridoxine nonresponders and pyridoxine supplementation for the roughly 50% of affected patients who are classified as pyridoxine responders.

Syndromes with extra Y chromosomes such as 47XYY or 48XYYY lead to tall stature in childhood and adult life, without any evidence of increased GH. Klinefelter syndrome (47XXY) may be associated with tall stature (see Chapters 8 and 9).

Endocrine Etiologies of Tall Stature

Pituitary gigantism is due to a GH-secreting adenoma in childhood; acromegaly occurs with the same type of tumor in an adult. Because the epiphyses are not closed in an affected child, height velocity is increased, although some of the coarse facial features of an acromegalic appearance also may be noted. Organomegaly may occur, and glucose intolerance or frank diabetes may result. Elevated fasting GH concentrations or IGF-1 (somatomedin) levels confirm the diagnosis. McCune-Albright syndrome may have, as one feature, pituitary gigantism due to autonomous GH secretion. Likewise multiple endocrine neoplasia 1 (MEN 1) may include excessive GH secretion, and if, as rarely occurs, it occurs before epiphyseal fusion, pituitary gigantism will result (see Chapter 14).

Precocious puberty of any etiology increases growth in childhood, but early epiphyseal closure and short adult stature will result (see Chapter 9).

One remarkable case of estrogen-receptor defect in a boy led to continued growth into the twenty-fifth year, with a bone age delayed so far that the epiphyses remained open, allowing continued growth.

Thyrotoxicosis increases height velocity and skeletal age advancement (see Chapter 6).

Increased insulin will increase growth rate. Infants of diabetic mothers are large at birth, but postnatal growth is normal. Fetal hyperinsulinism is the stimulus for the excessive fetal growth; neonatal hypoglycemia can be a serious complication, as the high maternal glucose concentration that led to the fetal hyperinsulinism is removed at the time of birth, but the insulin secretion continues. Children with β-cell adenomas may have continued rapid growth during their hyperinsulinemic state, but their hypoglycemia will most likely be the clinical condition that brings them to diagnosis.

Beckwith-Wiedemann syndrome (#130650 BECKWITH-WIEDEMANN SYNDROME; BWS imprinting at 11p15.5) leads to very large newborn length and weight, omphalocele (exomphalos), and macroglossia. Body size remains large throughout childhood, with an advanced bone age. Life-threatening hypoglycemia occurs because of hyperinsulinism due to pancreatic hyperplasia. In addition, hemihypertrophy, diastasis recti, hepatomegaly, and cardiomegaly are seen. A large fontanelle with a prominent occiput, a metopic ridge, coarse facial features, and linear ear lobe creases with posterior helical indentations occur. In addition, fetal adrenocortical cytomegaly and large kidneys with medullary dysplasia are found. Cryptorchidism is described, with a tendency to neoplasia including Wilms tumor, hepatoblastoma, adrenal carcinoma, and gonadoblastoma.

Diagnosis and Treatment of Tall Stature

Generally, the historical and physical manifestations of the conditions listed earlier are evident during the history and physical examination, so that these causes of tall stature can be investigated directly. Pituitary gigantism is one situation in which an IGF-1 concentration can be quite useful if it is remembered that during precocious puberty, IGF-1 concentrations increase higher than in age-matched controls. Basal GH concentration also should be elevated in pituitary gigantism when compared with the low concentrations seen in normal subjects (a situation in which a single GH determination may lead to a diagnosis). Pituitary giants also respond with GH secretion to agents that normally do not stimulate GH secretion, agents such as glucose (normally glucose suppresses GH), gonadotropin-releasing hormone (GnRH), and thyrotropin-releasing factor (TRF). Pituitary gigantism may be treated with transphenoidal microadenomectomy if the technical expertise is available.

SUGGESTED READINGS

Bell J. Tall stature. In: Finberg L, Kleinman RE, eds. *Saunders manual of pediatric practice.* Philadelphia: WB Saunders, 2002:827–829.

Cutler L. Growth hormone treatment. In: Finberg L, Kleinman RE, eds. *Saunders manual of pediatric practice.* Philadelphia: WB Saunders, 2002:846–848.

Drug and Therapeutics Committee of the Lawson Wilkins Pediatric Endocrine Society. Guidelines for the use of growth hormone in children with short stature. *J Pediatr* 1995;127:857–867.

Guyda HJ. Four decades of growth hormone therapy for short children: what have we achieved? *J Clin Endocrinol Metab* 1999; 84:4307–4316.

Hintz RL. Idiopathic short stature. In: Finberg L, Kleinman RE, eds. *Saunders manual of pediatric practice.* Philadelphia: WB Saunders, 2002:825–826.

Jones KL. *Smith's recognizable patterns of human malformation.* 5th ed. Philadelphia: WB Saunders, 1997:857.

Kaplan SL. Neonatal hypopituitarism. In: Finberg L, Kleinman RE, eds. *Saunders manual of pediatric practice.* Philadelphia: WB Saunders, 2002:843–844.

Parks JS. Hormones of pituitary and hypothalamus. In: Behrman RE, Kleigman RM, Jenson HB, eds. *Nelson's textbook of pediatrics.* Philadelphia: WB Saunders, 2002:1673–1680.

Reiter EO, D'Ercole AJ. Disorders of the anterior pituitary gland, hypothalamus, and growth. In: Rudolph CD, Rudolph AM, eds. *Rudolph's pediatrics*. New York: McGraw-Hill, 2002:2011–2024.

Reiter EO, Rosenfeld RG. Normal and abnormal growth. In: Larsen PR, Kronenberg HM, Melmed S, et al., eds. *Williams textbook of endocrinology*. Philadelphia: WB Saunders, 2003:1003–1114.

Rosenbloom AL. Growth hormone insensitivity: physiologic and genetic basis, phenotype, and treatment. *J Pediatr* 1999;135:280–289.

Rosenfeld RG. Growth hormone resistance (insensitivity) syndromes. In: Finberg L, Kleinman RE, eds. *Saunders manual of pediatric practice*. Philadelphia: WB Saunders, 2002:848–849.

Rosenfeld RG, Cohen P. Disorders of growth hormone/insulin-like growth factor secretion and action. In: Sperling MA, ed. *Pediatric endocrinology*. Philadelphia: WB Saunders, 2002:211–288.

Shalet ML, Toogood A, Rahim A, et al. The diagnosis of growth hormone deficiency in children and adults. *Endocr Rev* 1998;19:203–223.

Styne DM. Growth. In: Greenspan FS, Gardner DG, eds. *Basic and clinical endocrinology*. New York: Lange, 2001:163–200.

Styne DM. Constitutional delay in growth and adolescence. In: Finberg L, Kleinman RE, eds. *Saunders manual of pediatric practice*. Philadelphia: WB Saunders, 2002:838–839.

Styne DM. Acquired hypopituitarism. In: Finberg L, Kleinman RE, eds. *Saunders manual of pediatric practice*. Philadelphia: WB Saunders, 2002:844–845.

Styne DM. Evaluation of short stature. In: Finberg L, Kleinman RE, eds. *Saunders manual of pediatric practice*. Philadelphia: WB Saunders, 2002:946–949.

Vance ML, Mauras N. Growth hormone therapy in adults and children. *N Engl J Med* 1999;341:1206–1216.

6 ♣ Disorders of the Thyroid Gland

The thyroid gland produces hormones that have important effects on growth and development. These hormones exert actions on the central nervous system (CNS), regulate temperature, and influence many aspects of metabolism. Disorders of the thyroid gland are relatively common forms of endocrine disease in childhood. Many of the conditions, such as acquired hypothyroidism, may be appropriately evaluated and treated by a pediatrician or family physician, although some details of congenital hypothyroidism, hyperthyroidism, and certainly thyroid cancer are best approached with a pediatric endocrine consultation.

NORMAL THYROID PHYSIOLOGY AND ANATOMY

The thyroid gland originates from the embryonic pharyngeal floor and the fourth pharyngobronchial pouch at the site later identified as the foramen cecum, a pit at the back of the tongue. The normal thyroid gland descends to the normal location at the thyroid cartilage anterior to the trachea, but in some cases, it fails to descend far enough (sublingual or lingual thyroid is the result) or descends too far, sometimes ending up as far inferior as the mediastinum. Thus an ectopic thyroid gland may develop and may be too small or dysplastic to produce adequate thyroid hormone, resulting in hypothyroidism. A thyroid gland in the normal location also may be small (thyroid dysplasia or hypoplasia), or, in the most severe case, absent in athyrosis. One lobe may be absent, or an extra lobe, the pyramidal lobe, may develop, leading to asymmetry in appearance. Thyroid dysgenesis may be owing to abnormalities in the homeobox genes TTF-1, TTF-2, or PAX-8 in the approximately 2% of cases that are familial; most cases of thyroid dysgenesis occur sporadically.

The production of thyroid hormone by the thyroid gland is regulated by the hypothalamus and the pituitary gland (Fig. 6-1). Hypothalamic thyrotropin-releasing hormone (noted as TRH or thyrotropin-releasing factor or TRF in some publications), a three-amino-acid peptide, is released from the median eminence into the pituitary portal circulation. Although it has many functions in the CNS, for our purposes, it stimulates the pituitary gland to release thyroid-stimulating hormone (TSH) into the general circulation, whereby it reaches the thyroid gland and stimulates the production of endogenous thyroid hormones and release of thyroid hormone. In the absence of adequate thyroid hormone (primary hypothyroidism), TSH increases to very high levels, as in the presence of autonomous and excessive production or administration of exogenous thyroid hormone. The release of TSH is suppressed (as in Graves disease). Secondary hypothyroidism (the absence of pituitary TSH) and tertiary hypothyroidism (the absence of hypothalamic TRF) are differentiated from primary hypothyroidism by the measurement of serum TSH; in the former, serum TSH is nondetectable before or after TRF administration; in the latter, TSH is measurable and increases from low levels to an abnormally prolonged elevation after TRF.

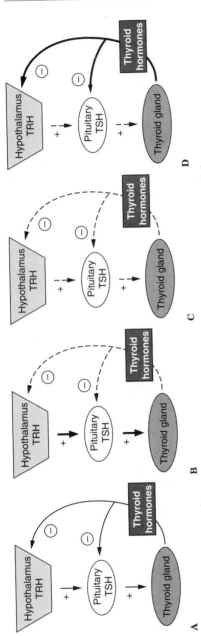

Fig. 6-1.   The hypothalamic pituitary thyroid axis. A: Normally a balance exists between thyroid hormones and thyroid-stimulating hormone (TSH). B: In primary hypothyroidism, insufficient thyroid hormones are produced to suppress TSH to normal. C: In secondary or tertiary hypothyroidism, insufficient TSH stimulates the thyroid gland to produce adequate thyroid hormone. D: In hyperthyroidism due to Graves disease, the autonomous production of thyroid hormone by thyroid-stimulating immunoglobulin (TSI) suppresses TSH to nondetectable levels.

Thyroid hormones are composed of two tyrosine molecules, an α and a β "ring," and a variable amount of iodine. They are synthesized in the following sequential steps:

1. Trapping of plasma iodide by the thyroid follicular cell;
2. Oxidation of iodide to iodine;
3. Organification of the tyrosine molecules (which are attached to the thyroglobulin molecule) by the addition of one iodine at the 3 position [causing the formation of monoiodotyrosine (MIT)] or two iodines at the 3 and 5 positions [forming diiodotyrosine (DIT)] by thyroid peroxidase;
4. The coupling of one DIT with one DIT to form $3,5,3',5'$-tetraiodothyronine (T_4) or one DIT with one MIT to produce $3,5,3'$-triiodothyronine (T_3).
5. The TSH-stimulated entry of thyroglobulin into the follicular cell, where it is metabolized, and iodine is subsequently released and reused in the process again.

Although both T_4 and T_3 are released from the thyroid gland, most of the circulating T_3 is derived from peripheral deiodination of the β-ring of T_4, except in the case of hyperthyroidism, in which excessive T_3 secretion from the thyroid gland may occur. T_3 is the metabolically active form of thyroid hormone. Reverse T_3 (RT_3) or $3,3',5'$ triiodothyronine is a metabolically inert product of the peripheral deiodination of the α-ring of T_4; this form is found in greater amounts in the fetus or during severe illness.

Circulating T_4 is bound predominantly to serum proteins; 75% is bound to thyroid-binding globulin (TBG), 20% to thyroxine-binding prealbumin (TBPA), and 5% to albumin, with only 0.02% to 0.06% present in the circulation as free thyroxine (FT_4); about 0.03% of T_3 circulates as free T_3 (FT_3). Free T_3 is the metabolically active form of thyroid hormone, whereas protein-bound T_3 and T_4 may be considered reservoirs of hormone in equilibrium with the metabolically active free hormone.

Laboratory Evaluation of Thyroid Function

In the past, total serum T_4 was the most common measurement available. However, the total T_4 value must be adjusted for the effects of available serum proteins on total T_4 measurement by the use of a resin T_3 assay or another surrogate test for the direct measurement of the free hormone. This complex procedure is now easily bypassed and replaced by the direct measurement of FT_4, usually by dialysis which does not require adjustment for protein values. Assays for FT_4 are now as generally available as is the assay of serum TSH. Serum TBG, thyroglobulin, and T_3 are other measures of interest in some of the conditions noted later.

New ultrasensitive TSH assays are now widely available to measure TSH accurately to 0.5 mIU/mL or less. Thus a patient with Graves disease will have a value of serum TSH below the normal range (often less than 0.5 mIU/mL) because of suppression by the autonomous secretion of thyroid hormones. A patient with secondary (pituitary defect lacking TSH production) or tertiary (hypothalamic defect due to lack of TRF production) hypothyroidism will also have a value below the limit of detection, whereas a normal patient will have a value between 0.7 and 6.4 mU/L (check the laboratory used for their exact standards for age, and refer to Chapter 17). In primary hypothyroidism or compensated hypothyroidism, serum TSH is elevated. The combination of serum FT_4 and TSH determination will allow the differential diagnosis of primary from secondary or tertiary hypothyroidism. Differentiation between secondary hypothyroidism and tertiary hypothyroidism may be difficult and may require a dynamic TRF test. A dose of 200 μg of TRF is given intravenously (i.v.) and TSH measured at 0, 10, 15, 30, 60, 90, 120, and 180 minutes (or at several of these times in some protocols). A normal response is an increase in TSH to at least 10 mIU/mL after about 15 minutes; in secondary hypothyroidism, no increase is seen in TSH; and in tertiary hypothyroidism, the increase may be delayed until 60 to 120 minutes, and the TSH may continue to increase during the 180-minute period. The TRF test also may be used in the diagnosis of hyperthyroidism, as no increase in TSH will occur after TSH with the autonomous thyroxine secretion characteristic of Graves disease. The TRF test is rarely invoked in Graves disease or other conditions with the development of other newer laboratory techniques.

Ultrasonographic scanning of the thyroid gland is useful to determine the location and size of a thyroid gland and to differentiate cystic from solid masses and the relation of the mass to neck structures. If a mass is solid, it is more likely to be carcinoma than if it is cystic. Ultrasonography also can be used to guide a biopsy needle, should this be considered advisable in a given case, but it must be ensured that if a needle biopsy is obtained, the pathology service can accurately interpret the results. Some suggest that, because excision may be indicated in the case of single cold nodules in any case, excision biopsy should be performed for both diagnosis and treatment of suspected cancer and that needle biopsy not be used. With features more strongly suggesting a malignancy, surgical excision biopsy is a better approach.

Radioiodine scanning of the thyroid gland and radioactive iodine uptake have limited roles in pediatric diagnosis compared with adult medicine. Imaging of a thyroid gland may be used in the differential diagnosis of nodules of the thyroid gland to determine whether they are functional or "hot" compared with nonfunctional or "cold" nodules. Imaging may be used for the localization of an ectopic thyroid gland. However, in a clear case of Hashimoto thyroiditis or Graves disease, little is added by a thyroid scan. The scanning of a neonate or infant presents particular problems; the radioactive tracer, which is administered orally or by nasogastric (NG) tube, may be spit up by the infant and may leave tracts of radioactivity on the skin, falsely suggesting thyroid tissue on imaging. Further, a neonate with primary hypothyroidism may have no detectable thyroid gland on scan just after birth, but after months to years, a normal gland may be detected; in several cases, this has been traced to the transient presence of thyroid-binding inhibitory immunoglobulin in the neonatal circulation that was passed from the mother (who may herself have symptomatic autoimmune thyroid disease) to the fetus. Application of iodine-containing cleaning compounds to the skin of the neonate may cause transient hypothyroidism. A congenital iodine-trapping defect will eliminate thyroidal iodine and suggest aplasia but will look the same as the transient condition on scan. The demonstration of an ectopic gland in a neonate on an acceptable-quality scan, however, is good evidence that the child has a permanent defect in thyroid metabolism. In the differential diagnosis of goiter, a perchlorate-discharge test may be used in which radioactive thyroid uptake is determined and then determined again, but after administration of potassium perchlorate, which causes the discharge of nonorganified iodine; if the turnover of iodine is much higher with perchlorate than without, an enzyme deficiency causing an organification defect is present.

An important consideration when performing thyroid-uptake determinations for hyperthyroidism is to measure the uptake early, such as at 4 hours, as well as at 24 hours, because a quick turnover of radioactive iodine, as occurs in Graves disease, may lead to a very high uptake at 4 hours but a low uptake at 24 hours, falsely eliminating hyperthyroidism as a diagnosis. Scanning is done with ^{123}I or technetium 99 pertechnetate; the former must be used before thyroxine is administered (if indicated), whereas the latter may be used even if thyroxine had already been administered. The ingestion of iodine or the use of contrast agents will decrease the ability to perform a scan with ^{123}I for a considerable period, so the iodine status of the individual may affect the results of the test.

DISORDERS OF THE THYROID GLAND

Goiter

An enlargement of the thyroid gland is a goiter; the affected patient may be euthyroid, hypothyroid, or hyperthyroid, so the finding of goiter does not indicate a diagnosis (Table 6-1). A goiter may be large enough to be visible to the patient or parent or may be subtle enough to be noted only on directed physical examination. Palpation usually is best accomplished with the examiner's fingers directed anteriorly around the neck while the examiner stands behind the patient. If the patient swallows water during the examination, the mobile nature of the thyroid gland should identify it as it rises and falls on swallowing. Hashimoto thyroiditis may be accompanied by a midline, pea-sized delphian node located 0.5 to 1 cm above the isthmus; the delphian node does not move with swallowing (delphian refers to the oracle that, in this case, indicates the presence of the condition). The margins of the goiter should be noted distinctly from the neighboring sternocleidomastoid muscle, and measurement should be recorded. The diagonal longest length of each lobe, the shortest diagonal length of each lobe, and the height of the isthmus may be recorded

Table 6-1. Etiologies of thyroid enlargement

Disorder	Goiter	Nodule	Free T_4	TSH	Other features	Inheritance
Autoimmune hypothyroidism (Hashimoto thyroiditis)	Usually	Usually not	Usually low but could be Nl or high	Usually low but could be Nl or low	Positive antithyroid peroxidase or antithyroglobulin antibodies	
Acute or suppurative thyroiditis	One lobe or overall enlargement				Painful	
Subacute thyroiditis	Usually				Painful	
Thyroid neoplasia		Yes				
Adenoma		Yes	High if functional or Nl if not	Low if functional or Nl if not		
Papillary carcinoma		Yes	Normal	Normal	History of radiation?	Sporadic (rarely familial)
Follicular carcinoma		Yes	High	Possibly low		Sporadic
Medullary carcinoma		Yes	Nl	Nl	Calcitonin high in basal, pentagastrin or calcium stimulated state; ret mutation positive even before calcitonin increases	Sporadic or familial (FMCT) and may be associated with MEN 2 or MEN 3

FMCT, familial medullary carcinoma of the thyroid; MEN, multiple endocrine neoplasia; Nl, normal.

for comparison at future visits to determine the effect of treatment. Some observers find it useful to trace the outline of the gland on a piece of tissue paper and to include it in the patient's record for future comparison. It is difficult to estimate the weight of the thyroid gland in children as is done in adult patients, but an estimation of the percentage the gland appears to be increased over normal size may be accomplished more easily (i.e., a slightly enlarged gland might be 25% to 50% increased, whereas an obviously enlarged gland may be 100% increased).

The thyroid functional status is next determined in a patient with a goiter. Most goiters in early childhood or infancy will be diagnosed by means of the newborn screening programs and will be owing to maternal ingestion of a goitrogen [such as propylthiouracil (PTU)] or an inborn error of thyroid biosynthesis. The majority of goiters in the late childhood through adolescent years will be because of euthyroid or hypothyroid Hashimoto thyroiditis, followed by a lower incidence of hyperthyroidism due to Graves disease. A minority of indeterminate goiters of mild degree may persist for years; these may be colloid goiters, a diagnosis that is established only after all other diagnoses are eliminated. Colloid goiter is not accompanied by an elevation in serum anti-microsomal or anti-thyroglobulin antibody levels, nor is there an alteration in thyroid function from normal. No real condition exists that was previously called "physiologic goiter of adolescence," so evaluation of all goiters is indicated, rather than accepting them as a normal variation.

A solitary nodule in childhood is unusual and worthy of careful attention and should not simply be considered a routine goiter. Serious consideration of thyroid cancer must arise if a solitary nodule is noted (see later). A thyroid scan may be used to determine whether the nodule is hot and functional, or cold and nonfunctional. A cold nodule is particularly worrisome, as it may indicate neoplasia (see later). A palpable nodule that is indistinguishable from the rest of the gland on thyroid scan may be followed up without immediate surgical intervention; thyroxine therapy may cause it to shrink, especially if the serum TSH is elevated.

Hypothyroidism

Neonatal Hypothyroidism

The detection and treatment of neonates with hypothyroidism should be considered a pediatric emergency (Table 6-2). If therapy is not begun soon after birth, certainly within weeks to months, developmental delay will result. Neonatal hypothyroidism is a relatively common disorder, with an incidence close to one in 4,000 live births. Routine neonatal screening has been instituted in all states in the United States and in most countries because of the difficulty in making a clinical diagnosis early enough, based on the history and physical examination. In most cases, samples of blood are collected from a heel-stick, placed on a filter paper, and

(text continues on page 92)

Table 6-2. Etiologies of congenital hypothyroidism

Disorder	Subtypes	Prevalence	Goiter	Free T$_4$	TSH	Other features	Inheritance
Thyroid dysgenesis		1:4000	No	Low	High	May be agenesis, hypoplastic or ectopia	Mostly sporadic, but recent evidence shows gene links in some (TTF-1, TTF-2, PAX-8)
Thyroid dyshormonogenesis		1:40,000					
	Iodine-transport defect		Yes	Low	High	Mutation of gene for sodium/iodine symporter. Treated with extra iodide	AR
	Organification defect	1:40,000	Yes	Low	High	Mutation of thyroid peroxidase. Positive perchlorate discharge test is diagnostic	AR
	Pendred syndrome	1:50,000	Yes	Low	High	Defect in pendrin gene. Deaf mute and positive perchlorate discharge test	AR
	Iodotyrosine deiodinase defect		Yes	Low	High	High RAIU but early discharge. High serum MIT and DIT	AR
Hypothalamic-pituitary abnormality		1:100,00	No	Low	Low		Mostly sporadic

	Incidence	Goiter	Serum T4	Serum TSH	Defect	Inheritance
Familial TSH deficiency		No	Low	Low	Abnormal TSH β gene	AR
Pit-1 or Prop-1 gene deficiency		No	Low	Low	Absence of GH and Prl secretion	AR
TSH unresponsiveness	Rare 1:40,000	No	Low	High	Mutation of TSH-receptor gene	AR
Transient hypothyroidism						
Maternal antibodies blocking TSH receptor		No	Low	High		
Goitrogens (medication such as maternal PTU or food such as certain cabbages)		Yes	Low	High		
Excess or inadequate iodine e.g., endemic cretinism		Yes	Low	High		
Thyroid hormone resistance	1:100,000	Yes	High	High	Mutation of thyroid-receptor gene. May be general (TSH may be normal), peripheral or pituitary resistance	AR, AD. Sporadic
Thyroglobulin defects	1:40,000	Yes	Low	High	Mutation of TG gene	AR

TSH, thyroid-stimulating hormone; AR, autosomal recessive; AD, autosomal dominant; PTU, propylthiouracil; RAIU, radioactive iodine uptake; MIT, monoiodotyrosine; DIT, diiodotyrosine; GH, growth hormone; Prl, prolactin. (Modified from Fisher DA. The thyroid. In: Rudolph CD, Rudolph AM, eds. Rudolph's pediatrics. New York: McGraw-Hill; 2002: 2059–2079.

sent to a centralized laboratory, where blood is eluted from the paper and analyzed for concentration of TSH (in some locations T_4 might be determined instead). A screening test is just that and should not be relied on for diagnosis and therapy without confirmation. However, if the TSH value is elevated, a diagnosis of presumptive hypothyroidism is made. If the result is intermediate, the centralized laboratory in some states might offer a repeated sample. However, a very high value of TSH on screening should suggest the wisdom of immediately obtaining a serum FT_4 and TSH by venipuncture in preparation for instituting therapy rapidly. If the TSH is low, it will not be detected on TSH-screening programs, and the diagnosis of secondary or tertiary hypothyroidism will be missed; in most cases, these diagnoses are accompanied by other deficits of the hypothalamus or pituitary, and the diagnosis will be indicated by these other conditions such as growth hormone or ACTH deficiency, which are likely to lead to neonatal hypoglycemia or even hypoglycemic seizures (see later).

It is important to view the normal developmental physiology of the fetus and newborn to understand the pitfalls of the neonatal screening program and interpretation of thyroid function in the days and weeks after birth. By 10 to 11 weeks of gestation, the human thyroid gland shows follicular organization and demonstrates the ability to concentrate iodine. By this time, TRF is demonstrable in the fetal hypothalamus, and TSH is found in the fetal pituitary and circulation. The pituitary hypothalamic portal system is developing around this time and is mostly mature by 20 weeks' gestation. Thus, most of the components of thyroid physiology are in place by the second half of gestation.

Serum concentrations of the thyroid hormones found in the fetus reflect this maturation, as little of the maternal thyroid hormones and virtually none of the maternal TSH crosses the placenta. However, untreated maternal hypothyroidism is reported to impair the intellectual development of the fetus, demonstrating the importance of the small amount of T_4 that does cross the placenta; cerebral palsy may develop in affected children of hypothyroid mothers as well. Serum TSH normally increases at about 20 weeks of gestation, the stage of gestation when TRF is able to reach the pituitary gland, and serum T_4 increases as a result. In the fetus, the vast majority of T_4 undergoes deiodination of the α-ring, leading to the formation of RT_3 (an inactive metabolite compared with T_3) in parallel with lower than postnatal concentrations of T_4. Late in gestation, β-ring deiodination of thyroxine increases, forming more T_3, and serum T_3 finally begins to increase as well. At term, fetal TSH and T_4 are slightly higher than those found in normal adult concentrations; fetal serum RT_3 is markedly higher than in the adult, and fetal serum T_3 is considerably lower. Thus the fetus is normally in a relatively decreased state of thyroid physiology compared with the postnatal state. Serum values of TBG and other thyroid-binding proteins increase with advancing gestation, as do other serum proteins.

After delivery, serum TSH quickly increases and peaks at 30 minutes; T_4 is secreted in response and increases by 24 to 72 hours to values equivalent to those found in adult hyperthyroidism, with a slow decrease toward adult normal values over the following weeks, months, and years. Serum T_3 exhibits a primary increase in the hours after birth because of increased β-ring deiodination of thyroxine and exhibits a secondary increase at 24 to 72 hours because of the increase in T_4; RT_3 decreases after birth because of the switch from α-ring deiodination to β-ring deiodination; TBG and therefore the RT_3U remain relatively constant after birth.

It is essential to understand this developmental physiology to diagnose congenital hypothyroidism properly. A normal term child will have serum T_4 concentrations in the adult hyperthyroid range during the 24 to 72 hours after birth, whereas a child with bona fide hypothyroidism will have serum T_4 either below the normal adult range or in the adult range. Healthy premature babies, interrupted before the normal end point of thyroid physiologic development at term, have a lower concentration of T_4, and premature babies with respiratory distress syndrome or others who are small-for-gestational-age will have T_4 values lower than do normal age-matched children. Thus, it should be clear that the gestational age of the neonate, the clinical condition, and the postnatal age are important in the interpretation of neonatal thyroid-screening tests. Age-adjusted normal ranges for these tests are essential.

The signs and symptoms of congenital hypothyroidism in its classic form include large tongue, coarse facies, umbilical hernia, a combination of lethargy and irritability, poor growth and weight gain, short extremities with a delayed or high upper- to lower-segment ratio, persistently open posterior fontanel, large anterior fontanel, and coarse voice. Further, pericardial edema can be noted on ultrasound study in infants left untreated for a prolonged time. However, these signs and symptoms take weeks to months to develop, and if suspicion of congenital hypothyroidism were to be triggered by physical stigmata alone, the majority of patients would have to wait until irreversible mental changes already were established before diagnosis was accomplished and therapy began. Although features such as prolonged gestation with large birth weight, persistent jaundice, temperature instability, lag in the time of the initial episode of stooling to more than 20 hours after birth, edema, and hypoactivity and poor feeding can be seen in hypothyroid patients in the neonatal period, most or all of these findings could be signs of other diseases as well and may not suggest the definitive diagnosis to the physician without the aid of neonatal screening.

Thus neonatal screening programs were established to diagnose patients uniformly before definitive symptoms occur. However, the signs and symptoms of congenital hypothyroidism must be remembered because the statewide screening programs are not infallible, and a few patients may miss screening because of home birth, early discharge from the hospital, long stay in the neonatal intensive care unit, transfer between hospitals, or even lost samples. If a suspicion exists that a newborn might have hypothyroidism, rather than waiting for the neonatal screening result, standard FT_4 and TSH determinations can be requested, and the results may be available even sooner than those from the screening program. Most screening programs will report results by age 7 days, quite a remarkable accomplishment.

The etiology of congenital hypothyroidism is usually athyrosis, hypoplasia of the thyroid gland (half to one third of cases), or a lack of descent of the thyroid gland from its initial site of formation to its normal mature location (thyroid ectopy or, by analogy to the term used for lack of descent of the testes, "cryptothyroidism"). These conditions were generally considered to occur in a sporadic pattern, but there is increasing evidence of inherited tendencies in some families (#218700 THYROID DYSGENESIS at 2q12-q14). The presence of thyroglobulin in the serum indicates the presence of at least some thyroid tissue. A ^{123}I thyroid scan is able to demonstrate ectopy, but an initial finding of athyrosis or hypoplasia on scan may be because of blocking antibodies, and may falsely suggest a permanent anatomic abnormality, when a transient condition is present (see earlier). Ultrasound examination of the area will help determine the presence of thyroid tissue in those infants with TSH receptor–blocking antibodies or a genetic iodine-trapping defect that will interfere with the demonstration of tissue on radioactive ^{123}I scan.

Endemic cretinism is found in areas of iodine deficiency, but with iodine supplementation of salt, bread, and other foods, the prevalence has decreased worldwide, and the condition is virtually nonexistent in the United States. Nonetheless, iodine deficiency is still the leading cause of congenital hypothyroidism worldwide, and it is all the more tragic because it is easily preventable.

Biochemical abnormalities of the thyroid gland are usually hereditary and often involve the development of a goiter. Possible diagnoses in patient with goiter include dyshormonogenesis, such as peroxidase defects (organification defects) (#274500 THYROID HORMONE ORGANIFICATION DEFECT II due to mutation in the thyroid peroxidase gene at 2p25) which may be a part of the Pendred syndrome (#274600 PENDRED SYNDROME; PDS at 1q21-q22, 10q11.2), deiodinase defects in which the individual cannot remove iodine from the DIT or MIT and therefore becomes iodine deficient from iodine loss in the urine (*274800 THYROID HORMONOGENESIS, GENETIC DEFECT IN, IV), and thyroglobulin defects causing lack of coupling of MIT and DIT (274900 THYROID HORMONOGENESIS, GENETIC DEFECT IN, V and *188450 THYROGLOBULIN; TG at 8q24.2-q24.3). A defect in TSH receptors (#275200 THYROTROPIN, UNRESPONSIVENESS TO At 14q3.1) and a defect in the transport of iodine into the thyroid gland (#274400 THYROID HORMONOGENESIS, GENETIC DEFECT IN, I at 19p13.2-p12) have been described with central and peripheral resistance to thyroid hormone and delayed speech development, attention deficit/hyperactivity disorder (#188570 THYROID HORMONE RESISTANCE at 3p24.3) with goiter, but euthyroid status due to increased secretion of thyroid hormone. Other kindreds have thyroid hormone unresponsiveness or Refetoff syndrome (#274300 THYROID HORMONE UNRESPONSIVENESS at 3p24.3) in which thyroid hormone and TSH concentrations are high; the patients are clinically euthyroid but may have exophthalmos, deaf-mutism, skeletal abnormalities, and goiter; a mutation in the gene for the β portion of the thyroid hormone receptor is found.

Rarely (fewer than one in 100,000 live births), isolated TSH deficiency or secondary hypothyroidism (#275100 THYROTROPIN DEFICIENCY, ISOLATED for the extremely rare familial form) or isolated TRF deficiency or tertiary hypothyroidism (*275120 THYROTROPIN-RELEASING HORMONE DEFICIENCY at 3q13.3- q21 for the rare familial form) may occur, but in most cases of TSH or TRF deficiency, other pituitary hormone deficiencies are present as well, which will likely manifest signs that will lead to the diagnosis. For example, TSH deficiency is found in Pit-1, Prop-1, or other autosomal genes or defects. Isolated TSH deficiency also is seen (see Chapter 3).

External agents can cause congenital hypothyroidism when they are administered to the mother. Radioactive iodine mistakenly given to a pregnant woman with Graves disease will immediately cross the placenta and damage the developing gland; if the dose is less than therapeutic, as in the aftermath of a nuclear accident, total destruction of the gland may not occur, but neoplasia may follow because of the damage to the fetal thyroid gland. PTU given to a pregnant woman with hyperthyroidism also will cross the placenta and can cause profound hypothyroidism if the maternal dose is too great; when the PTU is cleared after delivery, the baby will recover from the hypothyroidism caused by suppression by PTU, but the thyroid-stimulating immunoglobulin that was passed from the mother via the placenta will begin to exert its effect, causing transient but potentially clinically relevant hyperthyroidism. Paradoxically, excessive iodine given to the mother can suppress thyroid gland formation, as can a deficiency of iodine.

In several situations, thyroid-binding proteins are altered and thereby alter the serum T_4 and T_3 concentrations. Decreased TBG, or TBG deficiency (*314200 THYROXINE-BINDING GLOBULIN OF SERUM; TBG at Xq22.2), occurs in one of 10,000 live births in a sex-linked pattern. The serum T_4 and T_3 are decreased, the serum FT_4 is normal, but because serum TSH is normal, the child will be not detected by the newborn TSH-screening program. Most children are normal, but mental retardation also is reported in the literature. Familial dysalbuminemic hyperthyroxinemia (FDH) (*145680 HYPERTHYROXINEMIA, FAMILIAL) leads to increased T_4 but a normal serum T_3; the free forms of both hormones are normal, and the patient is asymptomatic.

With the receipt of a screening test result suggesting congenital hypothyroidism, another set of serum samples for confirmatory T_4 and TSH should be drawn, as the results of a screening test require proof. If the initial TSH was quite high, treatment with synthetic T_4 may be started while awaiting the results of the confirmatory tests. The decision to perform a thyroid scan is controversial because of the false positives noted earlier, but if the expertise is available, it may be helpful. A bone-age determination of the knee and foot is useful: the distal femoral epiphysis calcifies at 36 weeks of gestation; the proximal tibial epiphysis at 38 weeks; and the cuboid epiphysis at term. Thus a bone age of the leg and foot can be determined at the time of receipt of the screening results, and the finding of delayed lower extremity bone age for gestational age may strengthen the impression of congenital hypothyroidism (a hand bone age is useless at this age). Patients with congenital hypothyroidism may have epiphyseal dysgenesis or irregular multifocal calcification on radiograph when the epiphyses do appear after the institution of treatment.

Transient hyperthyrotropinemia, in which a child will have perfectly normal serum T_4 concentrations for age but a slightly elevated TSH (often in the range of 20 to 30 mIU/mL), may be confused with primary hypothyroidism. The natural history of such patients is a decrease in the TSH concentrations to normal by age 1 to 2 years in the absence of treatment. Children with laboratory values characteristic of transient hyperthyrotropinemia should be watched for evidence of decreasing thyroid function in case they have, instead of benign transient hyperthyrotropinemia, an ectopic or hypoplastic thyroid gland that, although functional enough at birth to allow a normal newborn screen, decompensates with time, and hypothyroidism develops. Patients with neonatal hypothyroidism will in some cases maintain a normal serum T_4 concentration at the time of the newborn screening at the expense of an elevated TSH; most will be detected, but some will have normal serum TSH at birth and for at least some time thereafter until the inadequate thyroid gland fails. Thus elevated serum TSH is a worrisome finding; the differential diagnosis in this case should be made by an experienced pediatric endocrinologist.

Treatment of congenital hypothyroidism should begin immediately after the diagnosis is established, as long as confirmatory tests beyond the neonatal screening tests are obtained. In those cases in which the screening results show an extremely high TSH, treatment can be started even before the confirmatory results return, as it will be most unlikely that a mistake in diagnosis has occurred. Presently, recommended dosage of synthetic thyroxine is 10 to 15 µg/kg for the newborn (a dose of 25 to 37.5 µg is the usual daily dose in term newborns) and less thereafter, on the basis of per kilogram body weight until a total dose of 100 to 150 µg is reached at the maximum in a teenager (Table 6-3). Thyroxine is most widely available in tablets and is crushed and administered in a small amount of formula in the newborn. Liquid thyroxine is available for parenteral use but is quite expensive; it has been used rarely for patients who are unable to take medications orally. T_3 is not now used for the treatment of hypothyroidism.

Table 6-3.   General doses of thyroxine by age in micrograms/kg: all must be adjusted by clinical state and serum thyroxine (and TSH after the newborn period)

0–3 mo	10–15
3–6 mo	8–10
6–12 mo	6–8
1–5 yr	5–6
6–12 yr	4–5
>12 yr	2–3

TSH, thyroid-stimulating hormone.

Children must be followed up carefully, with determination of growth rate, serum TSH and thyroxine, or free thyroxine at frequent intervals to make sure therapy is continuing and effective.

Some patients with primary hypothyroidism who have not had some elevation of the serum TSH during treatment to show that they have a permanent condition and who have no known anatomic defect in the thyroid gland may be carefully challenged at age 3 years to see if they have permanent hypothyroidism or a transient defect; in only those patients that have reliable families and can be counted on to return for follow-up, thyroxine can be discontinued for 2 to 4 weeks, with serum T_4 and TSH measured at 2 and 4 weeks to determine thyroid function. Most thyroid-dependent brain growth is completed by 3 years, so that the test is safer at this age than earlier, but it is not advisable to leave a hypothyroid child off thyroxine for long intervals, even at this age. Thus as soon as elevated TSH is seen, the trial off therapy is over, and the child deserves continued thyroxine therapy.

Neonates with congenital hypothyroidism may have elevated TSH concentrations for months or even years after the onset of appropriate therapy because of a persistent abnormality of feedback suppression; attempting to suppress these TSH concentrations to normal levels may lead to excessive thyroxine dosage. Thus the goal of therapy should be to maintain a normal serum thyroxine or free thyroxine concentration at the upper half of the normal range for age rather than to suppress the TSH to normal values for age. Overtreatment with thyroxine will cause advancement of the bone age and can lead to craniosynostosis. Further, the administration of full treatment dosages of thyroxine to infants with congenital hypothyroidism that were untreated for a period of months may cause the onset of congestive heart failure because of the rapid mobilization of fluid accumulated during the myxedematous state; in such children with late onset of therapy, it is preferable to work up to the full dose over a period of 7 to 14 days. Of course, excessively low dose of thyroxine for a long time may lead to an even poorer CNS result, so this titrating of the dose upward cannot be a prolonged process.

Patients treated early and appropriately with thyroxine are likely to have normal intelligence, according to follow-up studies. In rare cases on record, even therapy begun in the first week of life does not eliminate severe intellectual impairment, in a few patients, the prenatal thyroid deficit caused long-term problems not improved by postnatal therapy. This is exceptionally rare, as the institution of neonatal thyroid screening and neonatal treatment has markedly decreased the morbidity of this common condition. Parents should be reassured about the expected normal outcome.

Prenatal therapy of fetuses in families with proven genetic hypothyroidism is reported. This is presently considered an experimental procedure.

Acquired Hypothyroidism

Acquired hypothyroidism is not a rare disease. It is estimated that this group of disorders occurs in one in 500 school-age children.

Childhood hypothyroidism starting after age 2 years does not carry the risk of permanent mental retardation, as does neonatal hypothyroidism, but temporary, reversible behavior changes are frequent. Remarkably, children with acquired hypothyroidism may have a longer attention span, which may lead to improved grades in school; with treatment, their attention span is reduced and may even cause their grades to fall! Mild congenital abnormalities, such as an ectopic thyroid gland, may first manifest in the childhood period, although most will have been diagnosed by moderate elevations of the TSH level in the newborn screening programs. The addition of iodine to food in the United States has effectively eliminated endemic iodine-deficient goiter, although children born in many other countries are still at risk.

Symptoms of classic hypothyroidism include cold intolerance, constipation, and some weight gain due to myxedema. In spite of common perceptions that hypothyroidism is responsible for significant obesity, the weight gain does not occur to the extent of severe obesity. Skin is dry, and the hair is brittle and even sparse in hypothyroidism. Long-standing primary hypothyroidism may lead to enlargement of the pituitary gland due to increased TSH secretion: erosion of the sella turcica may appear to indicate the presence of a tumor on radiograph, so thyroid function should always be evaluated in the face of such a finding, if otherwise unexplained.

Hypothyroidism causes poor growth and results in short stature. Long-bone growth is diminished, and the upper- to lower-segment ratio is decreased for age, leading to immature proportions. The bone age is delayed, often significantly. Puberty is delayed or absent in teenage patients. Treatment will increase growth rate, advance bone age, and, if the child is old enough, precipitate pubertal appropriate development. However, if the condition is untreated for a long period, adult height will be compromised even with appropriate treatment.

Remarkably, premature sexual development occurs in some children with untreated primary hypothyroidism; girls have breast development, and boys have enlargement of testes and penis, but neither demonstrate premature development of pubic hair. Galactorrhea may be found because of increased secretion of prolactin in primary hypothyroidism, as TRF stimulates prolactin as well as TSH release.

Hashimoto thyroiditis (or chronic lymphocytic thyroiditis or autoimmune thyroid disease *140300 HASHIMOTO STRUMA at 8q23-q24) is responsible for the majority of cases of acquired hypothyroidism. This autoimmune disorder is found in a continuum with Graves disease, and both disorders may coexist in one family group; evidence of both disorders may be found in the same patient. In Hashimoto thyroiditis, there is formation of unsuppressed clones of thymus-dependent lymphocytes directed against the thyroid gland, causing lymphocytic infiltration of the gland. B lymphocytes, either through interaction with T lymphocytes or because of stimulation linked to the damaged thyroid cells, produce anti-thyroid antibodies, anti-thyroglobulin or anti-thyroid peroxidase antibodies (previously called anti-microsomal antibodies) that are characteristic of the disorder and are a cornerstone of the diagnosis.

Hashimoto thyroiditis is frequently associated with other disorders. Autoimmune polyglandular diseases may include Hashimoto thyroiditis:

Type 1 (*240300 AUTOIMMUNE POLYENDOCRINOPATHY SYNDROME, TYPE I at 21q22.3) consists of hypothyroidism with hypoparathyroidism, Addison disease, and mucocutaneous candidiasis, as well as hypogonadism and other features.

Type 2 (269200 SCHMIDT SYNDROME) consists of hypo- or hyperthyroidism, Addison disease, type 1 diabetes mellitus, with other features including candidiasis.

The term, type 3 autoimmune polyendocrinopathy, may be invoked to describe Hashimoto thyroiditis by itself.

Further, patients with Turner or Klinefelter syndrome are prone to Hashimoto thyroiditis, as are those with trisomy 21. Thus patients with any of these conditions should undergo surveillance for the development of this condition, usually annually.

Clinical characteristics of Hashimoto thyroiditis include goiter, a delphian node (a pea-sized, centrally located lymph node just above the thyroid gland), minimally to severely elevated TSH concentrations, and frequently a family history of thyroid disease. A characteristic pebbly surface to the gland is seen because of accentuation of the normal follicular structure of the gland. A positive titer of anti-thyroid peroxidase antibodies (or anti-microsomal antibodies in the older terminology) or anti-thyroglobulin antibodies or both are helpful in diagnosis; children more frequently have the former antibodies, whereas adults more usually have the latter. Lymphocytic infiltration of the thyroid gland occurs, with the formation of germinal centers on histologic study. No reason is known to perform a thyroid scan or uptake in a well-documented case of Hashimoto thyroiditis.

Normal to slightly elevated TSH concentrations with normal serum FT_4 indicate euthyroid goiter or compensated hypothyroidism. Elevated serum TSH and decreased FT_4 indicate obvious primary hypothyroidism. If the TSH is elevated, the treatment is clear: the administration of thyroxine until the TSH is suppressed to normal and the serum FT_4 increases to or stays at normal. If the TSH is not elevated and the goiter is minimal, the patient may be regularly evaluated for further deterioration in thyroid function during the following months and years. If the goiter is noticeable, thyroxine may be given for a period of 3 months to see if the goiter can be diminished; if the small goiter does not change, thyroxine may be stopped and the patient followed up until the thyroxine treatment may become definitively necessary.

Other causes for acquired hypothyroidism include a thyroglossal duct cyst (188455 THYROGLOSSAL DUCT CYST, FAMILIAL for the rare genetic form) in the midline of the neck. It may contain the complete complement of functioning thyroid tissue available to the patient; if any midline congenital defect of the neck is removed surgically, it may contain a thyroglossal duct cyst; the patient must be evaluated for the development of hypothyroidism, or alternatively, the patient should have a thyroid scan to confirm the presence of remaining thyroid tissue. Rare children are born with only one lobe of thyroid gland, usually the left. This tissue may undergo compensatory hypertrophy, and it has the usual chance of developing Hashimoto thyroiditis, causing a presentation of hypothyroidism with one-sided goiter. Internationally, iodine deficiency is the most common cause of acquired hypothyroidism as endemic cretinism. Excess iodine intake, (e.g., from kelp given by a naturopath) may suppress thyroid function and temporarily lead to hypothyroidism, as may the ingestion of certain drugs that impair thyroid function such as lithium or amiodarone. Infiltrative disease from Langerhans cell histiocytosis or lymphoma or hemochromatosis due to iron infiltration of the thyroid gland due to transfusions for thalassemia or cystinosis may cause primary hypothyroidism. Treatment for hyperthyroidism (e.g., surgery or radiation) may later lead to hypothyroidism. A liver hemangioma causing elevated activity of type 3 deiodinase that preferentially converts T_4 to reverse T_3 and T_3 to T_2, thereby decreasing available thyroid function, will lead to acquired hypothyroidism.

Any disease of the hypothalamic–pituitary area may decrease TSH secretion, leading to secondary or tertiary hypothyroidism (see Chapter 3).

Acquired hypothyroidism is treated with thyroxine in a variable dose, depending on age and based on weight, up to a maximum of 100 to 150 µg (see Table 6.3); older children require less thyroxine per kilogram body weight than is used in a neonate with hypothyroidism. Unlike some neonates with congenital hypothyroidism, older children can safely have the dose titrated until the serum TSH is suppressed to normal, unless severe myxedema and even pericardial effusion exist, in which case the dose should be slowly increased. No proven advantage is found in T_3 treatment over thyroxine treatment.

Abnormalities of TBG may be congenital, but also may be acquired. Thus increased TBG binding of thyroid hormones occurs with estrogen treatment or pregnancy or is the result of an inherited condition; decreased TBG binding of thyroid hormones occurs with androgen therapy, protein-losing conditions, phenytoin (Dilantin) therapy, and an X-linked genetic condition (see earlier).

Hyperthyroidism

Hyperthyroidism is usually due to Graves disease (#275000 GRAVES DISEASE), an autoimmune disease that may coexist with Hashimoto thyroiditis (Table 6-4). Thyroid-stimulatory immunoglobulin (TSI) antibodies (various laboratories use various abbreviations for this same test or similar ones, so check with the laboratories for the tests offered) are formed and directed toward the TSH receptor, leading to autonomous thyroid function and hyperthyroidism without the involvement of TSH. Other antibodies displace TSH from the TSH receptor but do not stimulate the thyroid gland (these are TSH binding-inhibiting immunoglobulins (TBIIs). T_3 is produced more efficiently in Graves disease than in the normal state, and both T_4 and T_3 exceed the TBG capacity, so that FT_4 and FT_3 increase. In some cases, the T_4 is normal, but the T_3 is elevated; in the diagnosis of hyperthyroidism, both should be measured, as both must be suppressed during therapy. Serum TSH is suppressed because of the autonomous formation of thyroid hormones.

Weakness, increased pulse rate, emotional lability (sometimes to the point of apparent psychiatric disease), hyperactivity, and lack of attention span, weight loss, and diarrhea are characteristic findings. Subtle or significant goiter may be found, possibly with a bruit. Exophthalmos may occur because of infiltration of glycosaminoglycan in the posterior area of the orbit. Increased autonomic tone can cause lid retraction and "stare." These two conditions may at first look similar but should be noted separately. Pretibial myxedema is found in some patients, although it is more common in affected adults (this is not to be confused with the myxedema of profound hypothyroidism, which shares the term, but means very different things). Signs also include tachycardia, systolic hypertension, and velvety (smooth) and moist skin. Deep tendon reflexes are brisk, even to the point of clonus.

Girls are more often affected than boys (5:1). Human leukocyte antigen (HLA)-DR3 and HLA-B8 predispose whites to Graves disease. The peak age at onset is near adolescence.

Laboratory findings in hyperthyroidism are elevated serum T_4 and T_3 (both in either the total or free determination) with nondetectable or suppressed TSH. If the TSH is not suppressed, the patient may have a TSH-secreting condition as the etiology, an exceptionally rare occurrence. A positive TSI titer may be found

Table 6-4. Etiologies of hyperthyroidism

Disorder	Free T$_4$	TSH	RAI uptake	Other features
Autoimmune Graves disease	High	Low	Early elevation	Thyroid-stimulating immunoglobulin positive
TSH-secreting pituitary tumor	High	High	NA	Look for pituitary tumor on MRI
Pituitary T3 resistance	High	High	NA	No sign of tumor as the TSH is secreted because of resistance to T$_3$ feedback
Nodular hyperthyroidism	High	Low	Hot nodule (nodule takes up ^{123}I, but the rest of the thyroid gland does not)	
TSH receptor–activating mutations	High	Low	NA	Could be isolated or part of the McCune-Albright syndrome

RAI, radioactive iodine; TSH, thyroid-stimulating hormone; MRI, magnetic resonance imaging; NA, not applicable.

(but check with the specific laboratory for the designation of this test, as noted earlier). Often positive titers of anti-thyroglobulin and anti-microsomal antibodies are seen; if the titers of anti-microsomal and anti-thyroglobulin antibodies are very elevated, the patient may have the hyperthyroid phase of Hashimoto thyroiditis (often called hashitoxicosis), which may be short lived and not require a permanent type of treatment. Thyroid growth-stimulating antibodies and thyrotropin receptor–blocking antibodies are found, as well as lymphocytic infiltration of the thyroid gland. It is usually not necessary to perform a thyroid scan or uptake if the constellation of symptoms is classic. If, however, a scan is used, an early (4-hour) determination of uptake should be made before turnover of the radioactive tracer occurs in this condition of increased thyroid metabolism. A complete blood count (CBC) is obtained to detect changes in the white blood cell (WBC) count due to the hyperthyroid state; the WBC count may already be decreased in untreated hyperthyroidism or may be decreased later by medical therapy for hyperthyroidism. Determination of antinuclear antibody (ANA) titer and SMA20 should be obtained if PTU is to be used as treatment to ensure that no abnormalities are present before medication is given; PTU may affect liver function or cause a lupus-like syndrome.

Three types of treatment for hyperthyroidism are used: medication, radiation therapy, and surgery.

1. Medication. PTU or methimazole are the medical therapies available in the United States. PTU blocks organification of iodine and decreases T_4 to T_3 conversion; it may inhibit the formation of the offending IgG of Graves disease, whereas methimazole demonstrates only the first activity. PTU is given in does of 150 to 450 mg/day (5 to 7 mg/kg/24 hours) divided into doses given every 8 hours; methimazole is give in approximately 5–10% of the PTU dose and may be given twice or even once per day in selected patients. The aim is to cause a sufficient suppression of the autonomous thyroid function to precipitate hypothyroidism and then to add replacement thyroxine to bring about a euthyroid state. The patient is followed up for shrinkage of the goiter, an essential finding if remission is to be expected. Remission has an incidence of 20% to 25% every 2 years for patients receiving medical therapy: thus, after 11 years of therapy, 75% of patients in one series achieved remission.

Side effects occur 5% to 20% of the time during PTU therapy. Serious side effects of PTU or methimazole are not common but can be life threatening. Lupus-like syndrome including arthralgia and glomerulonephritis or vasculitis, rashes possibly with urticaria, granulocytopenia or agranulocytosis, and hepatitis possibly leading to cirrhosis are generally idiosyncratic, occurring early in the course of therapy, and are usually reversible at the early stage. These drugs should be discontinued if serious side effects develop, and alternative methods of therapy should be used. Lack of compliance, unfortunately a common condition in the adolescent age group, also is an indication for surgical or radioiodine therapy. It must be emphasized that PTU can cause fatal complications, and its use must be carefully monitored.

Propranolol (2 to 3 mg/kg/day or 5 to 10 mg every 6 hours as a starting dose) can control symptoms of hyperthyroidism while awaiting another mode of therapy to exert its effects and is useful in short-term situations such as in preparation for surgery or in the face of thyroid storm; side effects of propranolol on respiratory (bronchospasm) or circulatory (hypotension) function are possible, so patients must be chosen carefully lest they have asthma or another condition in which propranolol is contraindicated. Studies have shown propranolol to be helpful for long-term management in adults, but it has not generally been used as such in children.

2. Surgery. Subtotal thyroidectomy is an alternative therapy. An experienced thyroid surgeon should perform the operation so that complications will be unlikely. Recurrent laryngeal nerve paralysis is an unusual but possible complication. Transient hypocalcemia can follow thyroidectomy because of postoperative edema of the parathyroid glands, or the condition could be permanent if the parathyroid glands are removed along with the thyroid tissue. Thyroid storm could develop after surgery. Preparation for surgery involves the use of medical management to control the hyperthyroid state. Some use supersaturated iodine solution (Lugol's, 8 drops/day) for the 10 days before surgery; the iodine will reduce the blood supply to the gland. Iodine has only a temporary effect in suppressing thyroxine secretion from the hyperthyroid gland; escape usually will occur after 2 to 4 weeks (the Wolf-Chaikoff effect). Although the surgeon may be able to remove the optimal amount of tissue to allow euthyroid function after surgery, hypothyroidism may develop in the years after surgery because of continued scarring and reduced function of the remaining thyroid tissue, according to some reports. Thyroid storm may develop during surgical therapy, especially in patients not yet under control, so propranolol therapy may be needed.

3. Nuclear medicine therapy. Radioactive iodine (^{131}I; RAI) therapy has been used in hyperthyroidism for more than 50 years and has proved safe in studies of adolescents who received this therapy. No cancers have been detected, although some adenomas were reported after therapy. No effects on offspring of adults treated with RAI were noted. Although no documentation of statistically increased risk is found, some still consider it ill advised to administer RAI to younger children for a potentially reversible condition. However, the Lawson Wilkins Pediatric Endocrine Society suggested that ^{131}I therapy may be beneficially used in younger patients; it is more commonly used now in adolescents. As one dose of RAI may

not cure the patient, another dose may be necessary. After the treatment, some patients may be euthyroid if just the correct amount of thyroid gland destruction occurs, but reports demonstrate the ultimate development of hypothyroidism because of continued scarring of the gland. Thyroid storm could occur during RAI treatment, especially in patients not yet under control, so propranolol therapy may be needed here as well.

Neonates can have bona fide Graves disease, but most newborns with hyperthyroidism have acquired it from transplacentally acquired TSI made by the mother. A minority of offspring of a mother with Graves disease will have signs of hyperthyroidism. As the mother has usually been diagnosed with hyperthyroidism and is receiving therapy with PTU, the child will necessarily receive a significant dose of PTU, which freely crosses the placenta. If the dose is excessive, the child may be born profoundly hypothyroid, with goiter, and can even have severe respiratory insufficiency because of pressure on the trachea exerted by the large goiter. The hypothyroid phase in the neonate will often trigger the statewide screening program to report the child as a presumptive positive hypothyroid child with a high TSH. After 3 to 6 days, as the PTU leaves the circulation, the child will bear the brunt of the TSI effect and, if this child is one of the few destined to respond unfavorably to the TSI, nervousness, diarrhea, shakiness, and tachycardia will be seen as indications of excessive thyroid function. Congestive heart failure due to supraventricular tachycardia and hepatosplenomegaly may occur. Digitalis or sedatives might be indicated. Owing to extreme manifestations in some, mortality is possible. The infant can receive Lugol's solution of iodine to suppress thyroid hormone output, propranolol to counter the effects of hyperthyroidism, or PTU if the condition seems severe and is predicted to last for several months. Ultimately the immunoglobulin leaves the circulation, and a euthyroid state develops, usually before 12 weeks and sometimes as soon as 3 weeks.

Thyroid storm is a rare complication in children and adolescents. Thyroid storm consists of acute onset of hyperthermia and tachycardia in a patient with underlying hyperthyroidism. Precipitating factors include surgery, infection, and diabetic ketoacidosis. It may occur during surgical or radioiodine therapy for hyperthyroidism. Symptoms include high fever, sweating, tachycardia, and reduced mental state ranging from confusion to coma. Immediate therapy is indicated for this severe condition.

Propranolol (2 to 3 mg/kg/day, divided into a dose every 6 hours as a starting dose) can control some symptoms of thyroid storm. Propranolol may be given intravenously at a dose of 0.1 mg/kg up to a total of 5 mg, but an intraatrial pacing catheter is a necessary precaution. Dexamethasone in a dose of 1 to 2 mg every 6 hours can reduce serum T_3. Intravenous NaI in a dose of 1 to 2 g/day may decrease the release of thyroid hormone from the thyroid gland; Lugol's solution of concentrated iodine can be given orally if the patient is conscious. A cooling blanket can help control the hyperpyrexia. PTU will not take effect for several days, but to plan for the possibly extended course of the disorder, 200 to 300 mg can be given every 6 hours by slurry, if necessary in larger children. Fluid management must be observed, and if tachycardia causes heart failure, digitalis may be necessary.

Hyperthyroidism rarely is because of a thyroid adenoma or carcinoma, subacute thyroiditis, or suppurative thyroiditis. These possibilities are covered elsewhere in this chapter.

Two rare instances occur when hyperthyroidism might be found with elevated serum TSH values. Selective pituitary resistance to thyroxine (#145650 HYPERTHYROIDISM, FAMILIAL, DUE TO INAPPROPRIATE THYROTROPIN SECRETION, autosomal dominant) leads to lack of feedback inhibition to T_3 feedback, so TSH increases, and hyperthyroidism results, as the rest of the body can respond to the increased secretion of thyroid hormone even if the pituitary gland cannot. Further, a TSH-secreting tumor might cause hyperthyroidism with elevated serum TSH and FT_4.

Hyperthyroidism may be caused by mutations of the TSH receptor, so that constitutive activation leads to uncontrolled thyroid hormone secretion. The McCune-Albright syndrome may demonstrate autonomous thyroid function because of mutations of the G protein (see Chapter 9).

Neoplasms

A single firm nodule of the thyroid gland is a more ominous finding in a child than is multiple nodular goiter. The majority of solitary lesions will be benign, but carcinoma can not be overlooked. Lack of concentration of ^{123}I on thyroid scan (a cold nodule) increases the likelihood of carcinoma more than does a functioning nodule (warm or hot nodule). Ultrasonographic evidence that the nodule is a cyst makes it less likely to be malignant, but carcinomas may be found in the walls of thyroid cysts, and the solid portion of a cyst is a target for fine-needle aspiration. The presence of enlarged anterior cervical lymph nodes, metastases on chest radiograph, or hoarseness all make the likelihood greater that the single thyroid nodule is malignant.

Carcinomas of the thyroid gland are rare in childhood (these constitute less than 1% of childhood cancers and less than 10% of all thyroid cancers), but certain historic features increase the likelihood of a thyroid mass being malignant. A history of irradiation of the thyroid gland (e.g., inadvertently while treating acne, enlarged thymus, or ringworm, as was done in the past, or due to a nuclear accident, as in Chernobyl) is significant, and if the irradiation was done for the therapy of another cancer (e.g., at the time of bone marrow transplant), the risk is higher. The risk of cancer is greatest if radiation occurs during childhood, but thyroid tumors appear even decades after irradiation. However, the local radiation used for the treatment of Graves disease appears not to be a etiology for thyroid carcinoma, as it kills the thyroid follicular cells while it controls the Graves disease. A patient with a family or personal history of one of the multiple endocrine neoplasia syndromes, type 2 or 2B, has a great likelihood of having medullary carcinoma of the thyroid gland (see Chapter 14).

Many areas and cell types of the thyroid gland may undergo neoplastic degeneration.

1. Medullary carcinoma of the thyroid (MCT) arises from parafollicular cells and is most often found in the MEN 2 syndrome (#171400 MULTIPLE ENDOCRINE NEOPLASIA, TYPE II; MEN 2 at 10q11.2 or #162300 MULTIPLE ENDOCRINE NEOPLASIA, TYPE IIB; MEN 2B at 10q11.2). These are autosomal dominant conditions. Isolated MCT can occur in an autosomal dominant condition. (#155240 MEDULLARY THYROID CARCINOMA, FAMILIAL; MTC at 1q21-q22, 10q11.2). Germ cell–line mutations in the *ret* oncogene are demonstrated in patients with MCT with or without MEN 2.

2. Papillary carcinoma may demonstrate enlarged lymph nodes as well as a thyroid nodule. This may be associated with Gardner syndrome (*175100 ADENOMATOUS POLYPOSIS OF THE COLON; APC at any of 5q21-q22, 1p34.3-1p32.1), which is transmitted in an autosomal dominant pattern and includes disorders of multiple systems including colonic polyps and other neoplasias; follow-up is necessary in case thyroid carcinoma develops in a patient diagnosed with Gardner syndrome. Abnormalities in the *ret* or *trk* oncogenes may be found. Autosomal dominant forms of papillary carcinoma exist (#188550 THYROID CARCINOMA, PAPILLARY associated with any of 17q23-q24, 14q, 10q21, 10q11.2, 8p22-p21.3, 1p13, 7q32-q34 loci).

3. Follicular thyroid carcinoma is usually found in a sporadic pattern but may be an autosomal dominant condition (188470 THYROID CARCINOMA, FOLLICULAR; FTC at 10q23.31). This neoplasm is found less frequently than the other two types listed.

The steps involved in the diagnosis of a solitary nodule are determination of structure by ultrasound scan, determination of function by radioiodine scan, and either needle biopsy or open surgical biopsy and excision. Needle biopsy is safe and has a low level of false-negative results, but the experience of the local pathologists in performing and reading needle biopsy specimens is important in making the choice. Even if a needle biopsy suggests a benign diagnosis, if the nodule fails to shrink on suppressive thyroxine therapy over the ensuing months, it may require open excisional biopsy as well. In the absence of experienced clinical help in the procedure of needle biopsy or in a situation heavily suggestive of a malignant diagnosis, open excisional biopsy seems best.

Measurement of calcitonin in the basal or calcium or pentagas-trin-stimulated (it is difficult to get pentagastrin at the time of this writing) state is indicated if there is suspicion of MCT, or the finding of a first-degree relative with a *ret* mutation. Evaluation for pheochromocytoma in affected individuals is important (see Chapter 14).

Total or near total thyroidectomy is performed if papillary or follicular carcinoma is found to minimize remaining neoplastic tissue. If radioactive uptake suggests that functional tissue sur-vives or metastases are present, radioactive ablation (^{131}I) of remaining tissue or metastases then follows until no suggestive tissue is left. Suppression of remaining tissue by replacement therapy with thyroxine administration is carried out thereafter. Serum thyroglobulin determination will indicate if there is any remaining thyroid tissue (normal or neoplastic) but must be mea-sured during times that T_4 is not being given. T_3 replacement may be used during periods that RAI scans or treatment is expected postoperatively because the short half-life of T_3 will allow the relief of symptoms of hypothyroidism without suppressing the thyroid tissue avidity for iodine uptake for a prolonged period and affecting the test.

Painful Thyroid Glands

Tenderness of the thyroid gland may indicate a viral infection (subacute thyroiditis) or a bacterial infection (suppurative thy-roiditis). Either of these conditions will be accompanied by an ele-vated sedimentation rate. Subacute thyroiditis may follow a viral illness. The course usually includes a phase of hyperthyroidism due to release of preformed thyroid hormone; during this phase the RAI uptake is decreased, so this is because of damage to the thyroid gland, which causes the release of preformed hormone. The course of the viral illness may last 6 to 9 months and sponta-neously improves. Suppurative thyroiditis might be accompanied by fever, sore throat, hoarseness, or dysphagia, most of which are absent in subacute disease. It is important to search for a pyriform sinus fistula by barium swallow, which may figure in the etiology of suppurative thyroiditis. The viral condition is accompanied by a lymphocytosis on CBC, and the bacterial form, by an elevated WBC count, with a "shift to the left." Bacterial infections are treated with appropriate antibiotics, and viral infections, with antiinflammatory medications until inflammation resolves.

SUGGESTED READINGS

Burman KD, Baker JR. Immunomechanisms in Graves disease. *Endocrinol Rev* 1985;6:183.

Dussault JH. Relation of basic and clinical research on fetal and neonatal thyroid pathology to neonatal thyroid screening. *Acta Paediatr* Suppl 1999;88:15–17.

Fisher DA. Congenital hypothyroidism. In: Rudolph CD, Rudolph AM, eds. *Rudolph's pediatrics*. New York: McGraw-Hill, 2002:882–885.

Fisher DA. The thyroid. In: Rudolph CD, Rudolph AM, eds. *Rudolph's pediatrics*. New York: McGraw-Hill, 2002:2059–2079.

Fisher DA. Disorders of the thyroid in the newborn and infant. In: Sperling MA, ed. *Pediatric endocrinology*. Philadelphia: Saunders, 2002:161–186.

Fisher DA. Thyroid disorders in childhood and adolescence. In: Sperling MA, ed. *Pediatric endocrinology*. Philadelphia: Saunders, 2002:187–210.

Fisher DA. Hypothyroxinemia in premature infants: is thyroxine treatment necessary? *Thyroid* 1999;9:715–720.

Fisher DA, Klein AH. Thyroid development and disorders of thyroid function in the newborn. *N Engl J Med* 1981;304:702.

Glaser N. Hyperthyroidism. In: Finberg L, Kleinman RE, eds. *Saunders manual of pediatric practice*. Philadelphia: Saunders, 2002:888–890.

LaFranchi S. Acquired hypothyroidism. In: Finberg L, Kleinman RE, eds. *Saunders manual of pediatric practice*. Philadelphia: Saunders, 2002:886–888.

LaFranchi S. Goiter. In: Finberg L, Kleinman RE, eds. *Saunders manual of pediatric practice*. Philadelphia: Saunders, 2002:836–837.

Zimmerman D. Thyroid cancer. In: Finberg L, Kleinman RE, eds. *Saunders manual of pediatric practice*. Philadelphia: Saunders, 2002:890–894.

7 ♣ Disorders of Calcium Metabolism

Calcium is necessary for skeletal integrity but also plays a role in the function of all of the cells of the body. Increases or decreases in serum and intracellular calcium concentrations may be caused by a wide range of etiologies and can lead to profound changes in organ function.

CALCIUM METABOLISM

The majority of the body's store of calcium resides in the skeleton, with about 1% in the recently deposited bone, a pool that can mobilize more easily, and only 1% in the serum. Calcium circulates in the ionized form, as ionized calcium, the form that causes physiologic changes; ionized calcium comprises about 50% of the total serum calcium. Of the remainder, 40% circulates bound to protein, albumin, and globulin, and thus total calcium must be interpreted in light of the amount of circulating protein, because in states of low protein, total calcium decreases while ionized calcium may be normal. Although the gastrointestinal (GI) tract can increase the efficiency of calcium absorption in states of diminished calcium intake, if oral intake is less than 200 mg/day, more excretion from stool than absorption occurs, leading to a net loss of calcium. An attempt is made by the GI tract to limit active calcium absorption if GI intake increases excessively, but passive absorption cannot be limited; thus excessive calcium intake can cause hypercalcemia (e.g., the milk alkali syndrome).

Serum calcium is regulated within close limits by several hormones that balance GI intake with urinary or fecal loss; the skeleton serves as a reservoir of calcium, so that calcium may be mobilized when needed or stored if necessary. In disorders of calcium metabolism, excessive calcium may be removed from the bone, or alternatively, deficiency in various factors may impair bone formation, leading to one of several bone diseases.

The factors that control calcium include (Fig. 7-1):

1. Vitamin D, which can be ingested from various vitamin D_2-supplemented dairy products (D_2 is known as ergocalciferol in this form) or other foods that may already contain vitamin D. However, endogenous vitamin D_3 (or cholecalciferol) can be considered a steroid hormone, which is produced from 7-dehydrocholesterol, a cholesterol metabolite, by the effect of sunlight on the skin. 25(OH)vitamin D is synthesized by 25-hydroxylation of either form of vitamin D in the liver. 25(OH)vitamin D values reflect the body's stores of vitamin D. 25(OH)vitamin D then undergoes 1-α-hydroxylation in the kidney to form 1,25-dihydroxy vitamin D (or calcitriol), the active factor in this sequence. 1-α-Hydroxylase is increased if serum Ca and phosphate are low and is also increased by parathyroid hormone (PTH), PTH-releasing protein (PTHrP), calcitonin, growth hormone (GH), prolactin and insulin-like growth factor (IGF)-1. Increased serum Ca and phosphorous and 1,25-dihydroxy vitamin D all decrease the activity of

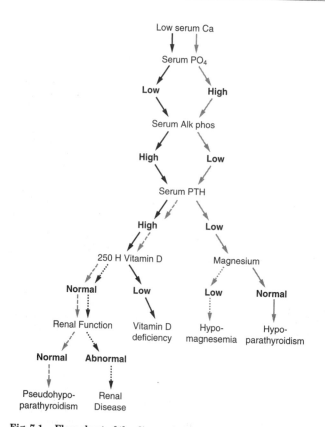

Fig. 7-1. Flow chart of the diagnosis of the etiology of hypocalcemia.

1 hydroxylase in a negative-feedback loop. Calcitriol decreases PTH synthesis and secretion by negative feedback.

1,25-Dihydroxy vitamin D increases absorption of calcium and phosphorous from the small intestine and assists PTH in the resorption of bone to increase serum calcium and phosphorus. This is accomplished by 1,25-dihydroxy vitamin D stimulating the production of osteoblasts, but it also assists in the mineralization of the skeleton by maintaining serum Ca and PO_4 within appropriate ranges. In addition, 1,25-dihydroxy vitamin D increases retention of calcium from the renal tubule to decrease the loss of calcium in the urine, while it decreases phosphorus retention from the nephron. Vitamin D circulates bound to a vitamin D–binding protein of 52 kDa.

2. PTH is produced in the four parathyroid glands formed by the third and fourth pharyngeal arches; a fifth parathyroid gland may be located within the thyroid gland in some individuals. PTH mobi-

lizes calcium from the skeleton by transforming osteoblasts into osteoclasts. PTH increases renal 1α-hydroxylation of 25-hydroxy vitamin D, which in turn increases intestinal calcium absorption. PTH increases calcium reabsorption in the distal nephron as well, whereas it decreases the reabsorption of phosphorus. PTH is secreted in response to a decrease in serum ionized Ca through the action of the calcium-sensing receptor (CaSR) of the parathyroid chief cell. PTH also is secreted in response to elevated phosphorus concentrations.

PTHrP shares some characteristics of the PTH molecule. PTHrP is formed locally in many tissues and acts in a paracrine manner on nearby tissue, in contrast to the endocrine action of PTH at a distance from the parathyroid gland. PTHrP may be produced in excess by neoplasms.

3. Calcitonin is secreted from the parafollicular cells of the medulla of the thyroid gland and decreases serum calcium by inhibiting the action of osteoclasts on bone and by restoring calcium into bone.

4. Magnesium is necessary for the secretion of PTH and, in turn, PTH increases magnesium resorption by the nephron. In states of magnesium deficiency, hypocalcemia may develop.

A complex feedback loop is found in this system, as an increase in serum calcium decreases PTH secretion, which in turn decreases the 1α-hydroxylation of 25(OH)vitamin D, limiting the production of 1,25(OH)vitamin D, and both limit further increase in calcium. Further, a decrease in serum calcium triggers a release of PTH, which increases 1,25(OH)vitamin D production and both of these factors increase serum calcium values.

HYPOCALCEMIA

A decrease in serum ionized Ca^{2+} leads to neuromuscular irritability, causing tetany (heralded by carpopedal spasm, causing the fingers to extend with ulnar deviation), muscle cramps, weakness, lethargy, paresthesias of the extremities, and in the most severe situation, convulsions and/or laryngospasm (stridor or complete closure of the larynx with the risk of death) (Table 7.1). Lengthening of the QTc interval may be seen on the electrocardiogram (ECG). Although presentation may appear similar to that of a grand mal seizure, in view of the tonic/clonic activity, no postictal phase occurs in hypocalcemia.

Hyperventilation causing respiratory alkalosis will reduce the ionized fraction of calcium by enhanced protein binding of ionized Ca, and this may precipitate tetany (this situation may occur in states of anxiety and is treated by rebreathing CO_2 (classically from a paper bag) to decrease serum pH, thereby freeing some calcium from the protein into the ionized state in the serum). Signs of long-term hypocalcemia include calcification of the basal ganglia, cataract formation, and poor tooth enamel formation. Hypomagnesemia will decrease PTH secretion and can precipitate a temporary phase of hypoparathyroidism, which is treated by remedying the deficit in magnesium rather than by administration of vitamin D or calcium.

Hypocalcemia may be demonstrated on physical examination by demonstration of

1. The Chvostek sign, in which tapping the facial nerve below the zygomatic arch causes a twitch at the angle of the mouth due to contraction of the perioral muscles, a demonstration of muscular irritability.
2. The Trousseau sign, in which a blood pressure cuff is inflated at least 15 mm Hg above the systolic blood pressure for 2 to 5 minutes; a positive response is indicated by carpopedal spasms in the arm to which the cuff was applied.
3. The peroneal sign, in which a tap on the peroneal nerve near the lateral tibial prominence causes plantar flexion (although tapping any nerve may lead to contraction of the associated muscle, other contractions may be more difficult to demonstrate).

Hypocalcemia in the Infant

Transient episodes of low serum calcium may occur during the first 3 days after birth in patients who are premature, have intrauterine growth retardation (IUGR), have sepsis, have asphyxiation, and in infants of diabetic mothers (the worse the control of blood sugar, the lower the Ca in the baby). Vitamin D deficiency may occur in an infant because of coexistent vitamin D deficiency in the mother. Breast milk is not a plentiful source of vitamin D, especially if the mother has a vitamin D–deficient diet, and thus supplementation of the neonate is customary. If hypocalcemia occurs after 5 days, it may be owing to hypoparathyroidism. Normal term infants have serum Ca greater than 8.5 mg/dL and ionized Ca more than 4.5 mg/dL. The normal values are controversial in premature infants, but as a guide, serum Ca may normally decrease to values as low as 6.5 mg/dL, and ionized Ca, to 3 mg/dL at some point. If a chest radiograph shows no thymic shadow or a cardiac defect of the great vessels is found, the diagnosis of DiGeorge syndrome is more likely than transient hypocalcemia (see later).

For the first few days after birth, the infant will have difficulty regulating serum calcium. During this period just after the infant separates from the maternal calcium supply and the maternal regulation of serum calcium, PTH secretion is often sluggish, so that transient and mild hypocalcemia and hyperphosphatemia may result; this is considered to be "physiologic hypocalcemia of infancy." Further, an infant has a low glomerular filtration rate that decreases phosphorus excretion and causes increased serum phosphorus, which further reduces serum calcium. Cow's milk contains more phosphorus than does human milk, even though the calcium content is higher: the load of oral phosphorus may enhance the physiologic hypocalcemia of infancy to symptomatic levels in infants fed with cow's milk formula. This is less common in breast-fed infants.

Therapy for symptomatic physiologic hypocalcemia of infancy consists of short-term intravenous (i.v.) calcium gluconate at 200 mg/kg/dose and long-term oral calcium lactate in the feedings

Table 7-1. Causes of hypocalcemia

Disorder	Serum Ca	Serum Ca^{2+}	Serum PO$_4$	Serum PTH	Alkaline phosphatase	pH	Other features
Vitamin D deficiency	Low or Nl	Low or Nl	Low	High	High	Nl	Serum vitamin D low, 1,25(OH$_2$) vitamin D may be normal
Hyperventilation	Nl	Low	Nl	Nl	Nl	High	Cured by rebreathing
Transient hypocalcemia of infancy	Low	Low	Nl	Low relative to Ca	Nl	Nl	Made worse with high-phosphorus feedings
Congenital hypoparathyroidism	Low	Low	High	Low relative to Ca	Low	Nl	May be part of DiGeorge syndrome
Autoimmune hypoparathyroidism	Low	Low	High	Low relative to Ca	Low	Nl	May be part of autoimmune polyendocrinopathy syndrome, type 1

Pseudohypo-parathyroidism	Low	High	High relative to Ca	Low	Nl	May be associated with Albright hereditary osteodystrophy
Magnesium deficiency	Low	High	Low relative to Ca	Low	Nl	May be part of Barter syndrome, mal-absorption, or renal disease
Calcium deficiency	Low	Could be low or normal	Elevated	Elevated	Nl	Rare in present day except for fad diets, vitamin deficiency with, possibly, sun avoidance
Renal disease	Low	High	High	High	Possibly acidotic	Tests of renal function are abnormal

PTH, parathyroid hormone; Nl, normal. (From: Fisher DA, ed. The Quest Diagnostics Manual: Pediatric endocrinology. San Juan Capistrano: Quest Diagnostics Incorporated 2000.)

to achieve a 4:1 calcium-to-phosphate ratio. ECG monitoring for arrhythmias or bradycardia is mandatory at any time i.v. calcium is administered.

PATHOLOGICAL HYPOPARATHYROIDISM

Nonautoimmune hypoparathyroidism may occur sporadically or in autosomal dominant (#146200 HYPOPARATHYROIDISM, FAMILIAL ISOLATED; FIH at 3q13), autosomal recessive (*241400 HYPOPARATHYROIDISM with sensineural deafness), or X-linked patterns (*307700 HYPOPARATHYROIDISM, X-LINKED; HYPX at Xq26–27). The Sanjad-Sakati (*241410 HYPOPARATHYROIDISM-RETARDATION-DYSMORPHISM SYNDROME; HRD at 1q42043) syndrome of fetal and postnatal growth retardation, seizures, developmental delay, and dysmorphic facial features is associated with autosomal recessive hypoparathyroidism. The Kenny-Caffey syndrome (*244460 KENNY-CAFFEY SYNDROME, TYPE 1; KCS at 1q42–43) may be inherited in an autosomal dominant, autosomal recessive, or even X-linked pattern and includes poor growth, stenosis of the bone marrow cavity, and thickened tubular cortical bones.

Hypoparathyroidism may occur from iron deposition of thalassemia (and its therapy) or hemochromatosis. Iron infiltration from Wilson disease will affect the parathyroid glands as well. Radiation to the area, trauma, or surgery also may cause acquired hypoparathyroidism.

Autoimmune hypoparathyroidism may occur as an isolated case or in association with type 1 polyendocrinopathy syndrome, which also includes chronic mucocutaneous candidiasis and ectodermal dysplasia (APECED *240300 AUTOIMMUNE POLYENDOCRINOPATHY SYNDROME, TYPE I). Other associated defects include Addison disease, autoimmune hypergonadotropic hypogonadism, diabetes mellitus type 1, autoimmune disease of the thyroid gland, pernicious anemia, vitiligo, alopecia, dental enamel hypoplasia, keratoconjunctivitis, malabsorption, chronic active hepatitis, and variable T-cell defects. A defect in the AIRE gene is seen at 21q22.3 in APECED.

The DiGeorge syndrome (*188400 DIGEORGE SYNDROME; DGS) results from disordered development of the third and fourth branchial pouches and first to fifth branchial arches derived from neural crest cells. This is usually found associated with microdeletions of chromosome 22q11.2. Physical findings include hypertelorism, short philtrum, micrognathia, malar hypoplasia, low-set ears, and sometimes cleft palate. Abnormalities of the aortic arch (such as truncus arteriosus or tetralogy of Fallot) and the thymus (immune defects related to T-cell defects and disordered cellular immunity) also are associated. Velocardiofacial syndrome (#192430 VELOCARDIOFACIAL SYNDROME at 22q11.2) has the same gene locus as DiGeorge syndrome and has, as well, high-arched or submucous cleft palate, retrognathia, short palpebral fissures, and VSD. The CATCH-22 syndrome is a general term encompassing many phenotypes caused by mutations at this locus; this syndrome may be composed as a cardiac defect, abnormal facies, thymic hypoplasia, cleft palate, and hypocalcemia. Thus any infant with tetany and hyperphosphatemia should have evaluation for cardiac and immune disease at the least.

Surgical hypoparathyroidism may occur after thyroid surgery. It may be transient because of inflammation of the area, or it may be permanent because of the removal of parathyroid tissue along with the thyroid tissue.

The diagnosis of hypoparathyroidism rests on demonstration of decreased serum ionized calcium and increased phosphorus, in the face of decreased serum PTH for the value of serum calcium. Low serum ionized calcium should, in the normal situation, cause elevation of serum PTH, and absence of such a response suggests inadequacy of PTH secretory ability; complete absence of serum PTH is not necessary for the diagnosis of hypoparathyroidism. Urinary calcium excretion is elevated (calcium/creatinine ratio greater than 0.2), phosphate excretion is diminished (tubular reabsorption of phosphate is greater than 88%), and cyclic adenosine monophosphate (cAMP) is low in the urine of hypoparathyroidism, as PTH normally stimulates the production of cAMP in the renal tubule.

Treatment of hypoparathyroidism must first address hypocalcemia. For severe symptomatic hypocalcemia, 10% calcium gluconate is given as a dose of 0.5 mL/kg up to a total of 10 mL, given with ECG monitoring (bradycardia and asystole are possible complications of an increase of calcium). During the administration of i.v. calcium, it is important to avoid extravasation, which may cause severe sloughing of the skin, possibly requiring plastic surgery. The infusion may be repeated if necessary for the relief of symptoms but is followed by 10% i.v. calcium gluconate at a dose of 500 mg/kg over a 24-hour period for neonates and 200 mg/kg for infants or older subjects. Long-term therapy is achieved by 1,25(OH)vitamin D (this form eliminates the need for 1 hydroxylation of vitamin D, which is impaired in hypoparathyroidism) given at a dose of 20 to 40 ng/kg/day (calculated as 0.25 to 0.75 g twice daily), with oral calcium supplementation adequate to maintain serum ionized calcium, if necessary. Urine can be tested for excessive calcium loss by determining urinary calcium/creatinine ratio (this normally should be less than 0.2) to evaluate the effects of therapy. Renal ultrasound examinations are administered at yearly intervals to search for nephrocalcinosis, which is a complication of vitamin D therapy. Phosphorus is restricted in the diet until serum phosphorus decreases to near-normal levels, which should occur when serum ionized calcium approaches normal. Serum ionized calcium should be measured regularly until stability is achieved to assure that serum calcium remains in the normal range. (For a discussion of emergency treatment of hypocalcemia, see Chapter 15.)

PSEUDOHYPOPARATHYROIDISM

Individuals with resistance to PTH, pseudohypoparathyroidism or PHO, have all the features of hypoparathyroidism except that PTH is elevated, although it is ineffective in controlling calcium values. In the classic form of PHO, an abnormality in the GNAS1 gene on 20q13,11 causes a G protein abnormality that makes the PTH receptor unresponsive. The phenotype known as Albright hereditary osteodystrophy, which consists of short stature, obesity, round facies, brachydactyly, and metacarpal or metatarsal hypoplasia resulting in shortened forth and fifth fingers and toes, often is found in pseudohypoparathyroidism type 1A (#103580 ALBRIGHT HEREDITARY OSTEODYSTROPHY; AHO at 20q13.2), although AHO also may be inherited in an X-linked pattern in an isolated form not associated with pseudohypoparathyroidism. It appears that if the mutated gene is derived from the father, only AHO results, a condition known as pseudopseudohypoparathyroidism, whereas if the gene is inherited from the mother, the child has type 1A PHO. Urinary cAMP excretion does not increase after PTH infusion if the defect is generalized (type 1A), and resistance to thyroid-stimulating hormone (TSH), antidiuretic hormone (ADH), and growth hormone–releasing hormone (GHRH) may occur in conjunction with PHO Basal ganglia calcifications are common on radiograph, and subcutaneous calcifications occur as well. Other subjects may have renal nonresponsiveness to PTH, but responsiveness of the skeleton to PTH, leading to the hyperparathyroid bone disease, osteitis fibrosa cystica. These subjects have type 1B pseudohypoparathyroidism (#603233 PSEUDOHYPOPARATHYROIDISM, TYPE IB at 20q13.3), in which the metabolic findings of hypoparathyroidism occur, but the general phenotype is normal, and no mutation is found in the GNAS1 gene. In pseudohypoparathyroidism type II, an autosomal recessive condition (203330 ALBRIGHT HEREDITARY OSTEODYSTROPHY; AHO), elevation of urinary cAMP is found, which, however, will not increase further with exogenous PTH administration: renal phosphate and serum calcium are unresponsive to PTH administration, and hypocalcemia occurs.

The therapy for pseudohypoparathyroidism is the same as that for hypoparathyroidism described earlier.

Magnesium Deficiency

Magnesium deficiency may result from renal disease (either with or without other tubular defects) or intestinal malabsorption (which may occur in an autosomal recessive or X-linked patterns #248250 HYPOMAGNESEMIA, PRIMARY 3q27). Bartter syndrome (#241200 HYPOKALEMIC ALKALOSIS WITH HYPERCALCIURIA at 1p36) also is associated with hypomagnesuria. Cisplatin, aminoglycosides, and loop diuretics can diminish urinary magnesium reabsorption and result in hypomagnesemia. Magnesium deficiency diminishes PTH secretion as well as PTH-mediated bone resorption. Replacement oral magnesium oxide given several times daily will reverse hypoparathyroidism hypocalcemia and tetany, as hypomagnesemia resolves.

Diagnosis of Hypocalcemia

The diagnosis of the etiology of hypocalcemia is accomplished by the measurement of various minerals, hormones, and often vitamin D. As noted on the flow chart (Fig. 7-1), the level of phosphorus gives much information, as if it is high, a deficiency of PTH effect is likely, and if low, a PTH effect is likely. The diagnosis may be complex and not always easy, so refer to Figs. 7-1 and 7-2 as well as to the descriptions of the various conditions.

RENAL OSTEODYSTROPHY

In significant renal disease, impaired 1 hydroxylation of vitamin D will lead to the hypocalcemia that triggers PTH secretion. The PTH will increase remodeling of the bone, and increased alkaline phosphatase results. The serum phosphorus remains elevated because of decreased urinary excretion caused by the renal disease. Thus renal osteodystrophy results in osteitis fibrosis caused by secondary hyperparathyroidism, as well as renal rickets or osteomalacia due to bone undermineralization. Bowing of the lower extremities, bone pain, and myopathy may occur. Therapy involves 1,25-dihydroxy vitamin D, which increases serum ionized Ca^{2+}, which in turn decreases PTH secretion. Oral calcium carbonate is given with meals to block intestinal phosphate absorption, and a low-phosphate diet is recommended. Because renal disease may be silent in some cases, evaluation of renal function is important in the evaluation of hypocalcemia.

CALCIUM DEFICIENCY

Hypocalcemia due to calcium deficiency, with or without rickets, is uncommon now. However, if an infant is raised on an inappropriate fad diet or even with a nondairy creamer instead of milk-based formula, an abusive situation that may be considered a form of urban kwashiorkor, hypocalcemia may result. Because calcium deficiency is the etiology and not vitamin D deficiency, serum $1,25(OH)_2D$ and PTH values are high.

RICKETS

Inadequate vitamin D intake or absorption during childhood will cause inadequate absorption of calcium and phosphorus, leading to hypocalcemia and hypophosphatemia (Table 7-2). These factors cause increased PTH secretion, which causes bone turnover and elevated serum alkaline phosphatase activity. Chondrocytes in the growth plate of long bones and osteoid, the collagen-containing organic matrix of the bone trabeculum, fail to mineralize normally in this situation, which causes rickets. Both rickets and osteomalacia are characterized by decreased mineralization of osteoid; the former occurs during periods of growth, causing abnormal form of long bones, ribs, and skull, and the latter occurs after growth ceases and leads to a tendency toward fractures. Radiologic evaluation of the bones shows undermineralization of the growth plate, an indistinct and ragged metaphysis, and bowing due to the influence of weight bearing on bones lacking tensile strength.

Findings in rickets include genu valgum (knock knees) or genu varum (bow legs) developing after the age of walking and usually associated with pain in ambulation. Bowing of the arms, classic

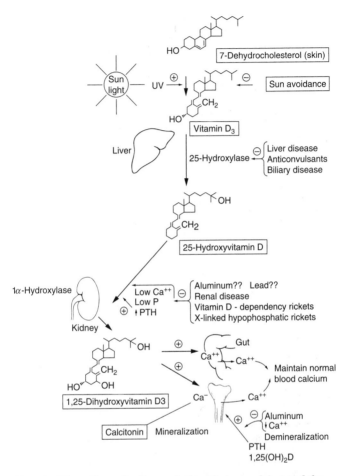

Fig. 7-2. The pathway for the regulation of serum calcium and the biosynthesis of 1,25(OH)$_2$ vitamin D. (From a figure by Chesney R, in Styne DM, ed. *Pediatric endocrinology: House officer series.* Philadelphia: Lippincott Williams & Wilkins, 1988, with permission.)

and often palpable widening of the metaphyses of the long bones, the "rachitic rosary," which is the prominence of the costochondral joints of the chest, Harrison groves or indentation of the lower chest wall, frontal bossing, and more rarely craniotabes are found. Appetite is poor, walking is delayed, and growth is decreased in many affected children. Radiographic findings of thin bones with cupping, widening, and irregular metaphyses are diagnostic after the condition is established. In those patients with hypocalcemia, all the findings listed earlier for low calcium may be found.

Nutritional Rickets

Milk and other food products have been fortified with ergocalciferol in the United States, whereas other areas of the developed world may provide vitamin D to children as a capsule, so vitamin D–deficiency rickets is rare today. However, not all dairy products are supplemented with vitamin D, and some children are given milk substitutes that have no vitamin D; inspection of the package is necessary to determine the vitamin D content. Further, fad or inappropriate religion-mandated diets may be deficient in vitamin D supplement. Alternatively, as breast milk has far less than recommended vitamin D content, especially if the mother herself is deficient, an infant raised on breast milk without vitamin D supplementation also may be deficient. If a child is not exposed to the sun (e.g., because of institutionalization or complete swaddling covering the skin), the conversion of 7-dehydrocholesterol to vitamin D_3 will be limited, and vitamin D deficiency results. Children with dark skin color living at northern latitudes, wearing opaque clothes, and mostly remaining indoors are at particular risk for developing rickets if not supplemented with vitamin D. Fat malabsorption due to a variety of conditions may lead to vitamin D deficiency and rickets. Calcium deficiency or, more rarely, inadequate dietary phosphate also can lead to rickets. Diets laden with phytates, found in some cereals, also will lead to calcium deficiency because they bind calcium in the GI tract and limit absorption.

The diagnosis of nutritional rickets is made by decreased serum Ca, PO_4, and increased alkaline phosphatase determinations, as well as a serum 25(OH)D value less than 8 ng/mL (normal, 15 to 60 ng/mL), which indicates inadequate vitamin D stores. Treatment of these children with conventional vitamin D at 800 to 2,000 IU (20 to 50 μg) daily is usually curative, although additional calcium intake may be required, and vitamin D is sometimes recommended on dosage up to 5,000 IU daily.

Hepatocellular Rickets

Liver diseases such as biliary atresia, neonatal hepatitis, some hereditary liver diseases, and rarely, cystic fibrosis cause several difficulties with vitamin D metabolism: (a) fat malabsorption due to inadequate bile salt in the small intestine decreases absorption of the fat-soluble vitamin D; (b) hepatic 25-hydroxylation may be decreased; and (c) because vitamin D is excreted in bile, the enterohepatic circulation of vitamin D may be interrupted.

Table 7-2. Types of rickets

Defect	Serum Ca	Serum PO$_4$	Serum alk phos	Serum 25(OH)D	Serum 1,25(OH$_2$)D	Serum PTH	Other features
Vitamin D deficiency	Normal at first, then low	Normal at first, then low	High to extremely high	Low	Low to normal	Normal at first, then high	Rare in the developed world owing to vitamin D supplementation. Occurs in fat malabsorption, infants breast fed with deficient maternal vitamin D, prematurity, sunlight avoidance
Hepatocellular rickets	Low	Low	High	Low	Low to normal	High	
Anticonvulsant-associated rickets	Low	Low	High	Low	Low to normal	High	Due to increased metabolism of 25(OH)D (e.g., from phenobarbital and hydantoins in addition to lack of sunlight exposure, usually in a poorly ambulatory individual)

Vitamin D dependency rickets type 1	Low	Low or normal	High	Normal	Low	High	Requires high doses of vitamin D. AR inheritance due to a loss of function mutation of the 1α hydroxylase gene
Vitamin D resistant rickets or vitamin D dependency rickets type 2	Low	Low	High	Normal	High	High	Might have alopecia, growth failure, dental hypoplasia. AR inheritance due to loss of function mutation of the vitamin D receptor
X-linked hypophosphatemic rickets	Normal	Low	High	Normal	Low	Nl to high	X-linked inheritance due to mutation of PHEX gene

AR, autosomal recessive; PTH, parathyroid hormone; Nl, normal. (From: Fisher DA, ed. The Quest Diagnostics Manual: Pediatric endocrinology. San Juan Capistrano: Quest Diagnostics Incorporated 2000.)

Therapy with 1,000 to 2,000 IU (25 to 50 µg) of vitamin D daily may cure this form of rickets, but the use of oral 25(OH)D may be necessary to treat children with biliary atresia. Exposure to the sun may be beneficial in such patients as well.

Anticonvulsant-associated Hypocalcemia

Anticonvulsants such as phenobarbital and hydantoins speed the metabolism of 25(OH)D to more inactive metabolites. Because some children taking these substances may be institutionalized, a decreased intake of dairy products fortified with vitamin D also may occur, as well as reduced sunlight exposure. These combined effects may lead to rickets or hypocalcemia. This complication is unusual in ambulatory children receiving anticonvulsants.

Treatment with 800 IU (20 µg) of vitamin D will assure correction of hypocalcemia and hypophosphatemia in these children, especially if calcium intake is assured.

Rickets of Prematurity

Very low birth weight preterm infants have not received the normal third trimester placental transfer of calcium (150 mg/kg body weight/day) or phosphate (75 mg/kg/day), and after birth, their intestine may not be adequate to absorb calcium to replace the interrupted placental function. Further, diminished 25-hydroxylation occurs because of liver immaturity, even if the mother was supplemented with vitamin D and the infant is not deficient in vitamin D. Hypocalcemia, hypophosphatemia, elevated alkaline phosphatase activity, rib and limb fractures, and rachitic changes at the diaphyses and metaphyses of long bones will result. Serum concentrations of $1,25(OH)_2D$ are extremely high as a compensatory mechanism, exceeding 120 pg/mL (normal values are 50 to 80 pg/mL), but these elevated values cannot resolve the defect. If the infants also have bronchopulmonary dysplasia and are receiving long-term loop diuretic therapy, they will lose more calcium through hypercalcuria.

Treatment consists of the use of calcium and phosphate supplements in the infant's milk, the use of high-mineral formulas, and additional vitamin D administration.

Inherited Causes of Rickets

Vitamin D–dependency rickets type 1 (*264700 PSEUDOVITAMIN D DEFICIENCY RICKETS at 12q14), also called pseudovitamin D deficiency rickets or 1α-hydroxylation deficiency rickets leads to inability to produce $1,25(OH)_2D$ by 1 hydroxylation. This condition may appear at age 12 to 16 weeks and is inherited in an autosomal recessive pattern. Patients with this condition require very large doses of vitamin D (200,000 to 1,000,000 IU daily) or physiologic doses (0.5 to 1.0 µg) of $1,25(OH)_2D$ to cure the rickets. The levels of 25(OH)D are normal or high, and of $1,25(OH)_2D$ are low; the latter do not increase during treatment with vitamin D.

Vitamin D–resistant rickets (277420 VITAMIN D–DEPENDENT RICKETS, TYPE II) or vitamin D–dependency rickets, type II, is owing to inactivating mutation of the vitamin D receptor, leading to a defect in the binding of $1,25(OH)_2D$ to its nuclear receptor. Rickets, hypocalcemia, enamel hypoplasia, and signs of secondary hyperparathyroidism are seen in these children. Other kindreds have these findings, and in addition, some also have short stature and total alopecia (#277440 VITAMIN D-RESISTANT RICKETS WITH END-ORGAN UNRESPONSIVENESS TO 1,25-DIHYDROXYCHOLECALCIFEROL at 12q12-q14). This condition is inherited in an autosomal recessive pattern. These patients have an extremely elevated serum concentration of $1,25(OH)_2D$ (exceeding 150 pg/mL; normal, 15 to 60 pg/mL), but endogenous and normal doses of exogenous $1,25(OH)_2D$ are ineffective. Treatment often requires remarkably high doses of $1,25(OH)_2D$, in excess of 10 µg/day.

The most common form of inherited rickets in the developed world is X-linked hypophosphatemic rickets (*307800 HYPOPHOS-PHATEMIA, X-LINKED at Xp22.2-p22.1), an X-linked dominant condition found in hemizygous males and heterozygous females. Affected children have a reduction in the amount of phosphate reabsorbed in the nephron and lose most phosphate in their urine. A reduction in the serum value of $1,25(OH)_2D$ also occurs. Affected children have hypophosphatemia, causing insufficient mineralization of the bone, even though their serum calcium is normal. By the time the child begins to walk, bowing of the lower extremities is seen, but unlike those with other forms of rickets, affected children do not have tetany, myopathy, a rachitic rosary, or secondary hyperparathyroidism. These children have inadequate dental enamel and frequent tooth decay. The disorder is usually due to a mutation in the PHEX gene on Xp22.1.p. Treatment involves oral phosphate supplements in up to five divided doses to attempt to maintain serum phosphate values within normal limits most of the day, although oral phosphate can precipitate diarrhea. $1,25(OH)_2D$ is also administered in doses of 0.25 to 0.75 µg every 12 hours, as the patients have inadequate serum $1,25(OH)_2D$ for the degree of hypophosphatemia. Some clinical studies used GH treatment in affected subjects, but the effect on adult height is not yet apparent.

HYPERCALCEMIC DISORDERS

Hypercalcemia is generally considered when calcium levels are greater than 12 mg/dL, at which stage, symptoms are usually noted (Table 7-3). Lethargy, weakness, inability to concentrate, and depression may develop. Many patients have nausea, vomiting, anorexia, constipation, and weight loss; the neonate may manifest gastroesophageal reflux, lethargy, decreased weight gain, and lack of growth in length. Because a high extracellular calcium concentration impairs the capacity of the distal tubule of the nephron to respond to ADH, hypercalcemic patients have polyuria and an inability to concentrate the urine; dehydration and azotemia may result. Signs on physical examination may include band keratopathy of the medial and lateral margins of the cornea (nonpurulent

Table 7-3. Causes of hypercalcemia

Condition	Serum Ca	Serum PO₄	Alk phos	PTH	25(OH) vitamin D	1,25(OH) vitamin D	Other features
Primary hyperparathyroidism	High	Low	High	High for Ca	Normal	Nl or high	
Familial hypocalciuric hypercalcemia	High	Normal, high or low	Normal or high	Normal or high	Normal	Normal	Urine Ca is low. Usually benign but in homozygosity, profound hypercalcemia and diffuse hyperparathyroidism develops as above. AD inheritance
Hypercalcemia of malignancy	High	Nl or low	High	Low	Normal	Nl	Due to secretion of PTHrP, which creates a state of hyperparathyroidism
Hypervitaminosis D	High	Nl or low	Nl or low	Low	High	Nl or high	Due to overtreatment or fad megavitamin diets

Renal insufficiency and secondary hyperparathyroidism	Low	Nl or high	Nl or high	High	Normal	Decreased	Could lead to tertiary autonomous (or tertiary) hyperparathyroidism
Increased 1 α-hydroxylation of 25 OH vitamin D	High	Normal	Normal	Normal	Normal	High	Occurs in granulomatous disease and neoplasms (lymphomas)
Immobilization hypercalcemia	High	Normal to low	High	Nl	Nl	Nl	
Hyperthyroidism	High		Nl	Low	Nl	Nl or low	
Adrenal insufficiency	High		Nl	Low	Nl	Nl or low	
Thiazide diuretics	High		Nl	Low	Nl	Nl or low	Urine Ca is low
Hypervitaminosis A	High		Nl	Low	Nl	Nl or low	

Nl, normal; PTHrP, parathyroid hormone–related peptide. (From: Fisher DA, ed. The Quest Diagnostics Manual: Pediatric endocrinology. San Juan Capistrano: Quest Diagnostics Incorporated 2000.)

conjunctivitis), shortening of the QTc interval on ECG) recording, hypertension, hypercalcuria and nephrolithiasis, pancreatitis, and peptic ulcer disease. Hypercalcemia also may lead to hypertension. Elevated calcium may be asymptomatic if serum concentrations remain less than 11.5 to 12 mg/dL. If serum calcium increases to more than 16 mg/dL, stupor and coma may develop.

Many nutritional and maternal causes of hypercalcemia in the newborn are seen. Thus excessive administration of calcium or, conversely, inadequate administration of phosphorus, as well as excessive vitamin D administration, causes elevation of serum Ca. Subcutaneous fat necrosis due to birth trauma or birth asphyxia elevates serum Ca.

PRIMARY HYPERPARATHYROIDISM

Sporadic primary hyperparathyroidism is rare in children, but one form is a variant of familial hypocalciuric hypercalcemia (*600740 HYPOCALCIURIC HYPERCALCEMIA, FAMILIAL, TYPE III; HHC3 At 19q13) caused by homozygous or compound heterozygous mutations at the CaSR, as described later. Some kindreds have neonates with extremely high levels of calcium (exceeding 18.0 mg/dL) who are seen in extremis along with massive parathyroid hyperplasia and bone erosions. These children require emergency parathyroidectomy as a life-saving procedure. Some affected subjects have a high set point for calcium regulation and seem to require little therapy, as they have few side effects. They may be helped with a high-phosphate diet or oral phosphate supplements, but some need no therapy. They will not respond to a low-Ca diet, for they will mobilize bone calcium to make up for the deficit and incur more complications of the skeleton.

Primary hyperparathyroidism causes increased absorption of ingested calcium and increased release of calcium from mobilized bone as well as increased urinary excretion of phosphorus and calcium. Thus hypercalcemia and hypophosphatemia occur, and ultimately, nephrocalcinosis develops. Mild hypercalcemia leads to constipation and polyuria, whereas in those with more significant manifestations, dysrhythmia, hypotonia to the level of respiratory compromise, and even fractures of the ribs and other bones occur. Bone pain, subperiosteal bone resorption, mainly of the distal phalanges, osteitis fibrosa, peptic ulcer, and hypertension are very rarely found in affected children. Because PTH stimulates the synthesis of $1,25(OH)_2D$ by 1 hydroxylation, serum $1,25(OH)_2D$ is elevated. This diagnosis is made if serum ionized calcium is elevated with inappropriately increased serum PTH, as PTH should be suppressed to nondetectable levels in a normal patient with elevated serum calcium. Imaging of the parathyroid glands is done with ultrasound, computed tomography (CT), or sestamibi scans.

Some infants with mild disease have remission or a mild course, but the usual treatment for a parathyroid adenoma is surgical extirpation. If hyperplasia of multiple glands is found, all of the glands may be removed, with a fraction of one reimplanted in the forearm, where it can be surgically reduced in size if hypercalcemia continues or recurs.

Parathyroid adenomas occur the multiple endocrine neoplasia syndromes (MEN 1, MEN 2) (see Chapter 14).

Transient hyperparathyroidism in the neonate may occur if the mother is hypocalcemic. Maternal hypocalcemia causes increased fetal PTH secretion to maintain a normal fetal serum calcium, but PTH secretion continues into the newborn period and causes elevated serum Ca in the newborn for a few days to weeks.

Familial hypocalciuric hypercalcemia (FHH #145980 HYPOCAL-CIURIC HYPERCALCEMIA, FAMILIAL, TYPE I; HHC1 at 3q13.3-q21) is an autosomal dominant condition due to inactivating mutation of the CaSR. Hypercalcemia, hypermagnesemia, hypocalciuria, and hypophosphatemia are found. Usually no symptoms occur, but pancreatitis and cholelithiasis, among other findings, are found in some subjects. This is a disorder of an abnormal set point of the calcium sensor and, as such, elevated calcium is seen by the sensor as normal and is maintained by increased PTH secretion, so that an equilibrium is reached at a higher than normal range of serum calcium (11 to 12 mg/dL is common) and ionized calcium. If, however, homozygosity of the inactivating mutation of the CaSR is found, profound and potentially fatal hypercalcemia (14 to 20 mg/dL) occurs, requiring immediate therapy. Urine calcium is inappropriately low (less than 4 mg/kg/day), and the calcium/creatinine ratio is usually less than 0.10 in spite of the level of hypercalcemia. Nephrolithiasis, ulcer disease, and band keratopathy seen in other causes of hypercalcemia are rare in this condition, although pancreatitis may be seen in older children. Parathyroid hyperplasia as a common finding in all affected family members.

Miscellaneous Causes

Hypercalcemia of Malignancy

Hypercalcemia may be caused in patients with malignancy by elevation of PTHrP. This may be found in children with leukemia, lymphoma, rhabdomyosarcoma, Ewing sarcoma, and other neoplasms. The treatment of the underlying malignancy usually reverses hypercalcemia.

Other Endocrine Disorders Causing Hypercalcemia

Hyperthyroidism leads to active bone turnover and enhanced resorption, causing mild hypercalcemia. Adrenal insufficiency allows increased intestinal calcium absorption and may lead to hypercalcemia. Replacement with glucocorticoids will reverse hypercalcemia in adrenal insufficiency.

Drug-Induced Hypercalcemia

Thiazide diuretics are natriuretic but not calciuretic and cause diminished urinary calcium and so may cause mild hypercalcemia.

Hypervitaminosis D may occur if excess vitamins are given a child in a mistaken confidence in megavitamin therapy. Alternatively, the therapy for any hypocalcemic disorders with excess vitamin D may cause the same outcome. Fat-soluble vitamin D [ergocalciferol (vitamin D_2) or cholecalciferol (vitamin D_3)] are stored for a long time, perhaps 6 months, so an overdose is quite significant. However, $25(OH)D$, $1,25(OH)_2D$, or dihydrotachysterol (Hytakerol) are all short acting, so that excessive dosage can be quickly corrected. Glucocorticoids (prednisone at 1 to 2 mg/kg/day) may be used to reduce intestinal calcium absorption in the condition. Children in England at the end of World War II frequently manifested hypercalcemia, apparently because of excess vitamin D intake.

Hypervitaminosis A increases bone resorption and causes hypercalcemia and may occur with megavitamin therapy. Usually vitamin A excess is found with vitamin D excess if caused by fad diets.

Individuals with renal insufficiency may have hyperphosphatemia, hypocalcemia, decreased $1,25(OH)D$ production, and therefore increase PTH secretion, causing secondary hyperparathyroidism. This may become autonomous (tertiary hyperparathyroidism). Thus even when calcium increases, it does not suppress PTH secretion. Calcium carbonate, lactate, or bicarbonate intake given to block intestinal phosphate accumulation in chronic renal insufficiency may lead to a form of the milk alkali syndrome, which includes hypercalcemia, hypocalciuria, alkalosis, and all the clinical signs and symptoms of hypercalcemia.

Granulomatous Disease

Disorders that demonstrate increased 1α-hydroxylation of $25(OH)$vitamin D to form $1,25(OH)_2D$ include granulomatous disease (sarcoid, eosinophilic granuloma, or various infectious granulomatous disorders) and neoplasms (lymphomas). Affected patients can experience hyperabsorption of dietary calcium and subsequent hypercalcemia. Sarcoid patients also may become hypercalcemic with small doses of vitamin D. With increased sun exposure, hypercalcemia is worse in sarcoidosis as serum $25(OH)D$ increases. Glucocorticoid treatment may be used to reduce intestinal calcium absorption, reduce serum calcium values, and decrease $1,25(OH)_2D$ values.

A child (or more usually an adolescent) who is immobilized, usually from a fracture and traction, will have enhanced bone resorption and diminished bone formation, leading to immobilization hypercalcemia. Intramuscular calcitonin (50 to 200 units) will block bone resorption, although ambulation is the best treatment.

William syndrome (#194050 WILLIAMS-BEUREN SYNDROME; WBS at 7q11.2) is a sporadic disorder consisting of short stature and developmental delay, supravalvular aortic stenosis, pulmonary arterial stenosis, and a pathognomonic facial appearance; it is owing to a mutation in the gene for elastin. "Elfin facies," consisting of a small head, protuberant ears, a cupid's bow lip with short philtrum, peg-like teeth, blue iris with whitish flecking, and frequent caries is the classic presentation. Subjects are hyperactive, with what is described as a "cocktail party patter" personality. They appear brighter than their full IQ scores would suggest, as they have a great discrepancy between their verbal and mathematics performance on testing. They have increased musical abilities on many instruments. About 20% of these children have hypercalcemia, hypercalciuria, nephrocalcinosis, and even renal impairment; the cause is controversial. A low-calcium diet or the use of glucocorticoids to block intestinal calcium transport may be indicated in those affected with the hypercalcemic portion of the disorder. Hypercalcemic children should not have full doses of vitamin D–containing compounds (such as multivitamins). Idiopathic hypercalcemia of infancy (143880 HYPERCALCEMIA, IDIOPATHIC, OF INFANCY) is a rare and usually self-limited condition that may represent a component of Williams syndrome. Usually normal serum $1,25(OH)_2D$ and $25(OH)D$ values are found. A low-calcium diet, using a meat-based formula, or even glucocorticoids may be prescribed, but most children are asymptomatic.

Fat necrosis with local dystrophic calcification leads to hypercalcemia and occurs in sick term or preterm infants who have had trauma, cold exposure, or hypoxia. The hypercalcemia can persist for several days to weeks, but generally resolves sooner without sequelae.

The therapy for acute hypercalcemia is increased hydration with sodium chloride–containing fluid and the use of furosemide (1 to 2 mg/kg/dose), which will increase urinary calcium excretion. In addition, sodium sulfate and sodium phosphate are administered during therapy. Oral phosphate may be administered to bind calcium in the intestine, but may result in diarrhea. Oral glucocorticoids decrease calcium absorption from the intestines and may be used in severe cases. (For a discussion of the emergency treatment of hypercalcemia, see Chapter 15.)

Osteoporosis

Mild decrease in bone mineral content is osteopenia (–1.1 to 2.4 SD below the mean for age and sex), whereas osteoporosis (–2.5 SD or more) is the diagnosis if the bones are so weak as to fracture pathologically. A peak increment of bone mineral accrual occurs in infancy and in late adolescence. The adolescent accrual occurs after peak growth rate, and it may be this imbalance of bone size to mineral content that causes the increased prevalence of fractures, even in normal adolescents. Inadequate calcium intake is endemic in the United States and elsewhere, and this factor increases the prevalence of thin bones. Further, ingestion of carbonated beverages serves the dual purpose of limiting calcium-containing dairy-product ingestion and limiting calcium absorption because of the phosphate content of the beverages or the pH achieved. Inadequate GH or sex steroids, excess thyroxine, PTH, or glucocorticoid all cause thinner bones, and any of the myriad conditions mentioned in this text that lead to those hormonal abnormalities must be considered a risk factor for diminished bone density. Immobilization reduces the ability of bone to reach normal density, and even the limited activity of children in our modern society has an effect of decreasing bone strength. Much of the determination of bone density is genetic, and those with a susceptible genetic background may already have more fragile bones at the time of puberty. Idiopathic juvenile osteoporosis is rare and appears a few years before puberty without family history; the cause is uncertain, as is therapy, but some subjects appear to resolve with the progression of puberty. Extremity fracture due to osteoporosis will cause the expected local pain and swelling; vertebral fractures, in addition, will diminish height.

Newborns are susceptible to osteopenia based on gestational age and nutritional status. Three fourths of the bone calcium content is accrued in the last trimester, so premature infants are deprived of much of this mineral. Further, abnormal GI function and absorption due to many disorders will limit calcium, phosphorus, and vitamin D intake. A limitation exists to the amount of calcium and phosphorus that can be infused in total parenteral nutrition, leading to greater risk of thin bones in subjects receiving such support.

Bone mineral density may be determined by DXA (dual-energy x-ray absorptiometry), but age-appropriate standards must be used. Most software in use has only the young adult standards, starting at age 20 years. This is not appropriate for children who have not yet reached peak mineral density; thus, many adolescents and children have the diagnosis of osteopenia or osteoporosis because of incorrect interpretation of the DXA results. Standards for children and adolescents by sex and divided by white, Hispanic, and Asian ethnic groups are available (see Bachrach, 1999, as listed in Suggested Reading). Determination of volumetric bone density (three-dimensional) is superior to determination of areal bone density (only two-dimensional), as thicker bones have higher calcium content but may not be any denser than smaller bones; this technique is not yet universally available.

Evaluation of the etiology after the establishment of the diagnosis of osteoporosis includes measurement of serum calcium, phosphorus, alkaline phosphatase, PTH, 25(OH)vitamin D, $1,25(OH)_2$ vitamin D, creatinine, and urinary calcium and creatinine. In appropriate cases based on history, serum thyroxine and sex steroids are useful.

Treatment includes ensuring that normal vitamin D levels are present, that calcium intake is at least at the normal level, if not more than recommended at basal levels, and activity is fostered as tolerated. Drug therapy by bisphosphonates is not approved for children as for adults, but clinical trials are under way, and references are found in the literature of successful use of bisphosphonates for osteogenesis imperfecta and osteopenia in childhood. Precipitating factors such as glucocorticoid therapy must be minimized in an attempt to balance the beneficial effects of these medications on the disease under treatment with the adverse effects of the medication on bones.

SUGGESTED READINGS

Bachrach L. Osteoporosis. In: Finberg L, Kleinman RE, eds. *Saunders manual of pediatric practice.* Philadelphia: WB Saunders, 2002: 924–925.

Bachrach LK, Hastie T, Wang M, et al. Bone mineral acquisitions in healthy Asian, Hispanic, Black and Caucasian youth: a longitudinal study. *J Clin Endocrinol Metab* 1999;84:4702–4712.

Diamond RB Jr, Root AW. Disorders of calcium metabolism in the newborn and infant. In: Sperling MA, ed. *Pediatric endocrinology.* Philadelphia: WB Saunders, 2002:97–110.

Markowitz ME. Hyperparathyroidism. In: Finberg L, Kleinman RE, eds. *Saunders manual of pediatric practice.* Philadelphia: WB Saunders, 2002:923.

Markowitz ME. Hypoparathyroidism. In: Finberg L, Kleinman RE, eds. *Saunders manual of pediatric practice.* Philadelphia: WB Saunders, 2002:920–921.

Markowitz ME. Neonatal hypocalcemia. In: Finberg L, Kleinman RE, eds. *Saunders manual of pediatric practice.* Philadelphia: WB Saunders, 2002:919.

Markowitz ME. Pseudohypoparathyroidism. In: Finberg L, Kleinman RE, eds. *Saunders manual of pediatric practice.* Philadelphia: WB Saunders, 2002:922.

Root AW. Disorders of calcium and phosphorus metabolism. In: Rudolph CD, Rudolph AM, eds. *Rudolph's pediatrics.* New York: McGraw-Hill, 2002:2142–2162.

Root AW, Diamond FB Jr. Calcium metabolism. In: Sperling MA, ed. *Pediatric endocrinology.* Philadelphia: WB Saunders, 2002:65–96.

Root AW, Diamond FB Jr. Disorders of calcium metabolism in the child and adolescent. In: Sperling MA, ed. *Pediatric endocrinology.* Philadelphia: WB Saunders, 2002:629–670.

8 ♣ Disorders of Sexual Differentiation

The appearance of ambiguous genitalia in a newborn must be considered a biologic and a psychological emergency: the former because of possible electrolyte and glucocorticoid abnormalities, and the latter because of the distress the parents will feel. This is a condition in which experience and careful consideration are essential; I recommend immediate consultation with a pediatric endocrinologist before making a diagnosis, assigning sex of rearing, or embarking upon a treatment plan. Much has changed in the management of this condition with recent insights derived from long-term patient observations.

NORMAL SEXUAL DIFFERENTIATION

Normal gender identity is based on genotype, which will determine gonadal sex, which leads to phenotypic sexual differentiation, which determines social sexual role. If something goes awry in this normal progression, an intersex situation results.

Genotype

Genotype or chromosomal sex is 46XY for a male and 46XX for a female (Fig. 8-1). The Lyon hypothesis predicts that one of the X chromosomes in a female is inactivated so that only one dose of each gene on the X chromosome is active. We now know that the entire X chromosome is not inactivated, as some genes remain active and are required for normal sexual differentiation. This "relatively" inactivated X chromosome appears as a Barr body at the periphery of the nuclear envelope on a stained preparation of cells scraped from the buccal mucosa (the buccal smear). Patients will have one fewer Barr body than the number of X chromosomes, so that those with more than two X chromosomes will have more than one Barr body (e.g., a patient with 48XXXY will have two), and those with only one X chromosome (45X Turner syndrome) will have no Barr bodies. Unfortunately, few laboratories are capable of performing buccal smears in a reliable manner, and few physicians have enough experience either to perform the buccal scrape correctly or to interpret the buccal smear results appropriately, and the information gained in the best situation is limited. Thus the buccal smear cannot be used as a definitive diagnostic technique; a karyotype determination is the only accurate approach to determining chromosomal sex, and even this is not adequate to determine the management of the child.

The Y chromosome contains the SRY gene, which directs the differentiation of the bipotential gonad in the early fetus into a testis. Active genes on portions of the distal arms of the Y chromosomes, the pseudoautosomal regions, can undergo meiotic recombination with the corresponding pseudoautosomal areas of the X chromosome. The SRY gene is located proximal to the boundary of the pseudoautosomal region of Y chromosome. The translocation of the SRY to an X chromosome can cause an XX individual, who inherited one normal X chromosome from the mother and

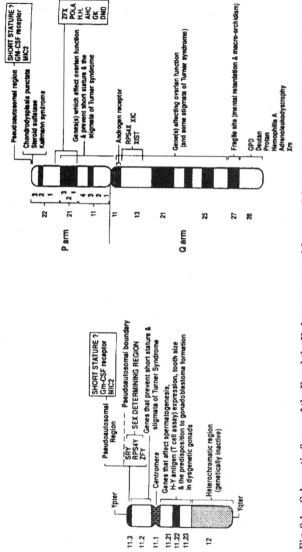

Fig. 8-1. Schematic figure of the X and the Y chromosomes with some of the genes indicated. (From Grumbach MM, Conte FA. Disorders of sexual differentiation. In: Wilson JD, Foster DW, Kronenberg HM, Larsen PR, eds. *Williams textbook of endocrinology*. Philadelphia: WB Saunders, 1999:1509–1626, with permission.)

one X chromosome with the SRY gene from the father, to develop testicular tissue; this is the origin of an XX male, an individual who would demonstrate some characteristics that could be found on a 47XXY male with Klinefelter syndrome. The SRY also can be transferred to an autosome, allowing an XX phenotypic male to result. Alternatively, 46 XY phenotypic females lack testicular development because of the loss of SRY from the Y chromosome inherited from the father. Other autosomal genes determine sexual differentiation; abnormalities of these regions also may lead to intersex conditions (Fig. 8-2).

Gonadal Sex

Gonadal sex is determined by the presence or absence of the SRY. Current theory holds that the indifferent gonad passively becomes an ovary (in the absence of SRY) or a testes in the presence of the SRY, although other genes are postulated to be necessary for ovarian development. If there is only one X chromosome and no SRY, the gonad will develop into an ovary during the fetal period and become laden with ova. The ova, however, will atrophy in the absence of a second normal X chromosome, and the ovary will degenerate into the "streak gonad" characteristic of Turner syndrome. Many other genes are involved in the creation of the gonad, so this schema must be considered a quite simple summary.

The steroid metabolism of the gonad involves several enzymes in the conversion of cholesterol into androgens or estrogens; several of the enzymes also are important in the biosynthetic activities of the adrenal gland, so that a genetic defect in an enzyme may affect both gonadal and adrenal function. Figure 8-3 demonstrates the action of the enzymes, their location in the cell, and the names of the genes that define them. Genetic probes in clinical practice or research laboratories may detect some of these defects.

Phenotypic Sex

Phenotypic sexual development involves the internal ducts and external genital appearance. These two areas may develop in alternative directions based on the effectiveness of androgens.

Internal sexual ducts (Fig. 8-4) are bipotential at first, but one set degenerates as sex is determined. Internal genital ducts are masculine if derived from the wolffian ducts or feminine if derived from the müllerian ducts. In the presence of the testicular peptide product derived from the Sertoli cells, müllerian duct inhibitory factor (MIF), the müllerian ducts will atrophy; in the absence of MIF, the uterus, oviducts, and the upper two thirds of the vagina will develop spontaneously into their basic form. Dysgenetic testes may have more Leydig cell function and testosterone production than MIF production, and some level of müllerian development may occur in a genetic male with impaired MIF production and dysgenetic testes. In the presence of high local concentrations of testosterone, the wolffian ducts will develop into the epididymis, vas deferens, and seminal vesicles. As the testosterone and MIF

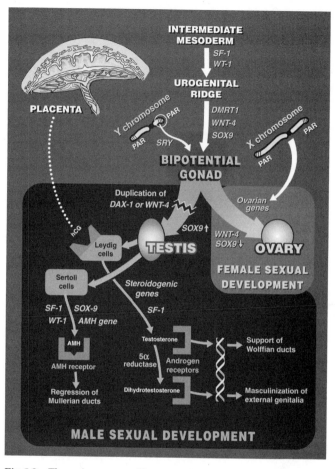

Fig. 8-2. The major genes and hormones in male sexual differentiation.
(Dennis M. Styne, M.D.)

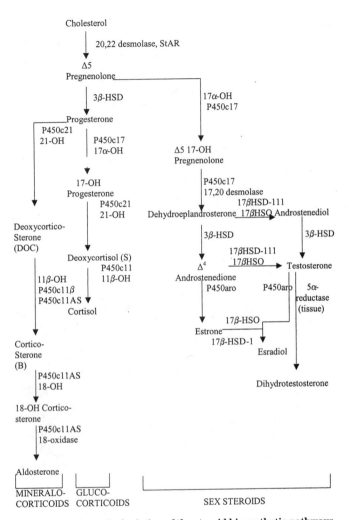

Fig. 8-3. A schematic depiction of the steroid biosynthetic pathways, with the enzymes and the genes involved in the process indicated. (From Styne DM. *Pediatric endocrinology: House officer series.* Philadelphia: Lippincott Williams & Wilkins, 1988, with permission.)

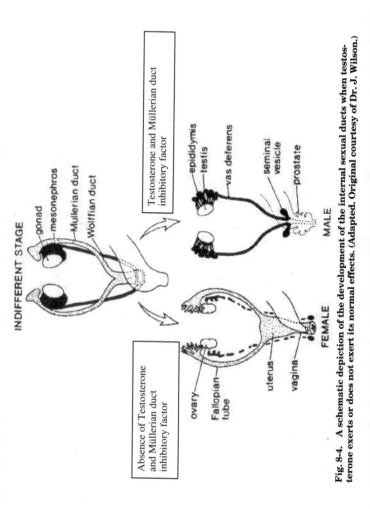

INDIFFERENT STAGE

gonad
mesonephros
Müllerian duct
Wolffian duct

Absence of Testosterone and Müllerian duct inhibitory factor

Testosterone and Müllerian duct inhibitory factor

epididymis
testis
vas deferens

seminal
vesicle
prostate

MALE

ovary
Fallopian tube
uterus
vagina

FEMALE

Fig. 8-4. A schematic depiction of the development of the internal sexual ducts when testosterone exerts or does not exert its normal effects. (Adapted. Original courtesy of Dr. J. Wilson.)

will come from a testis, a unilateral testis in a true hermaphrodite could produce müllerian regression and wolffian differentiation on the ipsilateral side, whereas a contralateral ovary could allow the development of contralateral oviduct and a hemiuterus. Thus in a true hermaphrodite, one side of the internal sexual ducts may appear similar to male, and the other, to the female, with any variation of this outcome possible.

External genitalia (Fig. 8-5) are bipotential until 8 weeks of gestation. Without intervention, the genital tubercle will become a clitoris, the urogenital folds will become the labia minora, and the labia majora will form from the labioscrotal swelling. In the presence of systemic circulating testosterone, which is locally converted into dihydrotestosterone (DHT) by the 5α-reductase enzyme in the sexual skin, and in the presence of normal androgen receptors (ARs), a boy will be virilized into a classic male appearance. With DHT, the genital tubercle will differentiate into a penis, with fusion of the urogenital slit to form a penile urethra, and with fusion of the labioscrotal folds to produce a scrotum.

The fetal testes must be functional to allow these steps of virilization to progress. In the first trimester, maternal human chorionic gonadotropin (hCG) stimulates the fetal testes to produce the testosterone necessary for male development, as fetal gonadotropins are not yet secreted from the fetal pituitary gland in substantial amounts. During the last two trimesters, fetal pituitary gonadotropins are secreted in the greater amounts that are necessary to stimulate testicular activity and cause further normal growth of the penis; if the fetal pituitary gland cannot produce luteinizing hormone (LH), the penis will be normally shaped (because of early hCG stimulation of the fetal testosterone production) but small because of lack of enlargement that should be stimulated by fetal LH, with a length likely to be less than 2.0 cm (which is –2.5 SD from the mean and is called a microphallus), as compared with a normal length of 4 cm at birth.

Any interruption of the normal progression toward masculine development in a 46XY fetus will result in the development of some degree of ambiguous genitalia. Any exposure to androgens at a sensitive time in development will cause a female fetus to virilize to some degree and also will cause ambiguous genitalia. If the female is exposed to the androgen after 8 weeks and before 13 weeks of gestation, the vaginal opening may fuse posteriorly to become slit-like, and the urogenital slit may enclose at least part of the urethra; androgen exposure after 13 weeks of gestation will only enlarge the length and thickness of the phallic structure, causing clitoromegaly without affecting the vaginal opening. Thus the appearance of the genitalia at birth reveals much about the physiology of the fetus.

Social Gender

Gender development may be thought to consist of (a) gender identity, the experience of one's self as female or male; (b) gender role, the behavior that identifies to others or self whether one is male

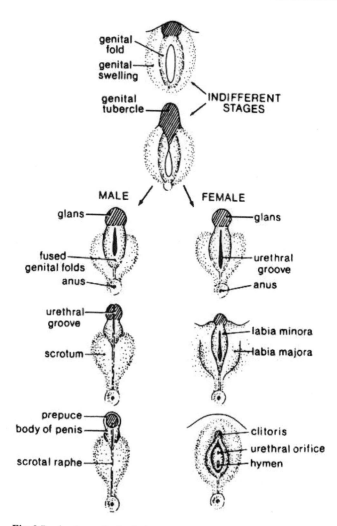

Fig. 8-5. A schematic depiction of the changes to the external genitalia when testosterone exerts its normal effects on the left by conversion to DHT and interaction with the androgen receptor in a normal male or does not in a normal female. Male development on the left proceeds with the presence of adequate amounts of dihydrotestosterone (DHT) and normal androgen receptors. (Courtesy of Dr. J. Wilson.)

or female; (c) sexual orientation, the choice of gender of sexual partners; and (d) the desire and capacity for parenting.

The classic view has been that gender identity is determined mainly by the surroundings of the growing child, but because the physical appearance of the child influences those interacting with the child, gender identity is affected by physical differentiation. Interactions with family and peers will teach the child how to act within the expected gender role. However, now a growing body of research demonstrates effects of prenatal androgen exposure on subsequent gender development, although human beings have a social overlay to the effects of prenatal androgens. For example, a girl exposed to prenatal androgens, because of virilizing CAH, if raised socially as a girl, will have a normal female gender identity but may demonstrate some male tendencies in play behavior and reasoning, and/or a male tendency in gender role. Conversely, males who are exposed to prenatal androgens but for some reason have inadequate male external genitalia and are raised as female, were recently shown to chose a male gender identity spontaneously in later childhood or adolescence in many cases. Thus in cases of male pseudohermaphroditism described later, decisions on sex of rearing are difficult, and recommendations are presently controversial and undergoing reconsideration. Patient groups have been forceful in suggesting that gender assignment and surgical reconstruction should await such time as the child can decide; others believe that this is unworkable, and gender should be assigned in an unambiguous manner early. All would agree that parents must be involved and that the best understanding of the biology of the condition must be considered. In the past, it has been generally considered difficult to institute change of gender successfully after age 18 months (except for the case of 5α-reductase deficiency seen later), and worry remains over the psychological effects of spontaneous or guided change in gender identity later in life.

DISORDERS OF SEXUAL DIFFERENTIATION
Diseases Causing Virilization of Genetic Females (Female Pseudohermaphrodite)
Congenital Adrenal Hyperplasia

An abnormality in any of the enzymes involved in the production of cortisol will, in the absence of feedback inhibition, allow increased adrenocorticotropic hormone (ACTH) secretion. The adrenal glands, unable to make the end product, cortisol, which will suppress ACTH, will become hyperplastic. Depending on the enzyme affected, the adrenal gland may make uncontrolled amounts of androgens to allow virilization of a female. Alternatively, a defective enzyme found in both the adrenal gland and the testes, which is essential for testosterone production, will cause inadequate virilization in the male. A defect of an enzyme in the pathway involved in the production of aldosterone will cause sodium loss and the retention of potassium, leading to hyponatremia and hyperkalemia, possibly to a life-threatening extent (see Table 8-1).

Table 8-1. Differential diagnosis of adrenal enzyme effects

Deficiency	Newborn phenotype	Postnatal virilization	Salt losing
StAR (previously thought to be 20, 22 Desmolase, also called lipoid congenital adrenal hyperplasia)	Infantile female	—	+
3β-Hydroxylase (3βHSD)	Ambiguous in XY	+	+
	Female or ambiguous in XX	+	+
17α-Hydroxylase (P450$_{c17}$)	Infantile female	—	*
11β-Hydroxylase (P450$_{c11β}$)	Male in XY	+	*
	Ambiguous in XX	+	*
21 Hydroxylase (P450$_{c21}$)	Male in XY	+	+(50%)
	Ambiguous in XX	+	+(50%)
18 Hydroxylase (P450$_{c11AS}$)	Normal	—	+

*HT, Hypertension.

21-Hydroxylase Deficiency (*201910 ADRENAL HYPERPLASIA, CONGENITAL, DUE TO 21-HYDROXYLASE DEFICIENCY at 6p21.3)

21-Hydroxylase deficiency, the most common type of CAH, is the most common cause of ambiguous genitalia, is the most common cause for virilization in a newborn female, and the nonclassic type of 21-hydroxylase deficiency is the most common type of genetic disease in human beings. The 21-hydroxylase enzyme is a P450-class enzyme with the gene (denoted as cpy 21OH) located on chromosome 6 in proximity to the human leukocyte antigen (HLA) genes. Progesterone is 21-hydroxylated into deoxycorticosterone (DOC) in the pathway toward aldosterone and 17-hydroxyprogesterone [17(OH)progesterone] is 21-hydroxylated to 11-deoxycortisol in the pathway toward cortisol. Thus because the production of cortisol is diminished at the 21-hydroxylation step, ACTH increases and stimulates the production of products of the adrenal gland proximal to this defect: the products are 17(OH)progesterone and its precursors. All affected patients have elevated 17-hydroxyprogesterone at diagnosis in the basal state in the congenital (severe) form or after ACTH stimulation in the late-onset (nonclassic) form discussed later. About 50% of patients with the congenital form have clinical salt loss and hyperkalemia because of impaired production of DOC. Within one family, if a proband has salt losing, other affected children also will be salt losers; further, the affected children within one family will share the same HLA types, allowing a possibility of prenatal diagnosis of future pregnancies.

Females with 21-hydroxylase deficiency will be virilized *in utero,* demonstrating any variation of clitoromegaly, posterior fusion of the labia majora into the appearance of an "empty scrotal sack," and lack of formation of the vaginal vesicular septum, causing a urogenital sinus. Thus a female will appear to be at any stage on the continuum from ambiguous genitalia to "male with undescended testes." A male infant with 21-hydroxylase deficiency will not appear obviously abnormal and may not be diagnosed until a metabolic emergency occurs, whereas a girl with ambiguous genitalia will usually receive immediate attention because of more immediate diagnosis caused by the unusual appearance.

Surprisingly, rarely are any electrolyte problems seen during the first days after birth in patients with salt-losing 21-hydroxylase deficiency. Salt wasting does not manifest until after several days of age. Likewise, hypoglycemia does not develop in the immediate neonatal period but may take a day or two to manifest. Thus, in these days of short-stay deliveries, a patient may actually be discharged from the hospital before biochemical complications develop. The initial signs of electrolyte disturbance may lead to vomiting and may appear as a case of viral gastroenteritis on casual evaluation. Boys who look normal may be mistakenly diagnosed as having pyloric stenosis and even undergo unnecessary surgery; one diagnostic difference is that patients with 21-hydroxylase deficiency have high potassium and often acidosis, whereas those with pyloric stenosis have low potassium and metabolic alkalosis. If untreated, salt loss can lead to sodium values in the 110 mEq/L or lower range and elevated potassium to the range greater than 9.5 mEq/L by age 3 to 4 weeks if the child survives that long with therapy. Vomiting can lead to weight loss, so that body weight decreases to a point lower than birth weight. Simple virilized patients have no obvious salt loss but may have elevated plasma renin activity (PRA), suggesting the need for extra salt or mineralocorticoid therapy.

Skin pigmentation may darken during the period that the patient is untreated because of extremely elevated ACTH secretion, but this will not occur in the immediate neonatal period. Androgen secretion will lead to incomplete sexual precocity in affected children, with the appearance of pubic hair, clitoral or penile enlargement, acne, deepening of the voice, muscular development, rapid growth, and bone-age advancement over months and years after birth if the child has the simple virilizing form and does not die of electrolyte disturbances in the neonatal period in the untreated state. Therefore, although the child will be large for age, the rapid bone-age advancement will lead to early epiphyseal fusion, and short adult stature will result. The testes will not initially enlarge in affected boys because the androgen that causes these changes comes from the adrenal gland rather than the gonads; later, adrenal rest tissue in the testes may enlarge under ACTH stimulation to form nodules in the testes in untreated or poorly treated boys. Remarkably, the advanced bone age and exposure to androgens will cause maturation of the hypothalamic-pituitary-gonadal axis. When glucocorticoid treatment is administered and adrenal androgen secretion decreases, the adrenal androgens that were suppressing gonadotropin secretion diminish, and true precocious puberty may develop (with pubertal testicular enlargement in boys). This secondary complication will further compromise final height by bone-age advancement; true precocious puberty after exposure to excess androgens can be treated with gonadotropin-releasing hormone (GnRH) analogues, as can any other cause of true precocious puberty (see Chapter 9).

Nonclassic or late-onset 21-hydroxylase deficiency is a more recently described condition characterized by normal phenotype at birth (i.e., no clitoromegaly or posterior vaginal fusion in girls), with virilization occurring years afterward in childhood, adolescence, or young adulthood. The serum 17-hydroxyprogesterone and other adrenal androgen concentrations will be elevated in the basal state or after ACTH stimulation, but not so high as in the congenital form. Female patients may complain of increasing facial or body hair. The incidence varies in ethnic groups, with an incidence in Ashkenazi Jewish women of 1 in 50 in some studies, making this disorder one of the most common genetic disease in human beings. Cryptic 21-hydroxylase deficiency appears to be a variant of the late-onset form; laboratory values are identical to those found in patients with the late-onset form, but for some as yet unexplained reason, the patient does not experience virilization. All four varieties of 21-OH deficiency are considered to be due to various combinations of alleles.

The diagnosis of 21-hydroxylase deficiency is made by elevation of serum 17-hydroxyprogesterone concentrations, the precursor of the enzyme that is deficient, in the basal state or 60 minutes after 250 g synthetic ACTH (1–24 ACTH or Cortrosyn) given intravenously. Serum concentrations of 17-hydroxyprogesterone are elevated in cord blood of normal infants because of the activity of the fetal adrenal and contributions from the mother's steroid metabolism, but values decrease to levels of 100 to 200 ng/dL within 24 hours after birth. A neonate with classic 21-hydroxylase deficiency will have concentration of 17-hydroxyprogesterone in the 1,000 to 10,000 ng/dL range or higher, allowing easy differentiation from normal infants. Methods of screening for 21-hydroxylase deficiency in heel-stick samples taken after birth are instituted in the newborn screening programs of many states. Prenatal diagnosis is available by measuring amniotic fluid steroid metabolite values or by matching the HLA type of the fetus (taken from amniocentesis or chorionic villus biopsy) to an affected proband sibling of known HLA type, by restriction fragment length polymorphism analysis of fetal tissue. Fetal treatment with glucocorticoid administered to the mother shows promise in diminishing virilization of affected females but is still considered experimental therapy and requires consultation with experienced practitioners of the method. Because an adrenal, testicular, or ovarian tumor may cause virilization in a child and because some metabolites are common to the adrenal gland and the gonads, the suppression of the offending androgens by glucocorticoid therapy is by itself a diagnostic test for an enzyme defect rather than a neoplasm.

Older methods of diagnosis, now superseded, include analysis of a 24-hour urine collection for 17-ketosteroid as a reflection of adrenal androgen secretion (primarily DHEA or dehydroepiandrosterone). Difficulties occur if a full 24-hour collection is not obtained; we have seen patients mistakenly considered normal on the basis of a 3-hour collection that was fallaciously low because of low volume and inadequate time of collection. A 24-hour urinary pregnanetriol determination, a reflection of 17-hydroxyprogesterone secretion, has the same reliance on a full 24-hour urine collection. It is now advisable to obtain a serum sample for 17-hydroxyprogesterone as well as other metabolites of the adrenal gland and to request that the laboratory treat the situation as a medical emergency; laboratories experienced with pediatric endocrine practice will comply with such a request and analyze the blood within a few days. These experienced laboratories will make determination on small samples of blood that are appropriate in a newborn rather than the large samples requested when diagnosing a young adult with hirsutism. New highly sensitive analyses of urinary metabolites of adrenal androgens are becoming available on spot collections and may further simplify diagnosis.

As salt loss is not usually manifested until after about age 5 days, vigilance must not be relaxed until after days to weeks of carefully observing the patient's electrolyte status. The increasing potassium value of a heel-stick sample obtained in such a patient should not be attributed to hemolysis alone, and a careful venous sample should be obtained. A PRA should be obtained to confirm salt loss, but the result of this test may not be available for several days, and immediate diagnosis cannot therefore rest on this test.

Radiologic evidence in the evaluation of 21-hydroxylase deficiency will include an advanced bone age if the child is untreated for a period of several months (a simple virilized child may survive this long, but a salt loser will become profoundly ill before this age) and an enlarging pituitary contour (due to basophil hyperplasia) on lateral skull radiograph if the patient is untreated for years. If an ultrasound examination in a newborn with ambiguous genitalia reveals a uterus, the patient will most likely be a female pseudohermaphrodite and therefore most likely be a female with 21-hydroxylase deficiency (confirm the diagnosis and do not simply guess, based on this statistic!). A vesicovaginogram with careful technique, using a rubber dam to contain the radiopaque dye, will reveal the anatomy of the internal vaginal structures and whether absence of the vesicovaginal septum is causing the development of a urogenital sinus.

For the differential diagnosis of adrenal enzyme defects, see Table 8-1.

Treatment of 21-Hydroxylase Deficiency

Virilizing 21-hydroxylase deficiency is treated with glucocorticoid replacement, and the best approach is the use of natural compounds such as hydrocortisone (cortisol). Synthetic glucocorticoids such as prednisone, prednisolone, or dexamethasone have their place in the treatment of older individuals, but growing children are more likely to maintain a better growth rate with the less-potent and shorter-acting natural glucocorticoid. The dose is variable among individuals, but for an initial dose, 13 to 18 mg/m^2 of cortisol is useful (this is greater than the normal secretory rate of cortisol, because the goal is not simply to replace the adrenal cortisol production but also to suppress abnormal product formation). Oral glucocorticoids are usually administered in doses every 8 hours. The dose should be titrated to the child as noted later. Some recommend that the greater portion of the dose be given at bedtime so the early-morning peak of ACTH will be suppressed and less androgen will be secreted (this is the reverse of the schedule for the treatment of adrenal insufficiency without CAH; see Chapter 10). If an emergency arises, subcutaneous, intravenous, or intramuscular hydrocortisone hemisuccinate (Solu-cortef) is appropriate. Intramuscular cortisone acetate takes hours to initiate effect and is not a medication to use in an emergency.

Many methods to follow the efficacy of treatment are proposed but the oldest, that of attention to growth rate and bone age, often is the final measure of adequacy of treatment; with too little a dose of glucocorticoid, the growth rate is excessive because of elevated androgens, whereas too much glucocorticoid quickly suppresses growth rate. Bone-age advancement is usually determined yearly; an increase of 1 year of bone age for each year of chronologic age is ideal. Serum 17-hydroxyprogesterone measured at a set time in the day after a dose of glucocorticoid (usually 2 hours after the morning dose in one scheme or at 8:00 a.m. before the morning dose in another scheme) and testosterone or androstenedione concentrations are frequently used to monitor therapy; a 17-hydroxyprogesterone concentration value will be above normal in most cases, but should be well below the untreated state, and age- and sex-appropriate testosterone or androstenedione concentration are the goals. Salivary steroid determinations have been used successfully to study some patients.

Mineralocorticoid therapy is administered to salt-losing patients in the form of 9-fluorohydrocortisone (Florinef) at 0.05 to 0.15 mg/day orally. Mineralocorticoids cause the retention of sodium and excretion of potassium at the proximal tubule level of the kidney. Extra salt also may be administered at a dose of approximately 1 to 2 g/day of sodium chloride; the parents may be given a few test tubes marked at the height 1 to 2 g of table salt would reach, so that they may measure the correct amount for the child. Blood pressure can increase high enough to cause hypertensive encephalopathy if too much salt or mineralocorticoid is given, whereas too little will precipitate hyponatremia and hyperkalemia. Inadequate mineralocorticoid also can cause elevation of ACTH and therefore cause increasing androgen concentrations. In such a situation, where the body interprets salt loss as stress, misinterpretation of the androgen levels may suggest the need for additional glucocorticoid, which would lead to growth suppression; if appropriate mineralocorticoid is given instead, the androgens will decrease, and growth will normalize.

At times of stress, glucocorticoid therapy must be increased threefold. Usually this will be necessary when an infectious illness causes a fever higher than 37.5°C or 101°F. If the patient is vomiting and cannot retain oral medications, the patient should be evaluated at the office or emergency room, but on the way, hydrocortisone-sodium succinate (Solucortef) can be given subcutaneously, intramuscularly or, in case of emergencies causing shock and poor perfusion, intravenously. A dose of 25 to 50 mg of hydrocortisone-sodium succinate for a child younger than 5 years and a dose of 50 to 100 mg for an older child will be an appropriate initial dose for most emergencies. Too much glucocorticoid in an emergency is not going to cause a problem, whereas inadequate dosage may be ineffectual in reversing the effects of adrenal insufficiency.

Patients with 21-hydroxylase deficiency require special preparation for surgery to avoid precipitating addisonian crisis. A dose of hydrocortisone-sodium succinate of 25 to 100 mg (depending on size) is given at the time of induction of anesthesia, and an infusion of the glucocorticoid is maintained during the procedure, or boluses are given every 4 to 6 hours to ensure a daily dose in excess of 45 mg/m^2, more than triple the secretory rate of the adrenal glands. This high-dose glucocorticoid therapy is maintained during surgery and in case of complications, but in most cases, the dose can be cut by degrees over the several days postoperatively. Because of the risks of hyponatremia and hypoglycemia, normal saline is infused during the operation and as needed thereafter and dextrose is infused in 5% to 10% concentrations.

Patients with 21-hydroxylase deficiency are treated in most ways as in any other child, but because they may develop complications of minor illnesses quite easily, they must be observed closely during illnesses. Frequent complications include hypoglycemia and hyponatremia in salt losers; any patient with 21-hydroxylase deficiency seen with acute illness must be considered to have these conditions until proven otherwise, and initial fluid management must include dextrose and salt. We strongly suggest that patients with 21-hydroxylase deficiency wear an identification bracelet or necklace (MedAlert or equivalent) and that they or their parents carry an identifying letter of emergency procedures from their doctor in case they require emergency treatment from an institution not familiar with this diagnosis. The treatment of hypoadrenal shock and hyponatremia are detailed in Chapter 15.

Other Types of Congenital Adrenal Hyperplasia Causing Female Pseudohermaphroditism

11-Hydroxylase deficiency (*202010 ADRENAL HYPERPLASIA, CONGENITAL, DUE TO 11-β-HYDROXYLASE DEFICIENCY At 8q21) leads to virilization, salt retention, hypokalemia, and hypertension; the enzymatic block leads to excessive 11-deoxy-cortisol (compound S), deoxycorticosterone (DOC, a potent min-eralocorticoid) production and, because ACTH is elevated in the absence of adequate cortisol and because no defect occurs in the formation of androgens, serum androgens also are elevated. Glu-cocorticoid therapy is necessary to stop virilization and reduce salt retention and hypertension. Conversely, mineralocorticoid is not used in this condition, as this is a disorder with excessive min-eralocorticoid production.

3-Hydroxysteroid-dehydrogenase deficiency (*201810 ADRENAL HYPERPLASIA II at 1p13.1) causes salt loss and virilization in genetic females but inadequate virilization in genetic males, because DHEA is a weak androgen and the only one made in the affected males. The genital appearance may be of tertiary hypospadias. The enzyme deficiency causes an increase in dehydroepiandrosterone and its sulfate (DHEA and DHEAS; and therefore elevated 24-hour urinary ketosteroids) while serum 17-hydroxyprogesterone is low or normal. Treatment is the same as that with salt-losing 21-hydroxylase deficiency.

Gonadal Conditions

Patients with both testicular and ovarian tissue are true hermaph-rodites, a rare condition. The tissue is more often combined in an ovotestes on at least one side rather than distributed laterally, with a normal ovary on one side and a normal testes on the other. Because of variable production of müllerian duct inhibitory factor and local and systemic testosterone, the internal ducts and exter-nal genitalia will be quite variable among individuals. Thus part of a uterus may be present on one side, with some male ducts on the contralateral side.

The patients most commonly have a 46XX karyotype, with the SRY present on some chromosomes (but not on the Y chromosome). Other cases may have the karyotype of 46XX/46XY chimeras or 46XY individuals with a presumed 46XX cell line in the gonads.

Fertility has rarely been described in hermaphrodites, but the ovarian tissue can produce some feminization at puberty in some cases. Conversely, the dysgenetic testicular tissue can undergo malignant degeneration and should be removed. Because of con-cerns over the difficulty of plastic reconstruction of the phallus, most patients are raised as girls.

Turner and Klinefelter syndromes are disorders of gonadal development and are discussed in Chapter 9 on puberty.

46 XX gonadal dysgenesis or 46 XY gonadal dysgenesis also are sometimes called pure gonadal dysgenesis. 46 XX gonadal dysge-

nesis has the phenotype of an immature female with internal müllerian ducts. The condition may be sporadic or follow an autosomal recessive pattern with deafness (*233400 GONADAL DYS-GENESIS, XX TYPE, WITH DEAFNESS)

46 XY gonadal dysgenesis, is also called Swyer syndrome, may result in an immature female phenotype if the dysgenesis is complete, or ambiguous genitalia if functional Leydig cells remain from the dysgenetic testes. Internal duct formation will depend on the amount of MIF produced from the dysgenetic testes. The etiology may be abnormalities of SRY function, autosomal mutations, or duplication of the DSS locus on the X chromosome. The condition may be sporadic or follow X-linked male limited (*306100 GONADAL DYSGENESIS, XY FEMALE TYPE; GDXY), autosomal dominant, or autosomal recessive patterns. The dysgenetic testes has a 20- to 46-fold increased potential for neoplastic formation and must be removed. If an affected subject feminizes at puberty, the cause might be estrogen formation from a gonadoblastoma formed within the dysgenetic testes and is a sign of concern rather than optimism that there is functional ovarian tissue.

External Sex Steroid Ingestion

Maternal ingestion of progestins of androgen derivation (present oral contraceptives do not contain these substances) can cause virilization of female fetuses in some cases. Diethylstilbestrol (DES) ingestion, no longer recommended, has been reported to decrease the masculinization of a male fetus.

Disorders Causing Inadequate Virilization of a Genetic Male (Male Pseudohermaphroditism)

An inability to produce testosterone, an inability to convert testosterone to DHT in the sexual skin, or a resistance to androgen action all can cause male pseudohermaphroditism.

Testicular Enzyme Defects

Testicular enzyme deficiencies include some disorders in which the same enzymes are deficient in the testes as in the adrenal glands.

StAR (steroid acute regulatory protein, which assists the entry of cholesterol into the gonadal or adrenal cell mitochondria for steroid synthesis) deficiency (#201710 LIPOID CONGENITAL ADRENAL HYPERPLASIA at 8p11.2) was previously thought to be because of 20–22 desmolase deficiency; the condition eliminates the production of all adrenal and gonadal steroid production, and large, lipid-laden adrenal glands develop, which may inferiorly displace the kidneys (the condition is also called lipoid adrenal hyperplasia. In the complete form, 46XX and 46XY individuals will have a normal female phenotype and no progression of secondary sexual development at puberty; in the incomplete form, 46XY patients will have some degree of ambiguous genitalia. Profound addisonian crisis will occur at 5 to 7 days after birth or earlier because of the complete absence of mineralocorticoids and glucocorticoids. Treatment is as for 21-hydroxylase deficiency, with the exception that glucocorticoid replacement dosage may be less because of the lack of necessity to suppress androgenic substances produced by the adrenal glands of the 21-hydroxylase–deficient patient. The condition is found in an autosomal recessive pattern and is most common in Korea and Japan.

17α-Hydroxylase deficiency (*202110 ADRENAL HYPERPLASIA, CONGENITAL, DUE TO 17-α-HYDROXYLASE DEFICIENCY at 10q24.3) eliminates the 17-hydroxylation of progesterone and pregnenolone and interferes with the production of both cortisol and sex steroids; 46XX and 46XY patients cannot produce cortisol or androgens or estrogens but make excessive mineralocorticoid in the form of desoxycorticosterone. The defect is in CPY17, which codes for both the 17α-hydroxylase and 17,20-lyase enzymes. Phenotype is of an immature female in the complete form, but some incompletely affected males may have ambiguous genitalia. Thus hypertension, hypokalemia, and elevated serum progesterone, pregnenolone, corticosterone, and DOC but decreased PRA, 17-hydroxyprogesterone, and aldosterone in an immature female are the clinical cornerstones. Primary amenorrhea may be the presentation if the subject is first diagnosed in adolescence.

Other Enzyme Deficiencies Involving the Testes but Not the Adrenal Gland in a 46 XY Genotype

17β-Hydroxysteroid dehydrogenase type 3 (or 17β-hydroxysteroid oxidoreductase deficiency or 17β-ketosteroid reductase deficiency) (#264300 17β-HYDROXYSTEROID DEHYDROGENASE III DEFICIENCY at 9q22) interferes with the conversion of androstenedione to testosterone and estrone to estradiol. Phenotype is infantile female or some degree of ambiguous genitalia. Internal ducts are wolffian because of the presence of müllerian duct inhibitory factor. The upper portion of the vagina is absent (as a müllerian derivative), and the testes are internal or labial; patients have had "hernias" repaired that contained the testes without the correct diagnosis being made. Gynecomastia or some virilization may occur at the time of puberty.

17,20-Lyase or desmolase deficiency (*202110 ADRENAL HYPERPLASIA, CONGENITAL, DUE TO 17α-HYDROXYLASE DEFICIENCY at 10q24.3) results from a mutation in the CPY17 gene, which interferes with the conversion of 17-hydroxyprogesterone to androstenedione and 17-hydroxypregnenolone to dehydroepiandrosterone and thereby limits the production of testosterone. This is the same enzyme that catalyzes the 17-hydroxylation of pregnenolone and progesterone, but this presentation is rarer. Phenotype is infantile female or ambiguous genitalia with undescended or labial testes. Some virilization may occur at puberty.

Defects in a 46 XY Genotype Not Involving the Testes

5α-Reductase deficiency (defect in SRDA2, the steroid 5α-reductase enzyme gene *264600 PSEUDOVAGINAL PERINEOSCROTAL

HYPOSPADIAS; PPSH at 2p23) causes reduction in the conversion of testosterone to DHT in the sexual skin, thereby causing the formation of chordee (ventral binding of the phallus by attached skin), small phallic structure, hypospadias, bifid scrotum, usually with undescended testes, and a urogenital sinus; this is described as pseudovaginal perinoscrotal hypospadias. The production of MIF ensures the absence of müllerian derivatives, but the presence of testosterone itself supports the development of wolffian structures. At puberty, possibly because of increasing production of testosterone or to the effects of normal SRDA type 1 activity located in the liver and other nonsexual skin, DHT-dependent effects such as enlargement of the penis, descent of the testes, and pigmentation of the scrotum occur, as well as increased muscle mass and deepening of the voice. No acne or male-pattern recession of hair occurs, however. Most remarkably affected patients from the Dominican Republic are initially raised as girls, but at the time of puberty and thereafter are considered male in social contexts. This phenomenon has been considered an example of the plasticity of human gender roles, but the children are usually known to have the condition in early life (known as *heuvodoces* for the descent of testes at puberty), and the situation is not so simple as an isolated change in gender. The condition is found in Papua New Guinea, known as *kwalatmala,* in which affected subjects also change gender role at puberty from female to male. It also is reported in Saudi Arabia, but patients are found elsewhere in smaller groupings.

The complete syndrome of androgen insensitivity (previously called testicular feminization; #300068 ANDROGEN INSENSITIVITY SYNDROME; AIS at Xq11-q12) results from mutation in the androgen receptor gene (AR) on the X chromosome. Complete androgen insensitivity is not actually seen as ambiguous genitalia, because in the absence of testosterone action, the phenotype is infantile female. Internal ducts are hypoplastic wolffian ducts. The vaginal pouch is blind because of the absence of the upper two thirds, normally derived from müllerian elements, which atrophies because of the normal production of MIF. At puberty, the unopposed estradiol causes normal feminization, but the lack of androgen action eliminates the development of pubic and axillary hair. The defect is transmitted as an X-linked trait and is characterized by a decrease in the testosterone and DHT receptors or a postreceptor defect in them. Patients have an unambiguous female gender role.

The incomplete syndrome of androgen insensitivity is because of a less severe deficiency or defect in AR. Phenotype may be normal male (with the only abnormality being infertility), may be an underdeveloped male with small but normally formed phallus, or may be ambiguous. Internal ducts are male because of normal production of MIF. At puberty, some degree of gynecomastia may be noted, and some pubic and axillary hair development should occur. Serum LH and testosterone concentrations are above normal. These patients experience some androgen effect *in utero,* and recent reports indicate a high degree of spontaneous reversion to the male gender role in individuals raised as girls.

Unresponsiveness to hCG and LH (*152790 LUTEINIZING HORMONE/CHORIOGONADOTROPIN RECEPTOR; LHCGR at 2p21) is associated with low testosterone production and ambiguous genitalia, because no Leydig cell function can occur.

The differentiation of anorchia from cryptorchidism is discussed in Chapter 9.

The Diagnosis and Treatment of Ambiguous Genitalia

Ambiguous genitalia in a neonate must be treated as an emergency. No suggestion of gender must be made to the parents until a diagnosis or plan of treatment is established. It is appropriate to talk about "the baby" instead of "he" or "she"; to not have the hospital print a card having any suggestion of gender on it, and to speak of "the gonads" rather than testes or ovaries. Never say that the baby is "partially girl and partially boy," as every child is either a girl or a boy. The parents can be told that the baby has a cosmetic problem, that the external genitalia are "unfinished," and that it is up to us, by the way of tests, to determine the sex of the baby. Even if the physician has a "gut'" feeling about the outcome of the diagnosis, the risks of incorrect assignment of diagnosis are great, and it is best to support the obviously concerned parents without giving them false direction.

Steps in the diagnostic process will vary, depending on whether the baby has palpable gonads or whether no gonads are palpable (see Figs. 8-6 and 8-7). Although a list of appropriate steps exists, it must be emphasized that in this situation, the help of an expert consultant is necessary, even if the child's life is not in immediate danger. The vagaries of the interpretation of the tests could allow an incorrect diagnosis, such as one in which a salt loser does not receive therapy or surveillance for hyponatremia ceases.

The mother must be queried for a history of unexplained deaths in the family (which would suggest CAH) or maternal androgen secretion or drug ingestion. The baby must be examined for phallic size (stretched length and width), chordee, the appearance of hypospadias, scrotalization of the labia (rugation and pigmentation of the skin to look like a scrotum), presence of palpable masses in the "labial" area, weight gain, and growth rate. An ultrasound study to determine the presence of a uterus or adnexa is useful if the ultrasonographer is experienced with the conditions noted earlier. In an older child, a bone-age examination as a reflection of androgen effect is useful, but in the infant, it may not help.

Laboratory determinations will include karyotype analysis performed as an emergency procedure (laboratories will hurry the process in most cases, so that an answer can be obtained in less than 5 days and perhaps in 2 to 3), but no reliance should be put on a buccal smear. Serum androgen metabolite determinations should be ordered, including at least 17-OH progesterone, androstenedione, DHEA, testosterone, and DHT. Serum LH and follicle-stimulating hormone (FSH), if markedly elevated to the castrate range, may

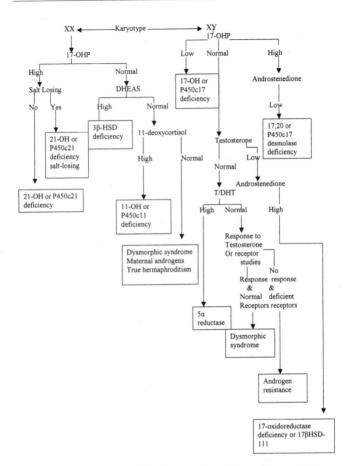

Fig. 8-6. Diagnostic algorithm for a patient with ambiguous genitalia in which no gonad is palpable. (From Styne DM. *Pediatric endocrinology: House officer series.* Philadelphia: Lippincott Williams & Wilkins, 1988, with permission.)

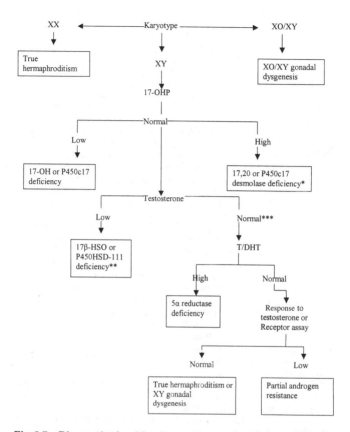

Fig. 8-7. Diagnostic algorithm for a patient with ambiguous genitalia in which gonads (possibly inguinal) are palpable. *Androstenedione is always low in 17,20-desmolase deficiency. **Androstenedione is always high in 17β-HSO deficiency. ***Androstenedione is always normal when testosterone is normal here. (From Styne DM. *Pediatric endocrinology: House officer series.* Philadelphia: Lippincott Williams & Wilkins, 1988, with permission.)

suggest dysgenetic gonads. Urinary collections for 17-ketosteroid and pregnanetriol are difficult because of the requirement of a 24-hour collection and should no longer be used. The serum tests will be done as an emergency if one of the few laboratories experienced in pediatric endocrine testing is used. The diagnosis should be relatively clear from the results, although an anxious several-day wait for the values will ensue, in even the best situations. If a question remains whether there is a functioning testis or what is the activity of 5α-reductase, an hCG stimulation test should be performed. The administration of hCG, 3,000 units/m^2 intramuscularly, should induce an increase in testosterone greater than 100 ng/dL (or an increase in other androgen metabolites of interest) within 72 hours in a cryptorchid newborn; if the patient is in mid-childhood or older, one injection of hCG may not be adequate to stimulate the quiescent Leydig cells. Thus hCG is given 3 times per week for 2 weeks, and then measurement of serum testosterone (or other appropriate androgens or precursors) is performed 24 hours after the last injection of hCG to determine whether testosterone secretion can be induced over this longer period of hCG administration. Serum levels of DHT as well as testosterone should be obtained if a reflection of the activity of 5α-reductase is desired. As another effect of the injections, if undescended testes are present, the testes may descend into the scrotum if the inguinal ring is not definitively too small to allow the passage. If there is a question of testosterone responsiveness of the phallus, 3 months of testosterone administration should be performed (as noted in Chapter 9). Sexual skin biopsy for androgen receptors or 5α-reductase activity may be sent to research laboratories for analysis, but now no commercial laboratory performs such testing.

The decision about sex of rearing in a patient with ambiguous genitalia depends on the diagnosis and on the wishes of the family. One consideration is to retain fertility, if possible, and another is to ensure that the external genitalia can be made compatible with the sex of rearing. However, an overriding issue is the effects of androgens on the fetal brain as the individual grows. Pediatric surgical or pediatric urologic procedures, performed by an experienced surgeon, are required if correction is considered for any patient with ambiguous genitalia. In female pseudohermaphroditism, the decision will usually be to raise the child as a girl in the conditions listed earlier. Most of these patients will have virilizing CAH, and although their external genitalia will be ambiguous, they will have normal internal ducts and should have the opportunity for fertility, if they wish, if correctly treated with glucocorticoids and mineralocorticoids. It is important to note that there is a decreased interest in childbearing by affected females with 21-OH deficiency owing to various factors, so in some cases, the preservation of fertility will not be important to the individual (although this knowledge may be clear only in retrospect). The clitoris will be enlarged, usually too much to appear as a normal variation, although there will be some shrinkage with time. The procedure of choice is clitoral recession with preservation of the glans and the nerve supply, in contrast to the clitorectomies performed before the last decades. However, if the clitoris is too large or if the patient is noncompliant and it enlarges further, a clitoral recession may be inadequate to avoid pain that may occur with erection of the tissue, and clitoral resection may be necessary. Clitoral recession is usually done by age 1 year to avoid allowing the child to be noticeably different from peers in the eyes of babysitters or child-care workers, because the child may not always be in the presence of the parents after the first few months. The vagina will have to be enlarged, and the posterior fusion opened in some cases. If there is a urogenital sinus, the anatomy will have to be repaired as well. The vaginal procedures may have to be done in stages, with the final steps done at the time of puberty.

Male pseudohermaphrodites have usually been raised as infertile females, except for 5α-reductase deficiency, when male gender role is the usual outcome after puberty. Those with severe testicular enzyme defects or dysgenetic testes will usually have basically female phenotypes and can never make adequate testosterone, whereas those with androgen resistance will never be able to respond to testosterone. Reconstruction of the phallus may be practically difficult or impossible. In all of these cases, the testes will be undescended or partially descended and will be subject to an increased risk of testicular neoplasm in a location where they cannot be regularly examined. Thus orchiectomy is the rule in all of these conditions. In testicular feminization, the testes will induce feminization at the time of puberty and may be left in until that time, although the unlikely risk of early testicular neoplasm in a location where it cannot be seen and the psychological considerations may suggest that early gonadectomy is best; the increased psychological difficulty of explaining the need for a gonadectomy to a teenage child will be encountered if orchiectomy is delayed. In 5α-reductase deficiency, a potential for fertility as a male remains, and many patients have been raised as males after correction of the chordee and hypospadias. It is important to recall that if the penis of a boy with microphallus is responsive to testosterone, the child can usually be raised as a male; patients with congenital hypopituitarism and microphallus will usually be able to achieve fertility with appropriate therapy.

The overall question presently under reconsideration is the decision of sex of rearing in a child with partial androgen insensitivity or with an anatomic defect that makes a male gender assignment far more difficult. In the past, these patients were raised as girls. However, increasing evidence indicates that exposure of the prenatal brain to androgens causes a tendency to a male gender role, making it more controversial to raise such affected children in a female gender, without regard for the possibility of reconstructive surgery creating an adequate penis. Several subjects were assigned to a female gender but self-reassigned to male gender in the prepubertal or the pubertal period. Again, the recommendation is to consult with a pediatric endocrinologist to assist in deciding on the sex of rearing until this situation is better understood.

SUGGESTED READINGS

Donohue PA, Saenger PH. Ambiguous genitalia. In: Finberg L, Kleinman RE, eds. *Saunders manual of pediatric practice.* Philadelphia: WB Saunders, 2002:872–875.

Grumbach MM. Abnormalities of sex determination and differentiation. In: Rudolph CD, Rudolph AM, eds. *Rudolph's pediatrics.* New York: McGraw-Hill, 2002:2079–2092.

Grumbach MM, Hughes IA, Conte FA. Disorders of sex differentiation. In: Larsen PR, Kronenberg HM, Melmed S, Polonsky KS, eds. *Williams textbook of endocrinology.* Philadelphia: WB Saunders, 2003:842–1002.

Kurzrock EA. Hypospadias. In: Finberg L, Kleinman RE, eds. *Saunders manual of pediatric practice.* Philadelphia: WB Saunders, 2002:878–880.

Lee P. Micropenis (hypogenitalism). In: Finberg L, Kleinman RE, eds. *Saunders manual of pediatric practice.* Philadelphia: WB Saunders, 2002:875–878.

Lippe BM, Saenger PH. Turner syndrome. In: Sperling MA, ed. *Pediatric endocrinology.* Philadelphia: WB Saunders, 2002:519–564.

Reiter EO, Saenger PH. Undescended testes. In: Finberg L, Kleinman RE, eds. *Saunders manual of pediatric practice.* Philadelphia: WB Saunders, 2002:880–881.

Styne DM. The testes. In: Sperling MA, ed. *Pediatric endocrinology.* Philadelphia: WB Saunders, 2002:562–629.

Witchel SF, Lee PA. Ambiguous genitalia. In: Sperling MA, ed. *Pediatric endocrinology.* Philadelphia: WB Saunders, 2002:111–134.

9 ♣ Disorders of Puberty

The striking physical changes of secondary sexual development during puberty are caused by remarkable changes in hypothalamic–pituitary–gonadal endocrine function. Puberty is best viewed as one stage in the continuum of reproductive function that begins during fetal life and extends through reproductive maturity and senescence. A secular trend of a decreasing age at onset of puberty of about 4 months each decade (using the recorded age of menarche as an indication) has been documented historically until about the 1950s in the United States. In spite of common perception, the age at onset of puberty has been stable until recently in the developed world, including the United States. However, with the increased prevalence of obesity in children in the United States, the age at onset of puberty, as reflected by the age of menarche, may be decreasing because of the advancement in physiological status caused by obesity.

PHYSICAL PUBERTAL DEVELOPMENT

The Tanner method of describing the stages of pubertal development is widely accepted (Sex Maturity Rating or SMR is an alternative term for Tanner staging in some texts). Objective description of physical development is essential to observe clinical progress:

Breast Development

B1: Prepubertal: elevation of the papilla only (Fig. 9-1).
B2: Breast buds are noted or palpable, with enlargement of the areola. This stage is quite subtle and may be missed. In obese children, breast development may be suggested by adipose tissue in the area with no true glandular development.
B3: Further enlargement of the breast and areola with no separation of their contours.
B4: Projection of areola and papilla to form a secondary mound over the rest of the breast.
B5: Mature breast with projection of papilla only.

Female Pubic Hair Development

PH1: Prepubertal: no pubic hair (Fig. 9-2).
PH2: Sparse growth of long, straight, or slightly curly minimally pigmented hair, mainly on the labia. This may be quite subtle and missed on cursory examination.
PH3: Considerably darker and coarser hair spreading over the mons pubis (above the vaginal opening).
PH4: Thick adult-type hair that does not yet spread to the medial surface of the thighs.
PH5: Hair is adult in type and is distributed in the classic inverse triangle.

No substantial enlargement of the clitoris occurs during puberty; significant enlargement would suggest an excess of androgen secretion rather than normal pubertal development.

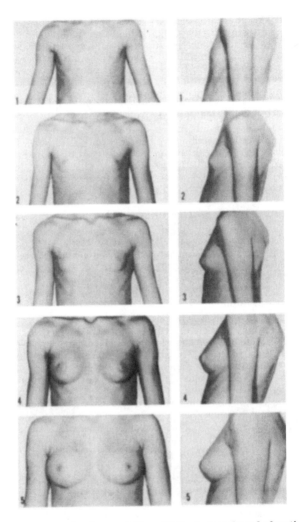

Fig. 9-1. Breast development. Stage B1 (top), prepubertal, elevation of the papilla only. Stage B2, breast buds visible or palpable with enlargement of the areola. Stage B3, further enlargement of the breast and areola with no separation of their contours (not shown). Stage B4, projection of areola and papilla to form a secondary mount over the rest of the breast. Stage B5 (bottom), mature breast with projection of papilla only. (From Tanner, Growth at Adolescence, 1962, Oxford, Blackwell Scientific Publications.)

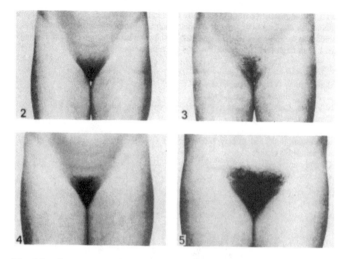

Fig. 9-2. Appearance of pubic and labial hair among girls. Stage PH1 (not shown), prepubertal, no pubic hair. Stage PH2 (upper left), sparse growth of long, straight, or slightly curly minimally pigmented hair, mainly on labia. Stage PH3 (upper right), considerably darker and coarser hair spreading over mons pubis. Stage PH4 (lower left), thick adult-type hair that does not yet spread to the medial surface of the thighs. Stage PH5 (lower right), hair is adult type and is distributed in the classic inverse triangle. (From Tanner, Growth at Adolescence, 1962, Oxford, Blackwell Scientific Publications.)

Male Genital Development

G1: Preadolescent.

G2: The testes are more than 2.5 cm in the longest diameter, excluding the epididymis, and the scrotum is thinning and reddening: No growth of the penis (Fig. 9-3).

G3: Growth of the penis occurs in width and length, and further growth of the testes is noted.

G4: The penis is further enlarged, and testes are larger, with a darker scrotal skin color.

G5: Genitalia are adult in size and shape.

The Prader orchidometer has ellipsoid standards representing testicular volume during puberty, which may be used to describe pubertal development.

Male Pubic Hair Development

P1: Preadolescent: no pubic hair (Fig. 9-3).

P2: Sparse growth of slightly pigmented, slightly curved pubic hair, mainly at the base of the penis. This stage is subtle and may be missed on casual examination.

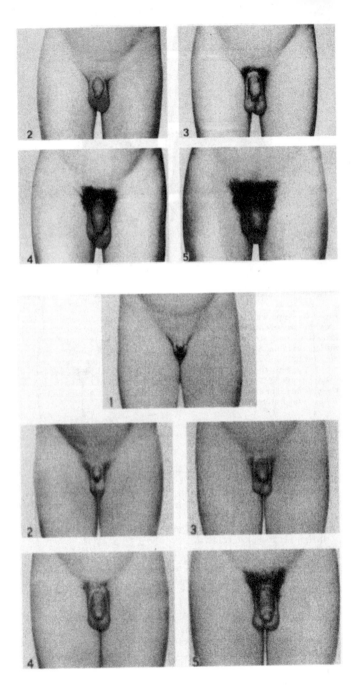

P3: Thicker, curlier hair spread laterally and to the pubic ramis.
P4: Adult-type hair that does not yet spread to the medial thighs.
P5: Adult-type hair spread to the medial thighs.

Pubertal Growth Spurt

At no time after the neonatal period does a child grow as rapidly as during the pubertal growth spurt. Both growth hormone (GH) and sex steroids add to this increase in linear velocity, during which girls gain an average of 25 cm, and boys gain an average of 28 cm. The difference in average adult height between men and women of 5 inches in the United States is partially because of the 2-year later age at onset of the pubertal growth spurt in boys compared with girls and partially to the difference in height attained during the process.

AGE AT ONSET OF PUBERTY

The normal age at onset of puberty in North America is 9 to 14 years in boys and has not appreciably changed in the last several decades, although recent data suggest that those boys with the greatest body mass index (BMI) values have the earliest age at onset of puberty and that this trend might be increasing. The determination of the age at onset of puberty in girls has become controversial. The previous range of pubertal development in U.S. girls had been stated to be 8 to 13 years. Recent reports suggest that an appreciable number of African American girls in the United States already have signs of puberty by age 6 years, and white girls have such signs by age 7 years. These findings do not necessarily indicate an earlier onset of puberty at the end of this century compared with the 1950s (when the last large data sets became available), because no data recorded the age of puberty in the United States in girls so young in the past with which to compare. Some find these data suspect and believe that the older limits are still appropriate. Nonetheless, reanalysis of the data from the 1997 study from which these conclusions emerged demonstrates that

----

Fig. 9-3.   Genital development and pubic hair growth among boys. Stage G1 (not shown), prepubertal. Stage G2 (upper left), enlargement of testis to >2.5 cm, appearance of scrotal reddening, and increase in rugations. Stage G3 (upper right), increase in length and to a lesser extent breadth of penis, with further growth of testes. Stage G4 (lower left), further increase in size of penis and testes and darkening of scrotal skin. Stage G5 (lower left), adult genitalia. Stage P1 (upper panel), preadolescent, no pubic hair. Stage P2 (middle left), sparse growth of slightly pigmented, slightly curved pubic hair, mainly at the base of the penis. Stage P3 (middle right), thicker curlier hair spread laterally. Stage P4 (lower left), adult-type hair that does not yet spread to medial thighs. Stage P5 (lower right), adult-type hair spread to medial thighs. (From Tanner, Growth at Adolescence, 1962, Oxford, Blackwell Scientific Publications.)

the earliest onset of puberty occurred in the girls with the greatest BMI values.

The following is proposed as a useful approach; if a girl appears to be otherwise healthy, without any evidence of neurologic or other chronic disease, and is showing breast or pubic hair development starting at 6 years if African American or 7 years if white, she might be carefully watched and not necessarily subjected to an extensive evaluation. However, consultation with a pediatric endocrinologist is strongly encouraged to determine which child fits into this observation category and which truly needs an evaluation. The time of transit from beginning to the end of puberty also is important. Rapid progression through the stages of puberty and very early onset of menses can indicate a disorder. Likewise a delay in progression after the initiation of puberty may indicate hypogonadism.

The average age at onset of puberty in the United States in girls is 10 years in white girls and 9 years in African American girls, whereas in boys, the mean is 10.5 years. Girls complete puberty in 1.5 to 6 years, with a mean of 4.2 years, whereas boys have a range of 2 to 4.5 years, with a mean of 3.5 years.

The age of menarche, being a single time point, is easier to establish than other stages of puberty and has been recorded for centuries. The age at menarche decreased 4 months per decade over the last 150 years, ceasing in the 1950s, with an age at menarche of 12.8 years in the United States. Remarkably a large cross-sectional study published in 1997 demonstrated an age at menarche of 12.2 years in African American girls and 12.9 in white U.S. girls, showing no appreciable change in the last 50 years. If indeed girls are now entering puberty at an earlier age, they appear to be spending longer in reaching the onset of menstrual periods.

ENDOCRINE CHANGES OF PUBERTY

The reawakening of gonadal function at puberty is known as gonadarche, and the increased adrenal androgen secretion of puberty is known as adrenarche. These processes are temporally related in the average child, but may be dissociated in, for example, premature adrenarche.

Gonadarche

The pituitary gonadotropins, luteinizing hormone (LH) and follicle-stimulating hormone (FSH), are secreted in response to hypothalamic gonadotropin-releasing hormone (GnRH). The GnRH is released episodically into the pituitary portal system in varying amplitudes and frequencies during different stages of development (and different stages of the menstrual cycle in females). If the pulsatile nature of GnRH secretion is altered to continuous secretion, the pituitary gonadotrope decreases its affinity for GnRH, and the number of GnRH receptors decreases, which leads to a decrease of gonadotropin secretion (downregulation). This phenomenon is used in treatment of precocious puberty with GnRH agonists.

LH stimulates the Leydig cells of the testes to secrete testosterone (T) in boys, and T exerts negative-feedback inhibition of LH secretion; LH has little effect in girls until after ovulation occurs, when it supports the corpus luteum. FSH stimulates ovarian follicle formation and estrogen secretion in girls, and estradiol (E_2) exerts negative feedback inhibition on FSH secretion. FSH has little effect in boys until spermarche (the onset of maturation of spermatozoa), when it supports the development of sperm. FSH also stimulates the development of the seminiferous tubules, which accounts for most of the enlargement of the testes at puberty, as Leydig cell stimulation has little effect on testicular size.

In addition to their steroid products, both ovaries and testes produce a protein (inhibin) that exerts negative-feedback inhibition on FSH secretion in both sexes. Inhibin is produced by the seminiferous tubules in males, whereas the follicle of the ovary produces inhibin in females. After ovulation, the theca cells of the ovaries secrete progesterone (P), and measurement of serum P may be used as a reflection of ovulation.

Hypothalamic GnRH and pituitary LH and FSH are present in the early fetus. By midgestation, when the pituitary portal system is formed and hypothalamic peptides can reach the pituitary, elevated GnRH secretion stimulates extremely increased secretion of LH and FSH, and serum levels are similar to those found in agonadal individuals. In the male fetus, testosterone increases [first because of stimulation by placental human chorionic gonadotropin (hCG), and by week 20 and after, by fetal LH] and is responsible for the enlargement of the penis in the second half of gestation as well as the normal suppression of pituitary LH secretion. Toward term, the gonadotropin concentrations decrease in the fetal circulation as the central nervous system (CNS) develops inhibitory influences on GnRH secretion.

After birth when the newborn is removed from the influence of maternal estrogen secretion, a period of instability occurs when LH and FSH concentrations increase in the newborn. Serum gonadotropin levels increase to elevated values characteristic of puberty in boys until age 6 months (or older) and in girls until 2 to 4 years. Elevated LH may stimulate T secretion in boys to concentrations greater than 150 ng/dL in the prepubertal range in the months after birth, and peaks of FSH may cause girls to have E_2 concentrations in the pubertal range during this period.

After infancy, gonadotropins and sex steroids are reduced to low concentrations until the peripubertal period (just before secondary sexual development begins). This midchildhood period is known as the "juvenile pause." The juvenile pause is caused by CNS suppression of gonadotropin secretion, but children without gonads or sex steroids, such as those with Turner syndrome, have elevated serum gonadotropin values during the juvenile pause in the absence of sex steroids, indicating the functional nature of negative feedback even before puberty.

Quantitative changes in gonadotropin secretion are noted in the peripubertal period. Gonadotropin concentrations increase during sleep because of increased amplitude of pulsatile secretion every 60 to 90 minutes. As puberty progresses, the peaks of gonadotropins occur throughout the day, until no diurnal variation remains in the adult. Gonadotropin values are higher in the adult than in the prepubertal child. The recent development of supersensitive third-generation gonadotropin assays allows single serum gonadotropin determinations to differentiate between puberty and prepuberty.

Sex-steroid secretion is more constant throughout the day than is gonadotropin secretion, but definite variation in estradiol levels is found, so that concentrations may vary from less than 10 pg/mL to 40 to 50 pg/mL within one 24-hour period. Assays with increased estradiol sensitivity are being developed, but commercial assays could be improved. Testosterone values are low in prepuberty and do not reach levels easily measured in standard testosterone assays until stage 3; sensitive testosterone assays are available in some commercial laboratories that specialize in endocrine conditions and should be used for accurate analysis in the diagnosis of early puberty (e.g., Quest Diagnostics, Exoterix, DSL Laboratories). More than 97% of sex steroids are noncovalently bound to sex hormone–binding globulin [SHBG, or testosterone-binding globulin (TeBG)]. SHBG increases in girls during puberty because of estrogen stimulation, but values of SHBG in boys decrease. Thus androgens in women are inactivated readily by SHBG, whereas androgens in men are relatively less bound, freer, and therefore more active. This difference in SHBG, in addition to the higher testosterone values in men, accounts for the greater androgenic activity of testosterone in men.

The increase in pituitary storage of readily releasable gonadotropin is reflected in the gonadotropin response to a bolus of exogenous GnRH. A 100 μg bolus of GnRH will cause an increase of LH greater than 16 mIU/mL in pubertal or adult subjects, whereas a far smaller increase is found in prepubertal subjects: thus the increase in LH after GnRH is a useful reflection of pubertal status. Girls of all ages release more FSH than do boys, so the FSH response to GnRH is not an adequate reflection of pubertal state. The GnRH test is more rarely used today because of the increased sensitivity of the gonadotropin assays and the limited supply of GnRH. Studies of the use of GnRH agonist as a test of gonadotropin secretion in delayed or precocious puberty suggest that this test substance may play an important role in diagnosis of disorders of puberty.

Adrenarche

An increase in adrenal androgens is noted several years before the onset of increasing gonadotropin secretion. The increase in the weak androgen dehydroepiandrosterone (DHEA) and its sulfate (DHEAS) occurs at 6 to 7 years in girls and 7 to 8 years in boys. The levels continue to increase through midpuberty. Control of adrenarche is separate from the mechanisms of gonadotropin stimulation; although adrenocorticotropic hormone (ACTH) must be present for adrenarche to occur, another as yet unknown factor also must be operative. The entire process occurs a few years earlier than normal in premature adrenarche, a condition classically considered mild and benign (see later for more complete discussion of the condition). Thus in premature adrenarche, serum DHEAS is higher than is age appropriate but is appropriate for the stage of pubic hair development. Now that puberty is recognized to start at an age earlier than considered appropriate in the past, the normal increase of DHEA at age 6 to 8 years may no longer hold true, and values may actually increase several years earlier than that in children destined to undergo puberty at the new lower boundary.

DELAYED PUBERTY (Table 9-1)

The term *delayed puberty* is applied to a boy who has not initiated secondary sexual development by age 14 years or a girl who has not done so by age 13 years. Because these are statistical limits set 2.5 standard deviations above the mean, it is still possible for the patient to be among the roughly 0.6% of the normal population who will enter puberty spontaneously at a later age, but by waiting until these limits to initiate a workup, the physician will limit the likelihood of performing an unnecessary evaluation. Abnormalities of the hypothalamic–pituitary–gonadal axis may allow a normal age at onset of puberty followed by a cessation of progression; thus patients who do not continue in their secondary sexual development after beginning also should be considered for evaluation.

Temporary Delayed Puberty

Constitutional Delay in Growth and Adolescence

Patients who are healthy but have a slower rate of development than average are said to have constitutional delay. These subjects will have a history of stature that is shorter than their age-matched peers throughout childhood, but their height will be appropriate for bone age. Their skeletal development usually will be delayed by more than 2.5 standard deviations. The body habitus will be thin. Although mental development will be appropriate for age, social development may lag behind if the patient has been treated as a younger child by family, teachers, and peers because of an immature appearance. Often a family history of constitutional delay is found, so mothers should be asked their age at onset of menarche or other aspects of puberty, and fathers, the age they started to shave or the age they ceased to grow in stature (mothers have been shown to be more accurate in their memory of their puberty than are fathers). Although considerable variation occurs, secondary sexual development generally occurs when a bone age of 12 is reached for boys and 11 for girls. It is rare for a patient to start puberty spontaneously after age 18 years, and usually a permanent gonadotropin deficiency is present if that age is reached without pubertal development occurring; cases of spontaneous pubertal development are rarely reported after age 20 years. Before that age, in the absence of a classic presentation of constitutional

Table 9-1.   Causes and classification of delayed puberty

Idiopathic (constitutional) delay in growth and puberty

Hypogonadotropic hypogonadism: delayed puberty related to
  gonadotropin deficiency

  CNS disorders

    Tumor
      Craniopharyngioma
      Germinoma
      Other germ cell tumors
        Hypothalamic and optic glioma
      Astrocytoma
      Pituitary tumor

    Other causes
      Langerhans histiocytosis
      Granulomatous and postinfectious lesions of the CNS
      Vascular abnormalities of the CNS
      Radiation therapy
      Congenital malformations especially associated with
        craniofacial anomalies
      Head trauma

  Isolated gonadotropin deficiency
    With hyposmia or anosmia: Kallmann syndrome
    Without anosmia
    Congenital adrenal hypoplasia (*DAX1* mutation)
    Isolated LH deficiency
    Isolated FSH deficiency

  Idiopathic and genetic forms of multiple pituitary hormone
    deficiencies
    Miscellaneous disorders
      Prader-Willi syndrome
      Laurence-Moon and Bardet-Biccil syndromes

  Functional gonadotropin deficiency
    Chronic systemic disease and malnutrition
      Sickle cell disease
      Cystic fibrosis
      Acquired immunodeficiency syndrome
      Chronic gastroenteric disease
      Chronic renal disease
      Malnutrition
      Anorexia nervosa
      Bulimia
      Psychogenic amenorrhea
      Impaired puberty and delayed menarche in female
        athletes and ballet dancers (exercise amenorrhea)
      Hypothyroidism
      Diabetes mellitus
      Cushing disease
      Hyperprolactinemia
      Marijuana use
      Gaucher disease

Table 9-1. *Continued*

Hypergonadotropic hypogonadism: delayed puberty related to
   gonadal failure
  Girls
    Syndrome of gonadal dysgenesis (Turner syndrome) and its
      variants
    XX and XY gonadal dysgenesis
      Familial and sporadic XX gonadal dysgenesis and its variants
    Other forms of primary ovarian failure
      Premature menopause
      Radiation therapy
      Chemotherapy
      Autoimmune oophoritis
      Resistant ovary
      Galactosemia
      Glycoprotein syndrome type 1
      FSH receptor gene mutators
      LH-hCG resistance
      Polycystic ovarian disease
      Noonan or pseudo-Turner syndrome
  Boys
    Syndrome of seminiferous tubular dysgenesis and its variants
      (Klinefelter syndrome)
    Other forms of primary testicular failure
      Chemotherapy
      Radiation therapy
      Testicular biosynthetic defects
      Sertoli only syndrome
      LH resistance
      Anorchism and cryptorchidism

CNS, central nervous systems; LH, luteinizing hormone; FSH, follicle-
stimulating hormone; hCG, human chorionic gonadotropin.

delay in puberty or neurologic symptoms related to gonadotropin
deficiency, it is difficult to differentiate temporary constitutional delay in puberty from permanent hypogonadotropic hypogonadism.

Various strategies of diagnosis are proposed to differentiate constitutional delay from isolated hypogonadotropic hypogonadism.
An increase in serum DHEAS and development of pubic hair at the
appropriate age of adrenarche in hypogonadotropic hypogonadism
is described without other secondary sexual development, whereas
both adrenarche and gonadarche are delayed in constitutional
delay in puberty. The increase in serum gonadotropins or sex
steroids after GnRH agonist is proposed to differentiate the two
conditions, as the increase is higher in constitutional delay. Unfortunately, none of these schemes has proven completely reliable in

all individual cases. After the elimination of serious disease (especially CNS disease), observation for physical changes of puberty with periodic sampling of gonadotropins and sex steroids at an established endocrine laboratory for elevation of pubertal levels is the standard method of diagnostic management.

Permanent Conditions of Sexual Infantilism

Hypothalamic Hypogonadism

Abnormalities of the hypothalamus or pituitary gland lead to lack of onset of pubertal development associated with low serum gonadotropins. If only gonadotropins are affected, the patient will be of normal height but may develop eunuchoid proportions (consisting of long legs and arms and an upper- to lower-segment ratio well below 0.9, the normal for adults). If GH is deficient as well, the patient's growth rate also will be decreased during childhood.

Isolated Gonadotropin Deficiency

In contrast to those patients with constitutional delay in puberty and those with GH deficiency, patients with isolated gonadotropin deficiency are of normal height until the adolescent age range when, because of an absent pubertal growth spurt, they fall behind normal subjects in growth rate; because of delayed epiphyseal closure, they may continue to grow and reach a normal or even increased adult height. They have characteristic eunuchoid proportions with long arms and legs for the size of their trunk, because epiphyseal fusion is delayed. Patients with midline defects may have congenital gonadotropin deficiency as well as other types of hypothalamic–pituitary disorders. The late acquisition of hypothalamic–pituitary deficiency must be considered a sign of a CNS tumor until proven otherwise.

Gonadotropin deficiency may manifest in several different manners. In the most severe form, puberty will not start or progress. However, puberty may start in some cases, and but the individual may fail to reach maturity, whereas some may progress throughout physical pubertal development but not achieve fertility. In some cases, constitutional delay in adolescence may coexist in the same family as Kallmann syndrome, suggesting a continuum between the two conditions.

Kallmann syndrome (*308700 KALLMANN SYNDROME 1; KAL1 at Xp22.3) classically consists of impaired sense of smell (hyposmia or anosmia) and gonadotropin deficiency. Within a family, some patients may have disorders of smell with normal gonadal function, and others may have abnormal gonadal function and normal sense of smell. The etiology of these cases is a lack of migration of GnRH neurons from the anterior region of the primitive nose in the early fetus to the normal postnatal location in the mediobasal hypothalamus, thus impairing the development of the control of gonadotropins, as well as the sense of smell. Inheritance may be X-linked because of mutation of the KAL gene, which codes for a neural cell adhesion molecule (anosmin) that is responsible for normal migration of the involved cells.

Kallmann syndrome may be associated with defects of the midline such as cleft palate, neurosensory hearing loss, and mirror extremity movements (synkinesia). Kallmann syndrome may follow an autosomal dominant pattern with mental retardation (*147950 KALLMANN SYNDROME 2; KAL2) and autosomal recessive (*244200 KALLMANN SYNDROME 3; KAL3) with midline defects, such as cleft palate or lip, as well as unilateral renal agenesis.

Other genetic causes of hypogonadotropic hypogonadism are

Mutations of the GnRH receptor (*138850 GONADOTROPIN-RELEASING HORMONE RECEPTOR; GNRHR at 4q21.2), as found in an autosomal recessive pattern.

Mutations of the FSH β gene (*136530 FOLLICLE-STIMULATING HORMONE, β-POLYPEPTIDE; FSHB at 11p13); gonadotropins are produced by the combination of α chains, which are identical in LH and FSH [as well as thyroid-stimulating hormone (TSH)] and β chains, which confer the specificity on the glycoprotein hormones.

Mutations of LH β (*152780 LUTEINIZING HORMONE, β POLYPEPTIDE; LHB at 19q13.32) may cause infertility in the pattern of the "fertile eunuch syndrome," with incomplete virilization, eunuchoid proportions due to impaired development of the Leydig cells; and development of the testicular seminiferous tubules and spermatozoa.

The absence of the DAX gene (*300200 ADRENAL HYPOPLASIA, CONGENITAL; AHC at Xp21.3-p21.2) leads to the combination of hypogonadotropic hypogonadism and adrenal hypoplasia (see later).

Abnormalities of the Central Nervous System

Central Nervous System Tumors

Gonadotropins, as well as all other pituitary hormones, may be affected by hypothalamic–pituitary tumors (also see Chapter 3). Late onset (as opposed to congenital onset) of pituitary deficiency, and particularly the combination of anterior and posterior pituitary defects, should suggest the diagnosis of a tumor of the CNS. Late onset of growth failure or cessation of pubertal development is of great concern.

Craniopharyngiomas are tumors of Rathke pouch originating in the pituitary stalk but spread to the suprasellar region as well as into the sella turcica. These tumors characteristically are diagnosed between ages 6 and 14 years. Usually, symptomatic patients may complain of headache, visual loss, polyuria, and polydipsia. On physical examination, the patient may be found to be short, hypothyroid, and sexually infantile, even if of pubertal age. In addition, papilledema or optic atrophy is found. However, indolent cases might be diagnosed with other evaluations (e.g., pituitary calcifications found on lateral skull radiograph done for other reasons or on orthodontic radiograph). Computed tomography (CT) will show flecks of calcium within the tumor in more than 80% of cases, but magnetic resonance imaging (MRI) scan with contrast will define the shape and size with better definition. The tumor may be cystic, and the sella may be eroded (irregular or enlarged sella might be seen on lateral skull radiograph, but MRI is far more sensitive). Transsphenoidal microsurgery can be used for excision if the tumor is intrasellar. Larger tumors usually cannot be removed completely without causing neurologic sequelae, but craniopharyngiomas are radiosensitive, and a combination of surgery and radiation is often used.

Other tumors of the CNS outside of the sella turcica, such as germinomas of the pineal, astrocytomas, and gliomas (which may be associated with neurofibromatosis), also may cause hypopituitarism. Intrasellar adenomas are rare but may impair pituitary function.

Histiocytosis X (Hand-Schüller-Christian disease) may cause only diabetes insipidus but also may affect other hypothalamic hormones. Granulomas of tuberculosis or sarcoidosis, postinfectious inflammation, and vascular lesions of the CNS all can impair hypothalamic–pituitary function. Trauma due to accidents, child abuse, or surgery for tumors near the area all can affect hypothalamic–pituitary function. Hydrocephalus may cause hypothalamic–pituitary deficiencies, as may any cause of increased intracranial pressure.

Congenital defects of the CNS should manifest in the neonatal period. Optic dysplasia, or the appearance of small pale optic disks usually surrounded by a dark margin, is associated with impaired vision and pendular (to-and-fro or horizontal) nystagmus: this condition should not be confused by acquired optic atrophy, an ominous sign of a tumor or other causes of increased intracranial pressure. Approximately 50% of patients with optic dysplasia have absence of the septum pellucidum, thus leading to the diagnosis of septooptic dysplasia (#182230 SEPTOOPTIC DYSPLASIA at 3p21.2-p21.1), which may be because of mutation of the homeobox gene HESX1. Some patients with septooptic dysplasia may be normal with respect to endocrine function, but any combination of anterior or posterior pituitary deficiencies can be manifest. Other midline defects, ranging from cleft palate to more severe anatomic midline defects, may be involved in hypothalamic–pituitary deficiencies.

Radiation treatment may cause GH deficiency or gonadotropin deficiency but also can cause precocious puberty in combination with GH deficiency.

Idiopathic Hypopituitarism

Congenital absence of any or all of the pituitary hormones may be found in idiopathic hypopituitarism. Because GH deficiency itself may delay the onset of puberty in an untreated patient, it may be difficult to determine which patient has gonadotropin deficiency until the teenage years. Familial hypopituitarism may follow an X-linked (*312000 PANHYPOPITUITARISM; PHP at Xq25-q26) or an autosomal recessive pattern (#262600 PITUITARY DWARFISM III at 9q34.3), sometimes with diabetes insipidus (241540 HYPOPITUITARISM, CONGENITAL, WITH CENTRAL DIABETES INSIPIDUS). Further, mutation in the pituitary transcription factor PROP1 (*601538 PROPHET OF PIT1, PAIRED-LIKE HOMEODOMAIN TRANSCRIPTION FACTOR; PROP1 at 5q) leads to hypopituitarism with absence of GHRH (see Chapter 3).

Newborn males with GH deficiency or gonadotropin deficiency may have microphallus (penile length less than 2.0 cm, which represents 2.5 standard deviations below the mean for term). The absence of GH or ACTH may lead to hypoglycemic seizures, and the combination of hypoglycemia and microphallus in a newborn boy should cause immediate concern over congenital hypopituitarism, especially if pendular nystagmus occurs in addition. The microphallus can be treated with low-dose testosterone therapy (25 mg intramuscularly every month for three doses) to enlarge the penis without causing advancement of the bone age; sex reversal is not appropriate in boys with congenital hypopituitarism with microphallus, as the penis can grow with treatment. It is important to note that later in childhood, obese boys are often brought to evaluation for microphallus, when in fact, their normal-sized penis is buried in the fat of the pubic area: if the adipose tissue is reflected away during the measurement of the stretched penis, the measurement will likely be normal, eliminating the diagnosis of microphallus and concern over hypogonadism.

Disorders and Syndromes

The Prader-Willi syndrome (#176270 PRADER-WILLI SYN-DROME; PWS at 15q12, 15q11-q13, 15q11) includes fetal and infantile hypotonia, short stature, obesity, and lack of satiety, almond-shaped eyes and characteristic facies, small hands and feet, mental retardation, and microphallus and undescended testes in boys or delayed menarche in girls. Rare patients are described as being of tall stature during childhood. The etiology is microdeletion of 15q11 in 70% of patients, which can be confirmed with fluorescent *in situ* hybridization (FISH), or caused by maternal disomy of the SNRPN gene in most others (see Chapter 5).

The Laurence-Moon (*245800 LAURENCE-MOON SYN-DROME) and Bardet-Biedl (#209900 BARDET-BIEDL SYN-DROME; BBS at 20p12, 16q21, 15q22.3-q23, 11q13, 3p13-p12, 2q31) syndromes share some features but are now considered two separate entities. Obesity, short stature, mental retardation, and retinitis pigmentosum can be associated with hypogonadotropic hypogonadism or hypergonadotropic hypogonadism. In the Laurence-Moon syndrome, spastic paraplegia is found, whereas the Bardet-Biedl syndrome includes polydactyly and other features of many organ systems; both syndromes follow an autosomal recessive pattern of inheritance.

Weight loss due to chronic disease, malnutrition, and even dieting to less than 80% of ideal weight can cause hypogonadotropic hypogonadism. Thus a host of diseases including poorly treated diabetes mellitus, gastrointestinal (GI) disorders causing malabsorption, and connective tissue diseases, among others, may cause delayed puberty.

A very severe example of weight loss and hypogonadotropic hypogonadism is anorexia nervosa, a psychiatric disorder of disturbed body image associated with avoidance of food, regurgitation of ingested food, and performance of rituals around food (e.g., some affected patients may ironically do all of the shopping and cooking for the family). Primary or secondary amenorrhea is frequently found in affected girls, and the onset of puberty may be delayed. Weight loss causes a reversion of gonadotropin-secretion patterns to prepubertal, low-amplitude pulsatile secretion. The psychiatric state may itself cause amenorrhea to persist, even after weight regain.

Athletic amenorrhea may occur with increased physical activity in the presence of weight loss, such as in ballerinas or gymnasts. However, athletic amenorrhea also may occur in spite of maintenance of normal body weight, such as found in swimmers or ice skaters; decreased physical activity allows the resumption of pubertal development or menses, sometimes with no change in weight.

Hypothyroidism will inhibit the onset of puberty and menses and, if hypothyroidism occurs after the onset of puberty, will stop the progression of puberty. Remarkably, severe hypothyroidism has been associated with some features of precocious puberty (see Chapter).

Hypergonadotropic Hypogonadism

Hypergonadotropic hypogonadism is synonymous with primary gonadal failure. Serum gonadotropins are elevated because of lack of feedback inhibition from the gonads.

The Turner syndrome of gonadal dysgenesis is the most common form of primary gonadal failure in a female phenotype; the incidence is between 1:2,000 and 1:5,000 live phenotypic female births. Turner syndrome is because of a loss or abnormality of one X chromosome or a portion of it. The SHOX gene (*312865 SHORT STATURE HOMEOBOX; SHOX at Xpter-p22.32) on the short arm of the X chromosome near the pseudo-autosomal region is absent, with the lack of its locus on the aberrant or absent X chromosome; this gene is related to the short stature of Turner syndrome and gives rise to the Madelung deformity of the wrist (see later). It has been estimated that the 45X karyotype occurs in one of 15 spontaneous abortions and that 99.9% of 45X fetuses do not survive longer than 28 weeks of gestation. Classic cases have a 45X karyotype (no Barr body on found buccal smear, but this test has been replaced by karyotype determination; the Barr body determination should no longer be used for diagnosis because of lack of reliability). Physical features of Turner syndrome include short stature (average adult height is 143 cm), streak gonads (a normal complement of ova are present at birth, but accelerated oocyte death leads to the abnormality of ovarian development), sexual infantilism, and a female phenotype. Other findings include fish-mouth appearance (down-turned edges of the mouth) with retrognathia and high-arched palate, ptosis and epicanthal folds, broad shield-like chest, the appearance of wide-spaced and hypoplastic nipples, short webbed neck with low hairline, short fourth metacarpals, Madelung abnormality of the wrist (radial shortening and bowing with dorsal subluxation of the distal ulna), wide carrying angle of the arms (cubitus valgus), knock-knee appearance (genu valgum), abnormalities of the shape of the kidneys (e.g., horseshoe kidneys or duplications), multiple nevi, spoon-shaped (hyperconvex) hypoplastic nails, lymphedema of the extremities, particularly in infancy, and left-sided heart anomalies (such as coarctation of the aorta). At birth, many patients have lymphedema of the extremities and loose skin folds around the neck, which later scar down into the classic webbed neck and account for the low-set ears. Patients usually have normal intelligence but may perform poorly on tests of visual-spatial perception and demonstrate other defects in memory and executive function. Frequent episodes of otitis media in childhood may lead to conductive hearing loss, although sensorineural hearing loss is possible, as well. Frequent urinary tract infections in those with abnormal kidney function also are a feature. A tendency exists toward keloid formation, which can complicate attempts to correct the webbed neck surgically. A tendency toward Hashimoto thyroiditis is found, as well as insulin insensitivity.

Variants of Turner syndrome occur with abnormal X chromosome or mosaicism (e.g., XO/XX). Such patients may have some gonadal function and a more normal female phenotype. Other variants of Turner syndrome include patients with mosaicism, such as XO/XY; because these patients may have dysgenetic testes rather than streak gonads and are at risk for malignant degeneration of the gonad, orchiectomy is indicated. Phenotype may be infantile female to ambiguous genitalia or phenotypic male. A FISH probe for Y chromosome material may be performed.

GH treatment increases stature in Turner syndrome, an approved indication for this medication. The age of estrogen replacement is of concern, for if it is offered too early and in high dosage, it will decrease the adult height achieved, even with GH therapy.

Affected girls require cardiac evaluation for left-sided heart defects and appropriate follow-up care. A renal ultrasound examination must be carried out to see if there is a renal anomaly and if it is significant.

Noonan syndrome (#163950 NOONAN SYNDROME 1; NS1 12q24.1), or pseudo-Turner syndrome, is a dominantly inherited condition with features similar to Turner syndrome (such as webbed neck, ptosis, short stature, wide carrying angle, and lymphedema), as well as features different from those of Turner syndrome (such as normal karyotype, triangle-shaped face, pectus excavatum, right-sided heart disease, and more commonly, mental retardation). Affected boys may have undescended, often impaired, testes.

XX and XY gonadal dysgenesis may be sporadic or familial. Stature is normal, and phenotype is sexually infantile female in the XX form (*233400 GONADAL DYSGENESIS, XX TYPE, WITH DEAFNESS) or may be ambiguous in the XY form (*306100 GONADAL DYSGENESIS, XY FEMALE TYPE; GDXY). Patients with an XY karyotype should undergo gonadectomy because of potential neoplastic degeneration of the dysgenetic testes (see Chapter 8).

Klinefelter syndrome, or seminiferous tubular dysgenesis, is the most common cause of testicular failure, with an incidence of 1 in 500 to 1,000 males. Because of variable Leydig cell function, serum testosterone levels in the adult patient vary from low to close to normal. Therefore the onset of puberty is often normal, but secondary sexual changes do not progress to the adult stage. Seminiferous tubular function is invariably affected, and impaired spermatogenesis is the rule. In puberty or in the adult, testes are hard and grow no longer than 3.5 cm, with histologic changes of hyalinization and fibrosis of the seminiferous tubules.

Stature is often taller than average. A significantly decreased upper- to lower-segment ratio (less than 0.9) is apparent, although arm span is not necessarily greater than height, as is found in patients with eunuchoid proportions. Serum LH and especially FSH are elevated to castrate levels. Gynecomastia is common, and breast cancer may develop (20-fold increased risk over a non-affected male). Germ cell tumors of the mediastinum also are more likely in affected males. Even before the onset of puberty, testes are small, upper- to lower-segment ratio is decreased for age, but arm span is equal to height, and these body proportions remain into adulthood.

Some patients come to evaluation because of personality disorders and learning disability in the prepubertal age range. For example, a verbal IQ disproportionately lower than performance IQ and expressive developmental defects in speech and language are found. A tendency toward explosive outbursts and difficulty in controlling anger are seen, even though the individuals otherwise tend to be passive. Thus the diagnosis should always been entertained in a child with any of these personality or learning problems.

Klinefelter syndrome results from nondisjunction of the sex chromosomes. It is more common with advanced maternal age. The karyotype is classically 47XXY. Variants of Klinefelter syndrome are reported, with mosaicism such as in XX/XXY, XXYY, XXXY, and XXXXY karyotypes. Other patients are reported with features similar to those of Klinefelter syndrome but with an XX karyotype (XX males); in these cases, transfer of the SRY from the Y to the X chromosome is the cause (see Chapter 8).

Cryptorchidism refers to unilateral or bilateral undescended testes and must be differentiated from anorchia, which is the complete absence of both testes. The testes develop in the abdominal cavity, but by month 7 of gestation, descend into the scrotum. Thus more than 97% of term and 79% of premature infant boys have descent of the testes. By age 9 months, 99.2% of testes are descended, with little progress there after. Thus by age 9 to 12 months, most testes that will descend spontaneously will have done so. Lack of descent is associated with a 10-fold increase in neoplasia, and the inability to examine undescended testes for changes makes the situation all the more worrisome. Thus, by age 1 year, all undescended testes should undergo orchiopexy or, if abnormal, orchiectomy. Although an increase in the incidence of carcinoma is noted if the testes are left in their undescended position, evidence exists that undescended testes have an intrinsic problem, as one third of carcinomas develop in cryptorchid testes after orchiopexy, and 20% of cryptorchid patients have carcinoma in the contralateral descended testes. A sequence of evaluations may determine whether bilateral cryptorchidism or anorchia is present. The administration of hCG, 3,000 units/m^2 intramuscularly (this is only one of several recommended dosages) should induce an increase in testosterone greater than 100 ng/dL within 72 hours in a cryptorchid neonate or infant, by interaction with the Leydig cell receptor. This response after only one dose of hCG in infancy is because of the priming effect of hCG stimulation of the testes during pregnancy. If the patient is in mid-childhood or older, one injection of hCG is likely to be inadequate to stimulate the Leydig cells, and a longer course of six injections of hCG separated by more than 2 weeks may be required (hCG is not to be given daily, or it will lose effectiveness because of downregulation of the LH receptor), with serum testosterone determined 24 hours after the last dose. Further, if hCG is given over a 2-week period, the testes may descend into the scrotum if the inguinal ring is not definitively too small, making orchiopexy unnecessary. GnRH or GnRH agonist has been used to promote testicular descent in some studies. It has been suggested that hCG and GnRH work only in cases of retractable or "yo-yo" testes, which travel up and down in the canal at various times during the day and in which surgery might not be indicated.

Orchiopexy is indicated at age 1 year if no descent of the testes occurs after hCG; it is thought that further testicular damage will occur if the testes are left in their warmer, intraabdominal location. If no increase in testosterone can be induced with one to six injections of hCG, the patient may have no Leydig cells and therefore has anorchia. Detection of inhibin indicates the presence of testicular tissue and can help to eliminate the diagnosis of anorchia. Elevation of gonadotropins above the normal for age indicates lack of testicular tissue. Ultrasound examination in experienced hands can reveal presence of the testes, but lack of visualization may not be definitive proof of absence of the testes. Exploratory surgery, which may lead either to orchiopexy if normal testicular tissue is found, or to diagnosis of anorchia if no testes are found, may be indicated. In anorchia, the testes were present during fetal life to allow the development of a normal male phenotype and normal wolffian duct structures, but the testes atrophied, possibly because of vascular insufficiency subsequent to genital development.

Survival is now possible in a wide range of childhood cancers. However, radiation therapy to the area of the gonads or chemotherapy may take a toll on gonadal function. Elevated gonadotropins suggest the diagnosis of gonadal failure after a period of follow-up. The damage to the gonads may occur whether the agents are administered during the pubertal or the prepubertal period.

Differential Diagnosis of Delayed Puberty

The first step in laboratory diagnosis of delayed puberty is to determine whether the patient has primary gonadal disease and hypergonadotropic hypogonadism or hypothalamic–pituitary disease and hypogonadotropic hypogonadism (Fig. 9-4). If the gonadotropins are high, consideration should be given toward a diagnosis that might be confirmed by karyotype, such as Turner syndrome or Klinefelter syndrome or their variants, even if the physical examination has not yet suggested these possibilities.

The most difficult part of diagnosis involves differentiation between temporary constitutional delay in puberty and permanent hypogonadotropic hypogonadism, both of which will have low serum gonadotropin values. If midline abnormalities are present or anosmia is present, the diagnosis is likely to be permanent impairment. If a compelling family history is found of delayed but ultimately spontaneous puberty (e.g., the father shaved later than his peers or mother's menarche was delayed), the diagnosis is likely to be constitutional delay in puberty. The presence of increased serum gonadotropin values into the pubertal range on third-generations assays, nighttime peaks of gonadotropins, a pubertal response of LH after GnRH or increasing a.m. serum testosterone values suggest that secondary sexual development will occur within a few months. Without these indications, the patient must be watched for signs of spontaneous pubertal development or an increase in sex steroid concentrations.

Other strategies to differentiate temporary from permanent conditions have been attempted: for example, an increase in adrenal androgens and the appearance of pubic hair without signs of gonadarche is reported at the usual age of puberty in hypogonadotropic hypogonadism, but a delay occurs in the increase in adrenal androgens and the appearance of all signs of secondary sexual development in constitutional delay in puberty. Alternatively, an increase in LH after GnRH agonist administration greater in constitutional delay than in hypogonadotropic hypogonadism is described. Unfortunately, these tests, and others, have proven to be less reliable in individual patients than in larger populations of study patients. Thus watchful waiting remains the main method of diagnosing delayed puberty: if a patient has not gone through the changes of puberty spontaneously by age 18 to 19 years, it is unlikely that he or she will do so.

If hypogonadotropic hypogonadism is suspected, with or without other endocrine anomalies, the underlying etiology must be investigated. Although hypogonadotropic hypogonadism might be an isolated finding, a CNS tumor could be present. Complete neurologic evaluation is performed and MRI considered if no other diagnosis or chronic disease is established.

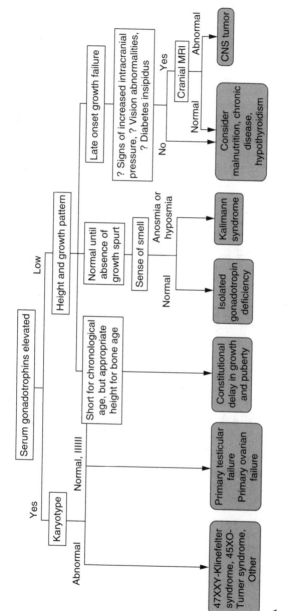

Fig. 9-4. A: Evaluation of absence of secondary sexual development among boys at 14 years and girls at 13 years.

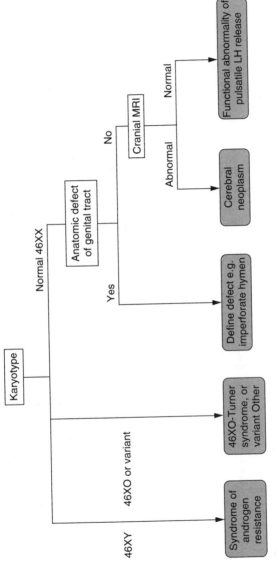

Fig. 9-4.(continued) B: Evaluation of primary amenorrhea with normal secondary sexual development. (Revised from Styne DM, Cuttler L. Normal pubertal development. In: Rudolph CD, Rudolph AM, eds. *Rudolph's pediatrics.* New York: McGraw-Hill, 2002:2093–2105, with permission.)

B

The differential diagnosis of primary amenorrhea with normal secondary sexual development may encompass the realm of chromosome anomalies, anatomic defects, or endocrine defects noted in this chapter. Historical and physical features may point the way to possible diagnosis, but Fig. 9-5 demonstrates the reasoning that may be used, based on the results of a karyotype determination after initial evaluation is complete.

Treatment of Delayed Puberty

It is less clear what psychological effects are caused by delayed puberty due to an immature appearance in subjects in the home environment compared with those who have chosen to be evaluated at the clinic, but no doubt exists that some patients have considerable stress with pubertal delay. As a general rule, boys are more distressed than girls. Certainly psychological status should be investigated and support offered if necessary, no matter what diagnosis is established.

Sex steroids are used to promote pubertal development in hypogonadotropic hypogonadism and also are useful temporarily in constitutional delay. If the difference between the two cannot be established, 3 months of low-dose sex steroid therapy can be used in patients feeling the pressure of an immature appearance who are not comforted by the thought of "waiting for nature to take its course." The goal is to cause some progression of secondary sexual development without advancing bone age and decreasing final height.

Individuals with hypogonadotropic hypogonadism have a risk of decreased bone density as adults; even those with constitutional delay in puberty have decreased areal bone density analysis, but when volumetric bone density is determined, the decrease is not apparent. Thus adequate calcium must be ingested at the very least; most teenagers do not get recommended doses of calcium anyway, so encouraging calcium is always wise. A genetic influence affects bone density, so sex steroid replacement may allow a closer approximation of the normal curve of bone density with age.

After age 14 years (the upper age at onset of normal pubertal development), boys may be given 100 mg of testosterone enanthate intramuscularly every month for 3 months. If no sign of spontaneous puberty occurs in the 3 months after the treatment, another course of testosterone can be offered after the interval. Patients with known hypogonadotropic hypogonadism will have to receive testosterone therapy continuously in increasing doses until the final dose of 250 to 300 mg/month is reached over a 6- to 12-month period. Often lower doses are given every 2 rather than every 3 to 4 weeks in higher doses. Some men will require hCG injections in addition to testosterone to promote pubic hair development and to achieve a more normal adult appearance. Testosterone may be administered by skin patches or even by the daily use of gel (under evaluation by the FDA for those under 16 years) if the patient wishes to avoid injections. However, no appropriate oral preparation is available, as methyl testosterone may cause liver damage.

(text continues on page 185)

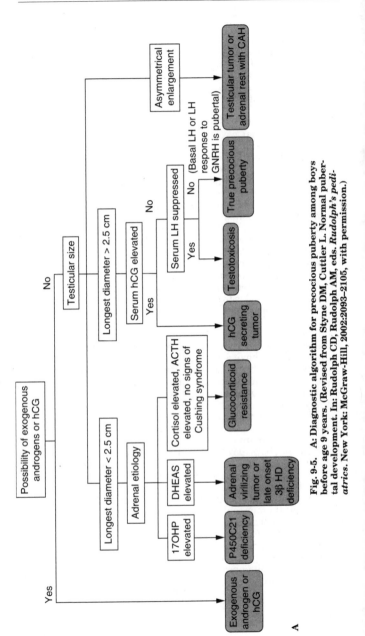

Fig. 9-5. A: Diagnostic algorithm for precocious puberty among boys before age 9 years. (Revised from Styne DM, Cuttler L. Normal pubertal development. In: Rudolph CD, Rudolph AM, eds. *Rudolph's pediatrics.* New York: McGraw-Hill, 2002:2093–2105, with permission.)

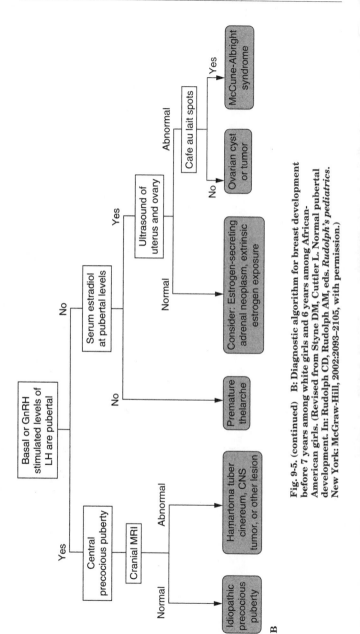

Fig. 9-5. (continued)   B: Diagnostic algorithm for breast development before 7 years among white girls and 6 years among African-American girls. (Revised from Styne DM, Cuttler L. Normal pubertal development. In: Rudolph CD, Rudolph AM, eds. *Rudolph's pediatrics.* New York: McGraw-Hill, 2002:2093–2105, with permission.)

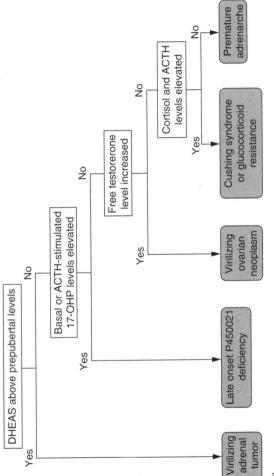

Fig. 9-5. (continued) C: Diagnostic algorithm for pubic hair before 7 years among white girls and 6 years among African-American girls. DHEAS, dehydroepiandrostenedione sulfate; 17α-OHP, 17α-hydroxy-progesterone; GnRH, gonadotropin-releasing hormone. (Reprinted from Styne DM, Cuttler L. Normal pubertal development. In: Rudolph CD, Rudolph AM, eds. *Rudolph's pediatrics.* New York: McGraw-Hill, 2002:2093–2105, with permission.)

Patients with GH deficiency who have been treated with GH regularly since an early age usually can receive the sex steroid treatment regimen described earlier. If they remain quite short or have not been treated before the teenage years, testosterone therapy may be withheld for a while and continued at lower dosage to ensure that maximal growth is reached before epiphyseal fusion eliminates the ability to respond to GH. Some investigators have even used GnRH analogue to delay the progression or onset of puberty to allow increased growth on GH as an experimental therapy. Girls with delayed puberty may be treated with low-dose estrogen therapy.

Ethinyl estradiol may be made into capsules and administered at 5 to 10 g/day for 3 months if the diagnosis is constitutional delay. If hypogonadotropic hypogonadism is proved, or if the patient has hypergonadotropic hypogonadism, treatment may continue and increase so that 10 to 15 g/day of ethinyl estradiol is given after feminizing effects are noted. After several months, and certainly after the appearance of breakthrough bleeding, estradiol is given only on days 1 to 21 of the month. If such small dose of ethinyl estradiol cannot be compounded, conjugated estrogen, 0.3 mg, might be used with care. Usually withdrawal bleeding will then occur regularly each month after the end of the estradiol administration. A progestational agent such as medroxyprogesterone acetate (5 mg) is given on days 12 to 21 of the cycle to achieve a more normal endocrine milieu and to decrease the risk of uterine neoplasia from the estrogen itself. Because of the suspected increase in uterine carcinoma with exogenous estrogen treatment, it is recommended that a girl taking estrogens have a pelvic examination yearly. Girls and parents must be warned about increased risk of breast cancer with estrogen therapy, especially in those with a family history of this disease. Similar to the case in boys, girls with GH deficiency should not receive long-term or higher-dose estrogen therapy until growth rate is normalized by GH administration.

Patients with Turner syndrome (the syndrome of gonadal dysgenesis) may benefit from new developments in the treatment of their growth deficiency. Previously these girls were not given estrogens until the late teenage years for fear of decreasing their final height; now, low-dose estrogens are started earlier to allow secondary sexual development at an appropriate age, such as 13 years, and to reduce psychosocial pressure. Growth rate can be increased in Turner syndrome with administration of GH. Final height is increased in most subjects. The addition of oxandrolone, a weak oral androgen, is reported to increase the effect of GH. Side effects of oxandrolone include pubic hair development, enlargement of the clitoris, and lowering of the voice, so this agent is added only after the age of onset of normal puberty, if at all. The combination of GH and estrogen has not increased adult height more than GH alone in studies when the estrogen is started early.

The infertility of Turner syndrome also has been addressed. With the appropriate endocrine support, a donated ovum may be fertilized, perhaps by an affected individual's partner by using the technique of *in vitro* fertilization, and transferred to a subject with Turner syndrome. Thus affected individuals may be able to maintain a pregnancy to term and give birth. Of course, adoption is a well-recognized option for an individual who wishes to be a parent.

SEXUAL PRECOCITY (Table 9-2)

If a boy develops secondary sexual characteristics before age 9 years, the condition is sexual precocity. The diagnosis is more controversial in girls, but when a girl has signs of puberty before 7 years if white or 6 years if African American, according to the new standards proposed earlier, the girl has precocious puberty. However, a girl younger than 9 years may still have a disorder advancing her pubertal development, particularly if she proceeds rapidly through puberty, if menarche occurs before age 9 years, or if neurologic or other signs of disease accompany such early puberty. In these cases and in any case in which concern arises, investigation for a disorder causing precocious puberty is warranted, rather than simply relying on the age criteria stated earlier. If the etiology of early puberty is the premature maturation of the hypothalamic–pituitary axis in boys or girls, the condition is central or true precocious puberty, which is a gonadotropin-dependent condition; if the etiology is autonomous secretion of sex steroids in boys or girls or autonomous secretion of hCG in boys, the condition is incomplete precocious puberty or pseudo-precocious puberty, a gonadotropin-independent condition. Patients of both categories will have rapid growth and skeletal maturation and, without treatment, may fulfill the paradox of the tall child who ceases growing early because of premature epiphyseal fusion and becomes a short adult.

Central (Complete or True) Precocious Puberty

Constitutional Precocious Puberty

Some children will normally begin puberty somewhat before the lower age limits of normal pubertal development described earlier, without evidence of an organic disorder. A family tendency toward this situation will point to the diagnosis. However, no signs of neurologic or other serious disease must be present, and the sequence of events and progression must be the same as in normal puberty to attribute this to a constitutional tendency. Early onset of puberty must be considered a disorder until proven otherwise.

Idiopathic Precocious Puberty

If no tumor or other definitive diagnosis is found, and if no family tendency exists, the diagnosis of exclusion is idiopathic precocious puberty. These patients manifest all of the endocrine findings of normal puberty, albeit at an earlier age. Their progress may be normal and continuous or slow and waxing and waning. Boys with this condition will first demonstrate symmetrical and progressive testicular enlargement, just as found in normal puberty. Girls are brought to evaluation of idiopathic precocious puberty more often than boys in the United States, probably as a reflection of differing parental concerns about girls compared with boys.

Table 9-2.   Causes and classification of sexual precocity

Complete isosexual precocious puberty (GnRH-dependent sexual precocity or premature activation of the hypothalamic pulse generator)
Familial or constitutional central precocious puberty
Idiopathic true precocious puberty

CNS tumors
   Craniopharyngioma
   Hamartoma of the tuber cincreum
   Craniooptic glioma associated with neurofibromatosis type 1
   Hypothalamic astrocytoma
   Ependymoma

Other CNS disorders
   Encephalitis
   Static encephalopathy
   Brain abscess
   Sarcoid or tubercular granuloma
   Head trauma
   Hydrocephalus
   Arachnoid cyst
   Myelomeningocele
   Vascular lesion
   Cranial irradiation

True precocious puberty after late therapy for congenital virilizing adrenal hyperplasia or other previous chronic exposure to sex steroids

Incomplete isosexual precocity (hypothalamic GnRH independent)
Boys
   Gonadotropin-secreting tumors
      hCG-secreting CNS tumor (e.g., chorioepithelioma, germinoma, teratoma)
      hCG-secreting tumors outside the CNS (hepatoma, teratoma, choriocarcinoma)
   Increased androgen secretion by adrenal gland or testis
      Congenital adrenal hyperplasia (CYP21 and CYP11B1 deficiencies)
      Virilizing adrenal neoplasm
      Leydig cell adenoma
      Familial testotoxicosis (sex-limited autosomal-dominant pituitary gonadotropin-independent precocious Leydig cell and germ cell maturation)
      Cortisol resistance syndrome
Girls
   Ovarian cyst
   Estrogen-secreting ovarian or adrenal neoplasm
   Peutz-Jeghers syndrome

Continued

Table 9-2. *Continued*

Both sexes
  McCune-Albright syndrome
  Hypothyroidism
  Iatrogenic or exogenous sexual precocity (including
    unintentional exposure to estrogens in food, drugs, or
    cosmetics)
Variations of pubertal development
  Premature thelarche
  Premature isolated menarche
  Premature adrenarche
  Adolescent gynecomastia of boys

CNS, central nervous system; hCG, human chorionic gonadotropin; GnRH, gonadotropin-releasing hormone.

Central Nervous System Disorders

Central precocious puberty occurs more often in girls than in boys. However, CNS tumors are found more often in boys with precocious puberty than in girls. In all cases of central precocious puberty, a CNS tumor must be considered the etiology; idiopathic conditions are diagnoses of exclusion.

Hamartomas of the tuber cinereum are composed of ectopic hypothalamic tissue and usually contain GnRH in the neurons. They function as a supplemental hypothalamus that operates outside of the normal inhibitory effects of the CNS on GnRH secretion. They have characteristic locations and appearances on MRI, so biopsy is rarely necessary. They are not neoplasms and do not enlarge, but are rather "tumors" in the sense that they are masses that take up space. Because of their sensitive location, hamartomas of the tuber cinereum are not amenable to surgical removal: medical therapy with GnRH agonists is the treatment of choice for this form of precocious puberty. However, because intractable gelastic (laughing) or other types of epilepsy may accompany the hamartoma, surgical treatment is rarely used for other reasons than precocious puberty.

More ominous CNS tumors include astrocytomas, ependymomas, and gliomas of the optic nerve or hypothalamus. Germinomas may secrete hCG and cause incomplete precocious puberty in boys (see later) or may activate the entire hypothalamic–pituitary axis and cause true precocious puberty. Germinomas are radiation sensitive. See Chapters 3 and 5 for more discussion of CNS tumors that affect growth.

Other CNS causes of true precocious puberty include most space-occupying lesions or causes of increased intracranial pressure, including granulomas, suprasellar cysts, hydrocephalus, or head trauma.

The McCune-Albright syndrome (#174800 MCCUNE-ALBRIGHT SYNDROME; MAS at 20q13.2) involves the triad of café-au-lait spots, fibrous dysplasia of the long bones (cysts are notable on radiograph or bone scan, and pathologic fractures are found), and either central or incomplete precocious puberty. Other syndromes exhibiting increased endocrine activity such as Cushing syndrome, hyperthyroidism, pituitary gigantism, and hypophosphatemic rickets are found in McCune-Albright syndrome. The wide-ranging effects of this condition are because of a somatic mutation in the Gα-stimulatory protein of the adenyl cyclase pathway. Thus the LH receptor and other membrane-based protein hormone receptors are constitutively activated and always functioning, even in the absence of the stimulatory ligand. Multiple tissues (e.g., skin, bone, Leydig cells, follicular cells, thyroid cells, adrenal cortical cells, and pituitary cells, as well as others) are activated in a random distribution in the body.

Severe hypothyroidism can cause delayed puberty or, paradoxically, precocious puberty. Any virilizing condition, when resolved, can trigger true precocious puberty, presumably because of maturation of the hypothalamic–pituitary axis. This may occur after glucocorticoid treatment is initiated for long-untreated virilizing congenital adrenal hyperplasia (CAH), after the removal of an adrenal androgen-secreting tumor, and after androgen therapy for various disorders, such as anemia.

Incomplete Precocious Puberty

Girls

Incomplete isosexual precocious puberty may develop in girls because of ovarian or adrenal secretion of, or ingestion of, estrogen. Serum gonadotropins are suppressed, whereas serum estradiol concentrations are elevated.

Ovarian follicular cysts can secrete enough estrogen to cause breast development, and when the cyst resolves, withdrawal bleeding can occur. Usually cysts are small and limited in effect, but some can secrete enough estrogen to cause serum estradiol concentrations to increase as high as those found in tumors. Cysts may occur only once, but recurrent cysts are possible. Surgical intervention is rarely indicated for simple cysts.

Estrogen-secreting tumors include granulosa cell tumors (the most common), gonadoblastomas (which can arise in streak gonads of gonadal dysgenesis), lipoid tumors, and ovarian carcinomas. The majority of granulosa cell tumors can be palpated by bimanual examination.

Exogenous estrogen exposure may occur through diet (chicken necks, beef, or veal may still contain estrogen because of improper estrogen treatment, although this is supposedly no longer likely), or by ingestion of medications that may include estrogen (perhaps given to mother or grandmother), or even by skin absorption after contact with estrogen-containing cosmetics or hair cream.

Boys

Boys can develop incomplete isosexual precocious puberty either by autonomous secretion of sex steroids or by tumor production of hCG, which will cause testosterone secretion from Leydig cells due to hCG interaction with the LH receptors. hCG production causes no endocrine or physical effects in girls.

Androgen secretion can occur because of 21-hydroxylase or 11-hydroxylase deficiency CAH, adrenal carcinomas, and interstitial cell tumors of the testes. With adrenal hyperplasia, the testes will usually be prepubertal size. However, an adrenal rest composed of ACTH-responsive tissue located in the testes, an ectopic location for adrenal tissue, may enlarge in response to increased ACTH secretion in poorly treated CAH. A Leydig cell tumor is seen with irregular enlargement of one or both testes. Serum LH and the LH response to GnRH will be suppressed because of autonomous testosterone secretion in incomplete precocious puberty.

Premature Leydig and germinal cell maturation (#176410 PRECOCIOUS PUBERTY, MALE-LIMITED at 2p21) is a rare condition but is instructive in the understanding of puberty, as it results from a unique error of biology. A mutation in the seven-transmembrane domain of the LH receptor causes the LH receptor to be constitutively activated so that testosterone is produced even in the absence of LH. Affected boys demonstrate androgen effects at an early age, and often a family history of affected fathers or uncles is found in this X-linked disorder. Remarkably, at the time of normal puberty, these boys switch from incomplete gonadotropin-independent precocious puberty, to normal pubertal physiology that ultimately can lead to fertility. Treatment is sometimes effective with an antiandrogen and an aromatase inhibitor in decreasing the effects of androgen secretion.

If hCG stimulates the testes to produce testosterone, the testes will be slightly enlarged (more than 2.5 cm) but will not be as large as found in true precocious puberty, because the seminiferous tubules, which are normally responsive to FSH, will not increase in size since no increased FSH secretion occurs. hCG-secreting tumors include hepatomas; hepatoblastomas; teratomas or chorioepitheliomas of the gonads, mediastinum, retroperitoneum, or pineal gland; as well as germinomas of the pineal gland.

Variations of Early Pubertal Development

Premature Thelarche

Premature thelarche is a benign condition of unilateral or bilateral breast development, usually in a girl younger than 3 years. Minimal or no other signs of estrogen effect are present [i.e., no dulling of the vaginal mucosa, little areolar (nipple) development or pigmentation, and no increase in growth rate]. Serum estradiol values are prepubertal, as the follicular cyst thought to cause this condition is often spontaneously resorbed by the time the patient comes to evaluation. Some evidence exists that FSH is higher in premature thelarche than in age-matched children without thelarche, but the serum LH and the LH response to GnRH are prepubertal. Some children with central precocious puberty may begin this condition appearing very much as if they have premature thelarche. Thus it is important to continue to observe children with premature thelarche over time.

Premature Adrenarche

Premature adrenarche is a benign self-limited appearance of a small amount of pubic hair, comedones, axillary hair, or odor, which usually occurs after age 6 years. The normal increase in adrenal androgens, including DHEA and its sulfate (DHEAS), occurs earlier in this condition than in an unaffected child, and the pubic hair then follows the increase in DHEAS. Thus a 6- to 8-year-old with Tanner stage 2 to 3 pubic hair may have a DHEAS value characteristic of a 12- to 13-year-old. The rest of pubertal development, such as testicular development in a boy or breast development in a girl, will occur at a normal age. A slight increase in growth rate may be noted, along with a slight advancement of bone age, but neither should be pronounced, or a more serious virilizing disorder is likely.

Late-onset CAH may have an initial appearance indistinguishable from that of premature adrenarche. Thus clinical follow-up is indicated, even if it appears that the child has the benign condition, premature adrenarche. If any doubt exists that the condition seems to be more severe than premature pubarche, or if a family history of the same condition is found, testing for CAH is indicated by using basal adrenal metabolite evaluation as well as measurement after ACTH stimulation (see Chapters 10 and 17). Polycystic ovarian disease also appears in some cases similar to premature adrenarche.

Gynecomastia

Gynecomastia is the appearance of breast development in a male. Physiologic or pubertal gynecomastia is a variation of normal that is seen in a boy who, usually, has reached Tanner stage 2 to 3 pubertal development. In the majority of cases, the condition disappears within 1 to 3 years, but in some cases, it may last longer and require surgical removal. The longer the tissue remains, the more likely it will not resolve, because scar tissue ultimately develops in the breast tissue. Obese subjects may have a reduction in this glandular tissue or its prominence by reducing their weight.

Pathologic gynecomastia will occur in Klinefelter syndrome, Reifenstein syndrome (#312300 REIFENSTEIN SYNDROME), or any form of partial androgen resistance, as well as in rare prepubertal boys with 11β-hydroxylase deficiency (*202010 ADRENAL HYPERPLASIA, CONGENITAL, DUE TO 11β-HYDROXYLASE DEFICIENCY at 8q21) or aromatase excess syndrome (139300 GYNECOMASTIA, HEREDITARY). Breast cancer may develop in the tissue affected by gynecomastia in Klinefelter syndrome. Only surgery is now available to treat persistent gynecomastia, but present clinical studies hold promise for medical treatment.

Differential Diagnosis of Precocious Puberty

A girl with early breast development may have estrogen secretion because of incomplete precocious puberty or gonadotropin-stimulated estrogen secretion due to true precocious puberty; however, if a girl has early breast development and an appropriate stage of pubic hair development for the degree of breast development, she probably has true precocious puberty. No other condition is likely to produce both estrogen and androgen in balanced amounts (Fig. 9-5). A boy who shows signs of virilization with symmetrically enlarging testes of homogeneous appearance is likely to have true precocious puberty: bilateral testicular tumors and gonadotropin-independent Leydig and germ cell maturation are alternative etiologies of enlarging testes, but it is unlikely that they will be symmetrical, homogeneous, and have regular surfaces. If the testes are not enlarging even though the patient exhibits androgen effects, an adrenal source of androgen products is suspected, such as an adrenal tumor or adrenal enzyme defect.

If significant isosexual pubertal development is noted (breast development in a girl or virilization in a boy), determination of sex steroid and serum gonadotropin concentration (in modern, sensitive third-generation assays) is performed. If sex steroids are elevated but gonadotropins are suppressed, autonomous sex steroid secretion is likely to be found. If hCG is elevated, an hCG-secreting tumor is suggested. An MRI is necessary to look at liver, CNS, mediastinum, or other locations for the hCG-secreting tumor. Serum gonadotropin concentrations and the GnRH test will reveal pubertal values in central precocious puberty, but the LH values will be prepubertal in precocious adrenarche or in precocious thelarche (see Fig. 9-5).

If the diagnosis is true precocious puberty, a search for a CNS abnormality is indicated, and an MRI is performed to determine whether a hamartoma of the tuber cinereum or an expanding neoplasm is present. Boys more often than girls will have a brain tumor as the cause of their true precocious puberty.

Treatment of True Precocious Puberty

Gonadotropin-releasing hormone analogues (GnRH-As) are extremely potent and have an extended time of action as compared with native GnRH. These agents cause downregulation of GnRH receptors, such would occur during a constant GnRH infusion, thereby decreasing episodic gonadotropin release. When GnRH-A suppresses gonadotropin secretion, sex steroid secretion decreases, the rate of bone-age advancement decreases, as does the rate of rapid growth, and the height prognosis of treated patients improves. The effects are reversible, as those whose therapy is discontinued increase gonadotropin secretion to pubertal values, following the same pattern as is usually found in the earliest stages of normal puberty. GnRH-As are commercially approved for the treatment of true precocious puberty in the form of monthly injections or daily subcutaneous injections. GnRH agonist therapy is not necessary to ensure an adequate final height in a patient who has slowly progressive precocious puberty that commences at an age only slightly younger than the normal age at onset of puberty.

Testolactone is an aromatase inhibitor that inhibits estradiol and estrone biosynthesis. It, or flutamide, a more potent form of the drug, is used in McCune-Albright syndrome in boys with incomplete precocious puberty and in familial gonadotropin-independent Leydig cell and germ cell maturation. Ketoconazole, an antifungal agent, causes a 17–20 lyase block in the testosterone biosynthetic pathway and can be used to decrease testosterone secretion in familial gonadotropin-independent Leydig cell and germ cell maturation; adrenal suppression is a side effect of such treatment. Newer agents are under study to determine whether they improve therapy. Incomplete precocious puberty can be followed by true precocious puberty if the condition has been uncontrolled for a long period and the sex steroids have exerted a maturational effect on the hypothalamic–pituitary axis.

Psychological support is helpful to both child and parents. Their larger size may make children with precocious puberty the center of unwanted attention. Children with true precocious puberty, if intellectually and socially appropriate, may be able to accept accelerated school placement so that they can be placed in a class with children whose size is closer to their own. Girls with premature menstrual periods should be prepared before menarche and supported through this difficult time. Of further significance is the possibility that the patient could be the target of sexual abuse, with the additional element of potential fertility. Boys with precocious puberty and high testosterone values will be prone to aggressive activity and may masturbate publicly, but are unlikely to seek out heterosexual activity in the absence of social maturation. In some cases, the treating physician can help the family through this stressful time, but psychological counseling should be considered in the more significant cases.

Early menarche is associated with a higher risk of breast cancer. Thus, affected girls should be regularly evaluated for this disease as they reach adulthood.

SUGGESTED READINGS

Boepple PA. Precocious puberty. In: Finberg L, Kleinman RE, eds. *Saunders manual of pediatric practice.* Philadelphia: WB Saunders, 2002:860–863.

Davenport M. Turner syndrome. In: Finberg L, Kleinman RE, eds. *Saunders manual of pediatric practice.* Philadelphia: WB Saunders, 2002:856–859.

DiMeglio LA, Pescovitz OH. Disorders of puberty: inactivating and activating molecular mutations. *J Pediatr* 1997;131:S8–S12.

Eugster E. McCune-Albright syndrome. In: Finberg L, Kleinman RE, eds. *Saunders manual of pediatric practice.* Philadelphia: WB Saunders, 2002:863–866.

Feuillan PP, Jones JV, Barnes K, et al. Reproductive axis after discontinuation of gonadotropin-releasing hormone analog treatment of girls with precocious puberty: long term follow-up comparing girls with hypothalamic hamartoma to those with idiopathic precocious puberty. *J Clin Endocrinol Metab* 1999;84:44–49.

Grumbach MM, Hughes IA, Conte FA. Disorders of sexual differentiation. In: Larsen PRKHM, Melmed S, Polonsky KS, et al., eds. *Williams textbook of endocrinology.* 9th ed. Philadelphia: WB Saunders, 2002:842–1002.

Grumbach MM, Styne DM. Puberty, ontogeny, neuroendocrinology, physiology, and disorders. In: Larsen PRKHM, Melmed S, Polonsky KS, eds. *Williams textbook of endocrinology.* 9th ed. Philadelphia: WB Saunders, 2003:1115–1286.

Herman-Giddens ME, Slora EJ, Wasserman RC, et al. Secondary sexual characteristics and menses in young girls seen in office practice: a study from the pediatric research in office settings network. *Pediatrics* 1997;99:505–512.

Hoffman P, Pescovitz OH. Premature thelarche. In: Finberg L, Kleinman RE, eds. *Saunders manual of pediatric practice.* Philadelphia: WB Saunders, 2002:831–833.

Lee P. Hypogonadotropic hypogonadism. In: Finberg L, Kleinman RE, eds. *Saunders manual of pediatric practice.* Philadelphia: WB Saunders, 2002:853–856.

Marshall WA, Tanner JM. Variations in pattern of pubertal changes in girls. *Arch Dis Child* 1969;44:291–303.

Marshall WA, Tanner JM. Variations in the pattern of pubertal changes in boys. *Arch Dis Child* 1970;45:13–23.

Paul D, Conte FA, Grumbach MM, et al. Long-term effect of gonadotropin-releasing hormone agonist therapy on final and near-final height in 26 children with true precocious puberty treated at a median age of less than 5 years. *J Clin Endocrinol Metab* 1995;80:546–551.

Rogol AD. Klinefelter syndrome. In: Finberg L, Kleinman RE, eds. *Saunders manual of pediatric practice.* Philadelphia: WB Saunders, 2002:859–860.

Rosenfield RL. Hirsutism and hyperandrogenism in adolescent girls. In: Finberg L, Kleinman RE, eds. *Saunders manual of pediatric practice.* Philadelphia: WB Saunders, 2002:866–872.

Rosenfield RL. Puberty in the female and its disorders. In: Sperling MA, ed. *Pediatric endocrinology.* Philadelphia: WB Saunders, 2002: 455–518.

Saenger PH. Premature adrenarche. In: Finberg L, Kleinman RE, eds. *Saunders manual of pediatric practice.* Philadelphia: WB Saunders, 2002:833–835.

Saenger PH. Gynecomastia. In: Finberg L, Kleinman RE, eds. *Saunders manual of pediatric practice.* Philadelphia: WB Saunders, 2002: 835–836.

Seminara SB, Hayes FJ, Crowley WJ. Gonadotropin-releasing hormone deficiency in the human (idiopathic hypogonadotropic hypogonadism and Kallmann's syndrome): pathophysiological and genetic considerations. *Endocr Rev* 1998;19:521–539.

Sher ES, Migeon CJ, Berkovitz GD. Evaluation of boys with marked breast development at puberty. *Clin Pediatr (Phila)* 1998;37: 367–371.

Styne DM. New aspects in the diagnosis and treatment of pubertal disorders. *Pediatr Clin North Am* 1997;44:505–529.

Styne DM. Constitutional delay in growth and adolescence. In: Finberg L, Kleinman RE, eds. *Saunders manual of pediatric practice.* Philadelphia: WB Saunders, 2002:838–840.

Styne DM. Normal and abnormal age of onset of secondary sexual development. In: Finberg L, Kleinman RE, eds. *Saunders manual of pediatric practice.* Philadelphia: WB Saunders, 2002:829–831.

Styne DM. The testes: disorders of sexual maturation and puberty. In: Sperling MA, ed. *Pediatric and adolescent endocrinology.* 3rd ed. Philadelphia: WB Saunders, 2002:562–629.

Styne DM, Cuttler L. Normal pubertal development. In: Rudolph CD, Rudolph AM, eds. *Rudolph's pediatrics.* New York: McGraw-Hill, 2002:2093–2105.

Styne DM, Grumbach MM. Puberty in boys and girls. In: Pfaff DW, ed. *Hormone, brain and behavior.* Amsterdam: Elsevier, 2002: 661–716.

10 ♣ Disorders of the Adrenal Gland

Disorders of the adrenal gland can lead to effects as disparate as abnormal sexual differentiation, decreased or increased growth velocity, and life-threatening endocrine emergencies. Diseases can arise from abnormalities within the gland itself, from abnormalities in the control of the gland, or from the ingestion of exogenous steroid compounds, even if these are prescribed for the appropriate treatment of diseases.

NORMAL ADRENAL GLAND PHYSIOLOGY

The paired adrenal glands sit above the kidney (which accounts for their archaic name, the suprarenal glands) and are composed of two major components derived from different embryonic tissues (Fig. 10-1). The adrenal cortex is derived from mesenchyme and produces steroid compounds synthesized from the cholesterol molecule; the adrenal medulla is derived from neural crest tissue and produces catecholamines.

The median eminence of the hypothalamus secretes corticotrophin-releasing factor (CRF), a 41-amino-acid peptide that stimulates the release of adrenocorticotropic hormone (ACTH) from the anterior pituitary gland. ACTH is cleaved from the precursor molecule, pro-opiomelanocortin (POMC), which also plays a role in appetite regulation, among other important functions. ACTH increases the activity of the enzymes of the adrenal cortex to facilitate the production of cortisol (compound F or hydrocortisone), which, through negative-feedback inhibition of the central nervous system (CNS), reduces the secretion of ACTH until an equilibrium is reached. Cortisol is considered a glucocorticoid that stimulates gluconeogenesis, maintains blood pressure, and affects mood. Cortisol circulates in association with a protein, cortisol-binding globulin (CBG), so that most is bound, although it is the free fraction that is active. If excess glucocorticoid is produced, as in Cushing disease, free cortisol will overwhelm the available CBG and spill over into the urine as urinary free cortisol.

The production of the weak adrenal androgen, dehydroepiandrosterone (DHEA), is dependent on the presence of ACTH, but it is produced in increased quantities at the time of normal puberty because of other controlling factors that are poorly characterized.

Aldosterone, the main mineralocorticoid of the adrenal cortex, under normal conditions is regulated by the renin–angiotensin axis but can be secreted in response to abnormally high concentrations of ACTH, as found in ectopic ACTH-secreting tumors. If there is ACTH deficiency, mineralocorticoid function will still remain normal. However, with lowered total body sodium or hypotension, renin, an enzyme produced in the juxtaglomerular apparatus of the

(text continues on page 200)

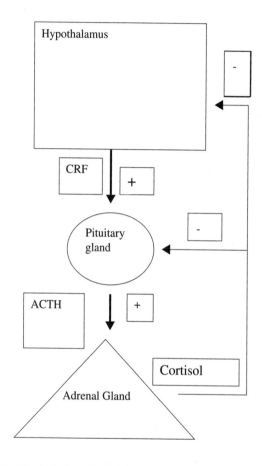

A

Fig. 10-1. Normal adrenal physiology.

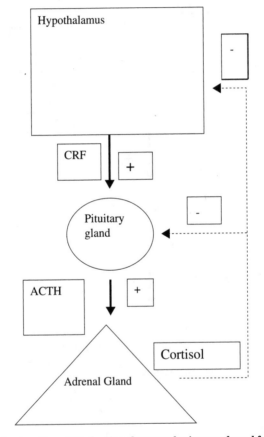

Fig. 10-1. (continued) Endocrine changes of primary adrenal failure.

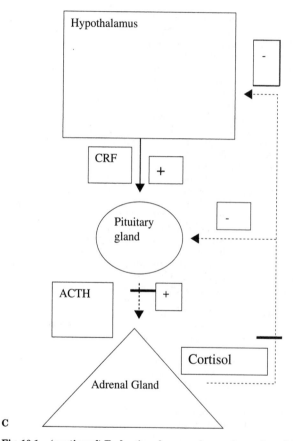

C

Fig. 10-1. (continued) Endocrine changes of secondary adrenal failure.

kidney, acts on angiotensinogen to form angiotensin I; angiotensin I is transformed by the converting enzyme of blood and lung to form the octapeptide, angiotensin II. Angiotensin II (and its metabolite angiotensin III) stimulate aldosterone production and secretion from the zona glomerulosa of the adrenal cortex. Aldosterone stimulates the reabsorption of sodium and chloride from the proximal convoluted tubule, as, to a lesser extent, does its precursor, deoxycorticosterone (DOC), another potent mineralocorticoid. When DOC is produced in excess, as in 17-OH deficiency, congenital adrenal hyperplasia (CAH), an increased mineralocorticoid effect will be noted, renin will be suppressed, as will aldosterone. Without mineralocorticoid effect, serum sodium decreases, and serum potassium increases, whereas in states of excess mineralocorticoid, total body sodium increases, serum sodium increases to high normal, and blood pressure increases. DOC also is produced in the zona fasciculata, an ACTH-responsive region that produces mainly cortisol. Thus when ACTH is extremely elevated, as in ectopic ACTH syndrome, mineralocorticoid increases, causing hypokalemia, possibly with alkalosis, and blood pressure increases because of sodium retention.

Serum ACTH normally increases in the morning, about 6:00 to 8:00 a.m., in a person on a normal daily schedule, and serum cortisol increases thereafter in response. Serum concentrations of both ACTH and cortisol decrease in the afternoon and evening as part of the normal diurnal rhythm of adrenal activity. If a person changes to another sleep–wake cycle, after a period of approximately 7 days, the diurnal rhythm will adjust to the new schedule; thus a person waking at night and sleeping during the day will have the peak of ACTH and cortisol phase shifted to increase just before awakening at night. Because ACTH concentrations vary considerably because of the episodic nature of ACTH secretion, a single serum ACTH determination may not be a valid reflection of the ACTH–cortisol axis. Serum cortisol concentrations are more stable than those of ACTH because of protein binding by CBG and other proteins, but can be quickly elevated by stress; unless serum samples for cortisol are obtained under relaxed conditions or unobtrusively obtained through an indwelling intravenous catheter, a high value may be specious. Serum cortisol concentrations, when abnormally elevated for time of day, are considered a reflection of stress or excessive secretion (as might be seen in Cushing disease).

DISORDERS OF THE ADRENAL CORTEX

Hypoadrenal States

The most common causes of decreased cortisol production are the CAH syndromes discussed in Chapter 8. In these conditions, ACTH is elevated with reduced production of cortisol. Increased cortisol secretion is not produced in response to the elevated ACTH because of enzymatic defects in the adrenal gland, and abnormalities of adrenal sex steroids or mineralocorticoids occur.

Addison disease exhibiting glucocorticoid and mineralocorticoid deficiency is rare in pediatrics, but the findings may be found in some salt-losing forms of CAH or other congenital defects. Tuberculous infection of the adrenal gland was more common in previous generations and gave rise to most of the earlier reports of Addison disease. Autoimmune disease is responsible for the majority of cases of Addison disease at present, and often other associated autoimmune disorders are found. Antibodies to adrenal enzymes are measurable, and lymphocytic infiltration of the adrenal glands occurs.

Types of autoimmune syndromes include

1. Type 1 polyglandular syndrome (*240300 AUTOIMMUNE POLYENDOCRINOPATHY SYNDROME, TYPE I) includes Addison disease as well as hypoparathyroidism, pernicious anemia, and chronic mucocutaneous candidiasis, among other features.
2. Type 2 polyglandular syndrome (269200 SCHMIDT SYNDROME), or Schmidt syndrome, includes thyroiditis and/or diabetes mellitus type 1 and, later, ovarian failure, in addition to adrenal insufficiency. A relation is seen to human leukocyte antigen (HLA) type DR32 and DR4 in this condition.

A rare form of mutation of the gene for cholesterol esterase that limits cholesterol entry into the steroidogenic pathways is described. Wolman disease (*278000 WOLMAN DISEASE 10q24-q25) is an autosomal dominant disorder that manifests with vomiting, diarrhea, steatorrhea, hepatosplenomegaly, hepatic fibrosis, esophageal varices, and intestinal malabsorption. Diffuse particulate adrenal calcifications are seen on radiograph. Laboratory evaluation reveals acid cholesteryl ester hydrolase deficiency; disseminated organ foam cell infiltration; normal or moderately elevated plasma lipids with hypercholesterolemia; foam cells in the bone marrow and vacuolated blood lymphocytes; xanthomatous changes in liver, adrenal, spleen, lymph nodes, bone marrow, small intestine, lungs, and thymus; and slight changes in skin, retina, and CNS.

Adrenoleukodystrophy, sometimes called bronze Schilder disease (*300100 ADRENOLEUKODYSTROPHY; ALD at Xq28) is an X-linked disorder that combines degeneration of nerves and of the white matter of the brain (causing CNS changes, ultimately leading to dementia) and glucocorticoid deficiency; some individuals also demonstrate mineralocorticoid deficiency. Blindness, hyperpigmentation, degenerative neurologic disorder, slurred speech, spastic paraplegia, and peripheral neuropathy are seen, and ultimately impotence and sphincter disturbances and limb and truncal ataxia. Elevated long-chain fatty acids are found in plasma, fibroblasts, amniocytes, and chorionic villi because of peroxisomal lignoceroyl-coenzyme A (CoA) ligase deficiency. Primary adrenal failure and gonadal failure develop late in childhood. On radiographic examination, atrophy of pons and cerebellum are seen on CT scan. A defect in the metabolism of very long chain fatty acids is noted, and serum hexicosanoic acid (c26) is elevated, leading to an abnormally high ratio of c26/c22 fatty acids.

CAH (*300200 ADRENAL HYPOPLASIA, CONGENITAL; AHC at Xp21.3-p21.2) may cause an Addison-like condition, occurring in an X-linked pattern, with a histologic pattern of cytomegaly; this may be accompanied by hypogonadotropic hypogonadism. The X-linked form is due to mutations in the DAX-1 gene and occurs with glycerol kinase deficiency and muscular dystrophy. An autosomal pattern of inheritance is described as well (202150 ADRENAL HYPOPLASIA, CONGENITAL, WITH ABSENT PITUITARY LUTEINIZING HORMONE), which is seen with a miniature adult cortex and complete lack of the fetal cortex at birth; this also is associated with absence of pituitary LH.

Congenital unresponsiveness to ACTH is seen with glucocorticoid deficiency but not mineralocorticoid deficiency. This may be found in an autosomal recessive or sex-linked pattern. Symptoms are those of primary adrenal insufficiency without abnormal electrolytes or dehydration. This syndrome may combine with alacrima, achalasia, and autonomic symptoms to cause Allgrove syndrome due to a mutation in the ALADIN gene (#231550 ACHALASIA-ADDISONIANISM-ALACRIMA SYNDROME; AAA at 12q13 with the gene described in *605378 ALADIN; AAAS). Adrenal hemorrhage in the newborn may lead to calcifications within the adrenal gland and a flank mass, but rarely leads to compromise of adrenal function. Cysts and tumors of the adrenal cortex and medulla also may lead to calcifications within the adrenal gland. The Waterhouse-Friderichsen syndrome of adrenal hemorrhage associated with meningococcemia or other bacterial sepsis is rare but devastating, leading to shock and, if untreated, death.

Symptoms of chronic glucocorticoid deficiency include weight loss or lack of adequate weight gain, weakness and lethargy, fatigue, hypoglycemia, and anorexia, whereas mineralocorticoid deficiency is heralded by hyponatremia with hyperkalemia, hypotension, low-voltage electrocardiogram (ECG) with small heart on radiograph, tachycardia, and acidosis. Metabolism of ACTH to melanocortin leads to hyperpigmentation of exposed skin, especially of flexural or injured surfaces, as well as hyperpigmentation of the gum line. A decrease in urine output due to the inability to excrete a water load may be seen. Salt craving may be noted on questioning. Monilial lesions of the skin or nails will occur in the syndrome of mucocutaneous candidiasis and adrenal insufficiency, which combines an immune defect with an autoimmune disorder of the adrenal glands. In mineralocorticoid deficiency, postural hypotension or an increase in pulse rate on standing may be seen; a decrease of blood pressure of 10 mm Hg or an increase in pulse rate of 20 is considered significant.

Acute adrenal crisis can lead to hypoglycemic seizures, abdominal pain, fever, vomiting, and even shock and death. Fluid volume, sodium, and glucose are necessary therapy along with glucocorticoid replacement. Serum sodium will be low, and serum potassium will be high if mineralocorticoid secretion is low; replacement of sodium and mineralocorticoid is appropriate therapy. Glucose/insulin infusions or oral potassium-retaining resin may be necessary to allow rapid decrease in extremely elevated serum K if ECG changes suggest hyperkalemia (peaked T waves).

Deficiency of pituitary ACTH (secondary adrenal insufficiency) or hypothalamic CRF (tertiary adrenal insufficiency) may occur from a congenital defect or a hypothalamic–pituitary tumor; usually an associated deficiency of other anterior pituitary hormones is noted (see Chapter 3).

Diagnosis of Hypoadrenal States

Laboratory evaluation of primary adrenal failure will demonstrate elevated ACTH concentrations at any time of the day and decreased cortisol concentrations when measured in the morning hours (because values are already low in the evening, measurement then may not differentiate between normal and abnormal values) (Fig. 10-2). Reduced cortisol reserve is noted on ACTH stimulation testing or insulin-induced hypoglycemia (we do not recommend insulin-induced hypoglycemia if the physician has no previous experience in performing the test in children). The ACTH test is accomplished by the administration of 0.25 mg of intravenous (i.v.) synthetic 1–13 ACTH at or before 8 a.m. and measuring cortisol at 0 and 60 minutes; an increase of 100% and a baseline of more than 10 μg/dL is considered normal. A metyrapone test is accomplished by using 300 mg/m^2 every 4 hours for a total of six doses over a 24-hour period, for a total dose of no more than 3 g. Metyrapone administration leads to an 11-OH block so that, in a normal subject, cortisol decreases while ACTH and 11-OH deoxycorticosterone increase (as do urinary 17-OH corticosteroids), indicating normal ACTH reserve. Thus an 8 a.m. serum cortisol, 11-deoxycortisol, and ACTH are determined, and a 24-hour urine for 17-OHCS is collected the day before and the day after the metyrapone is given. Older children are given 30 mg/kg at midnight (with food), and a blood sample is taken the morning before the metyrapone and the morning after. Other signs of autoimmune phenomena, such as Hashimoto thyroiditis or diabetes mellitus, may be found if an autoimmune syndrome is occurring.

Treatment of Hypoadrenal States

If adrenal function is inadequate, the goal is the replacement of glucocorticoid, or if necessary, mineralocorticoid, in physiologic dosage (see Chapter 15 for discussion of acute adrenal insufficiency). This is difficult in view of the episodic secretion of cortisol and diurnal variation. In general, natural glucocorticoid, cortisol, is preferable during the growing years, but the stronger,

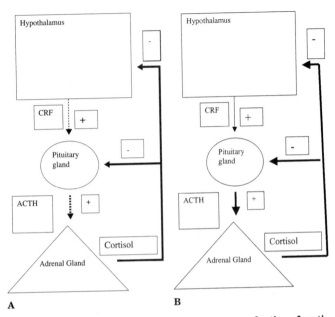

Fig. 10-2. (A) Endocrine changes of autonomous production of cortisol. (B) Endocrine changes of increased ACTH secretion escaping from feedback inhibition as in Cushing disease or ACTH secreting pituitary adenoma.

longer lasting glucocorticoids, such as prednisone, are used after growth has ceased, mainly because of the ability to cut dosage to twice per day. Table 10.1 shows the difference in potency of various preparations as to glucocorticoid or mineralocorticoid effects. Note that prednisone must be converted to prednisolone, and cortisone must be converted to cortisol for biologic activity, and these medications are therefore given in higher dosage than the more active forms. In the past, the daily production rate of cortisol was stated to be 12.5 mg/m^2, but recent data indicate that the true secretory rate is 6 to 7 mg/m^2. Because oral absorption is half the parenteral absorption, the rate is doubled and administered orally 3 times per day, with most given in the morning, unless the problem is virilizing CAH, when the time of administration may change (see Chapter 8). Thus for a 1-m^2 child, the oral dose would be 12 to 14 mg, but because five or ten mg tablets are the only available oral form, 15 mg is used, with 5 mg t.i.d. or 7.5 mg in the morning, 7.5 mg at noon, and 5 mg at bedtime preferable, or 10 mg at 5 mg, 2.5 mg, and 2.5 mg, respectively. The correct dosage cannot be measured by labora-

Table 10.1. Glucocorticoid preparations

	Glucocorticoid effect (based on antiinflammatory effect with cortisol = 1.0)	Mineralocorticoid effect [fludrocortisone (Fluorinef) = 1.0]	Time of biologic action (hr)
Cortisol (hydrocortisone)	1	0.005	8
Cortisone	0.8	0.005	8
Prednisone	4	0	18
Prednisolone	4–5	0	16–36
6α-Methylprednisolone	5–8	0	16–36 est
Dexamethasone	27–66	0	36–54
9α-Fluorocortisone	15	1	

tory methods, but if the child feels well, is not gaining too much weight or decreasing the growth rate, the dosage is likely to be appropriate (see Chapter 8 for dosage in virilizing CAH). In times of stress, fever, or surgery, accidents, but not usually psychological stress, the dose is doubled or tripled until the condition is resolved. Injectable glucocorticoid in the form of Solucortef in a Readivial© that combines diluent and powdered medication is easiest to use; 25 mg for infants, 50 mg for smaller children, and 100 mg for adolescents is the rough dose to be given immediately before the child is taken to the emergency department (ED) at times of emergency (severe accident or shock) when the child is not able to take medication orally. No danger occurs in giving the medication in one dose inappropriately, but not giving the dose when needed can be serious or fatal. Intramuscular (i.m.) cortisone takes hours to work and should never be used as emergency treatment. The child should wear a MedAlert bracelet or necklace stating the steroid dependence and a letter, telling any ED doctor the problem, should be carried when possible. In the ED, sugar, fluid, glucocorticoid, and, if salt losing is part of the problem, salt and mineralocorticoid are given immediately.

Mineralocorticoid is given as 9α-fluorohydrocortisone, or Florinef. Dosage is meant to keep body sodium in an adequate range so the plasma renin activity (PRA) is kept in the normal range; Florinef is increased if PRA is too high and decreased if PRA is too low, with a similar observation of serum sodium. Florinef is given once or, more usually, twice per day, because Florinef retains salt. Oral sodium supplementation may be needed to keep the Florinef dose in the 0.05- to 1.5-mg/day range. Usually older children will self-select the correct amount of salt to meet their needs, but infants may need added salt. Sodium chloride or table salt is given as measured by the teaspoon or by a test tube marked to hold 1 g or more. Note that cortisol and cortisone have some mineralocorticoid effect (Table 10.1), whereas the more potent glucocorticoids do not; if switching from one preparation to the other, watch for a change in sodium balance or adjust/add mineralocorticoid to the regimen. Shock is a real possibility if mineralocorticoid deficiency or sodium deficiency develops.

It is imperative that if hypothyroidism and glucocorticoid deficiency coexist, the glucocorticoid be instituted before or with thyroid hormone, or the minimal glucocorticoid that may be present endogenously will be more rapidly metabolized, leading to acute glucocorticoid-deficient crisis.

Steroid Withdrawal

Iatrogenic glucocorticoid deficiency is caused by the abrupt discontinuation of glucocorticoids. This may occur after therapy for a glucocorticoid-responsive disease or after the removal of a tumor, causing Cushing syndrome. Generally, more than 7 to 10 days of glucocorticoid therapy will lead to suppression of endogenous ACTH secretion and some degree of atrophy of the adrenal gland. This process must be reversed before the individual is able to mount a response to stress. Depending on the dose, potency of the glucocorticoid, and the length of therapy, it may take months for ACTH to increase and more months for cortisol to follow suit. Nighttime administration of exogenous glucocorticoid is more likely to affect the peak of ACTH secretion and cause longer suppression, whereas every-other-day glucocorticoid administration has less effect. The tolerance of a patient for glucocorticoid discontinuation is difficult to define, but it is prudent to wean the child off slowly rather than cutting the therapy immediately if any question of adrenal suppression is seen. Symptoms of the steroid-withdrawal syndrome that occurs if weaning is too rapid include headache, myalgia, arthralgia, and fever, although patients receiving glucocorticoids for specific diseases may experience resurgence of symptoms of those diseases and confuse the situation. Many schemas exist for weaning an individual off glucocorticoids; the following is only one possibility. The dose of glucocorticoid may be decreased rapidly until the physiologic range is reached. Normal endogenous production is about 6 to 8 mg/ m^2/day, but oral medication is probably only 50% absorbed, and so the physiologic ranges starts at double this secretory rate [e.g., for a child taking 20 to 30 mg of prednisone divided into two doses per day (which is equivalent in bioactivity to about 120 to 160 mg of cortisol) for more than 1 month, the dose may be cut to 15 mg of prednisone for 1 week, to 10 mg for 1 week, to 5 mg for 2 weeks, and then switched to 20 mg of hydrocortisone (divided into two doses per day) for 1 week, 10 mg for 1 week, and then the medication may be given only in the morning until the a.m. cortisol is demonstrated to be greater than 10 µg/dL].

An a.m. serum cortisol greater than 15–20 µg/dL indicates adequate basal adrenal function, but the subject may not yet have adequate reserves of ACTH for stress. Thus an ACTH-stimulation test using 0.25 mg i.m. or i.v. cosyntropin, with a measurement of serum cortisol in 60 minutes greater than 20 µg/dL indicating good reserve. Stress dosage of glucocorticoids (2 to 3 times normal basal secretion of 8 mg/m^2/day given orally or parenterally if the child cannot swallow or is vomiting) must be administered if the child has an illness or accident or if surgery is required before adrenal reserve returns (see Chapter 8 concerning CAH). It is useful for the child to wear a MedAlert bracelet to notify of reduced adrenal reserve.

Hyperadrenal States

Cushing Syndrome

Cushing syndrome refers to the general class of disorders with increased cortisol effect, including those due to exogenous glucocorticoid intake. The specific causes include endogenous hyper-cortisolism secondary to increased pituitary ACTH secretion (Cushing disease), ectopic ACTH secretion, and autonomous cortisol secretion by the adrenal gland. Before age 7 years, the usual cause of Cushing syndrome is an adrenal tumor, whereas thereafter, pituitary ACTH secretion becomes a more common etiology. Hypercortisolism has wide-ranging effects on the body, including decreased growth rate; weight gain in a truncal or centripetal pattern, leading to the characteristic buffalo hump on the back; a characteristic round face (moon facies); osteopenia or osteoporosis; muscle weakness, especially in the distal regions, leading to thinning of the extremities while weight gain progresses; thinning of the skin, leading to purple striae; hypertension; and insulin resistance. Because the min-eralocorticoid receptors respond to cortisol (although such activity is usually minimized by the 11β-hydroxylation of excess cortisol to cortisone, which is inactive), an excess of cortisol overwhelms the system and leads to salt retention and hyper-tension. If the cause of the excess glucocorticoid is excess ACTH, hyperpigmentation will be found, as described earlier for Addison disease.

An abnormal regulation of the pituitary-adrenal axis leads to the specific diagnosis of Cushing disease (called bilateral adrenal hyperplasia, because of the enlarged appearance of both adrenal glands, even though the etiology is in the hypothalamic–pituitary axis). The original report by Cushing describes a patient with a basophilic adenoma and physical signs of hypercortisolism, but it was not until 50 years later that the primary importance of the pituitary microadenomas in these patients was proven by the technique of transsphenoidal microadenomectomy. The fact that some patients appropriately treated with pituitary microadenomectomy have recurrences suggests that hypothala-mic CRF may be the etiologic agent for the formation of some microadenomas.

Cushing disease in childhood first manifests with growth fail-ure and is quickly followed by weight gain in the truncal or centripetal pattern, with thin and weak extremities. Other fea-tures may include the classic cushingoid appearance of a buffalo hump of adipose tissue on the back of the neck; purple striae of the trunk due to thinning of the skin and exposure of the cap-illaries; sometimes, but not invariably, pigmentation of the flexural surfaces and gums; weakness and lack of energy; and the early appearance of acne or pubic hair. The personality of patients with Cushing disease may be abnormal, and some describe the children as obsessive. The diastolic and systolic blood pressure may be elevated. Because of the small size of the usual lesion, neurologic symptoms or signs are not found in Cushing disease unless it has progressed markedly. If the adrenal glands are removed in an attempt to treat the disease, enlargement of the unsuppressed pituitary gland leads to pressure effects on the surrounding tissue, including the optic chiasm; this is known as Nelson syndrome.

Autonomous cortisol secretion may be seen in single or multiple autonomous nodules of the adrenal gland(s) or in adrenal carcinoma. Nodular adrenal hyperplasia is characterized by areas of active secreting adrenal tissue interspersed with areas of quiescent gland on histologic examination. A carcinoma of the adrenal gland often is difficult to differentiate from a benign tumor of the gland; pathologic criteria are available, but often, clinical observation is necessary to define the difference between a carcinoma and an adenoma. Carcinomas of the adrenal gland may have defects in 3β-hydroxylase and secrete large amounts of DHEA as well as cortisol, leading to a greater amount of virilization than found with the other causes of Cushing syndrome. Testosterone may be produced directly by such tumors, and severe virilization has been seen; the differential diagnosis should include virilizing ovarian tumors in girls. Feminizing tumors of the adrenal gland have been rarely reported in childhood.

Ectopic secretion of ACTH is exceedingly rare in childhood but has been reported in Wilms tumors and in islet cell carcinoma of the pancreas. Serum ACTH may be measured greater than 1,000 pg/mL, although modest elevations may be seen at first. The exceptional elevations can stimulate mineralocorticoid production, leading to salt retention and potassium excretion; hypertension, hypokalemic alkalosis, and subsequent muscle weakness will result. It is rare to see such excess mineralocorticoid production in Cushing disease.

Differential Diagnosis of Cushing Disease

Serum ACTH is not necessarily strikingly elevated in Cushing disease; the finding of a concentration of ACTH more characteristic of the morning (higher) in the afternoon (i.e., ACTH concentration is too high for the time of day) associated with a value of cortisol too high for the afternoon or evening is suggestive of abnormality in the regulation of the ACTH-cortisol axis (Fig. 10-3). It must be remembered, however, that stress or even depression will elevate both ACTH and cortisol levels and can falsely suggest Cushing disease. As most patients with Cushing disease are obese, the differential diagnosis is often between exogenous obesity and Cushing disease. The urinary 17-OHCs and urinary free cortisol may be elevated for age in exogenous obesity because of the changes in glucocorticoid metabolism of obesity, but in Cushing disease, the values will be higher when corrected for body surface area than those found in obesity (24-hour urinary 17-OHCs greater than 4.5 mg/m² and urinary free cortisol greater than 60 g/m² are highly suggestive of hypercortisolism). The great variations in urinary values from day to day and the difficulty in collecting a full 24-hour sample of urine in childhood mandate

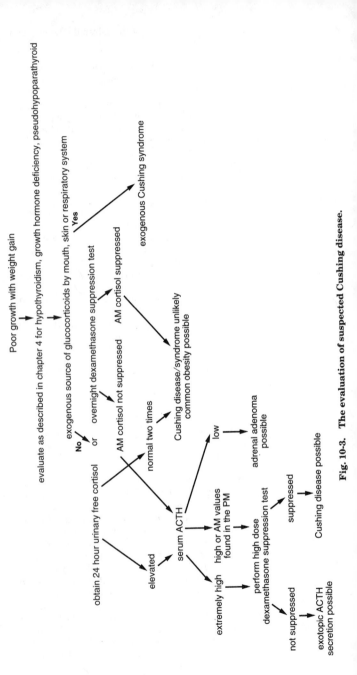

Poor growth with weight gain

evaluate as described in chapter 4 for hypothyroidism, growth hormone deficiency, pseudohypoparathyroid

exogenous source of glucocorticoids by mouth, skin or respiratory system

No or **Yes**

overnight dexamethasone suppression test

AM cortisol suppressed → exogenous Cushing syndrome

AM cortisol not suppressed

AM cortisol suppressed → Cushing disease/syndrome unlikely common obesity possible

obtain 24 hour urinary free cortisol

normal two times

elevated

serum ACTH

low → adrenal adenoma possible

high or AM values found in the PM

extremely high

perform high dose dexamethasone suppression test

suppressed → Cushing disease possible

not suppressed → exotopic ACTH secretion possible

Fig. 10-3. The evaluation of suspected Cushing disease.

that at least two baseline urine collections are evaluated and collected for glucocorticoid determinations.

An overnight dexamethasone-suppression test may be used to screen patients for Cushing disease, but this test has a high incidence of false-positive results, although the rate of false negatives is low; 1 mg of dexamethasone (or 15 μg/kg body weight for smaller children) is given orally at midnight, and a serum sample is analyzed for cortisol at 8:00 to 9:00 a.m. the next morning. In presumptive Cushing disease, plasma cortisol will not suppress below 5 μg/dL, whereas in exogenous obesity, the values decrease. If the results are negative, Cushing disease is unlikely, but if the results are positive, the following tests are considered.

The classic tests for the differential diagnosis of Cushing syndrome are the dexamethasone-suppression tests. The low-dose dexamethasone-suppression test uses 1.25 mg/m²/24hr of dexamethasone, divided into four doses per day for 2 days; if the urinary 17-OHCs on the second day of the test decrease 50% from the two baseline collections (or if the 17-OHCs is less than 1 mg/m² and the urine free cortisol less than 25 μg/m²), the patient is likely to have exogenous obesity because they are easily suppressible. It is useful to collect serum ACTH and cortisol concentrations during the baseline and dexamethasone suppression phases of the test to see if serum values also are affected (e.g., if the cortisol is suppressed to less than 5 μg/dL and the ACTH to less than 25 pg/mL). If the suspicion of Cushing syndrome remains because the results are abnormal, a high-dose dexamethasone suppression test is performed to differentiate between Cushing disease and Cushing syndrome of other causes. In the high-dose dexamethasone suppression test, 3.75 mg/m²/24 hr of dexamethasone is divided into four doses a day for 2 days, and urinary 17-OHCs excretion on the second day is compared with the two baseline collections; in Cushing disease, complete suppression of urinary 17-OHCs and free cortisol will occur, whereas in the ectopic ACTH syndrome or with autonomous cortisol secretion, no suppression will be seen over baseline levels.

CRF infusion also may be used for the differential diagnosis between Cushing syndrome and Cushing disease. A patient with autonomous cortisol secretion will have low basal ACTH and will not have an increase in ACTH with CRF administration. A patient with ectopic ACTH secretion will have a high basal ACTH concentration and will not have an increase in ACTH with CRF, whereas a patient with Cushing disease will have a large increase in ACTH, demonstrating the CRF-responsive nature of the microadenoma.

Invasive sampling procedures more often are applied in adult patients than in children; if the technical expertise is available, however, these techniques may be applied in pediatrics. Adrenal venous sampling for cortisol or other metabolites may be used to evaluate further patients suspected to have an adrenal etiology of Cushing syndrome and can indicate whether a unilateral adrenal tumor is responsible for the cortisol secretion. For the evaluation of Cushing disease, petrosal sinus sampling for ACTH may indicate the side and location of a pituitary or extrapituitary source for the ACTH to narrow the surgical approach necessary for treatment.

Noninvasive radiologic procedures meet with mixed success, especially in the CNS. CT scanning or MRI with gadolinium of the pituitary region may not be helpful because of the small size of some microadenomas, and the presence of silent adenomas in many normals may confuse the issue. The adrenal glands may both appear enlarged on abdominal CT scans in Cushing disease, whereas a solitary nodule or tumor or nodular adrenal hyperplasia may be identified on high-quality computerized scans or MRI. Exploratory laparotomy may yet be required to localize the tumor.

Treatment of Cushing Syndrome

If the diagnosis of Cushing disease is established, the treatment may be medical, radiotherapy, or surgery. Transsphenoidal microadenomectomy is a useful method of curing the patient of the microadenoma that causes the problem and leaving the rest of the pituitary gland intact. Experience with this particular tumor is a must if the surgeon is going to remove the appropriate part of the gland. Recurrence is possible, but reoperation can be performed if necessary. In the right hands, this procedure appears the treatment of choice. Previous studies demonstrated the utility of o,p'-DDD, an adrenolytic agent, to diminish the adrenal function, but other methods have supplanted its use in all but inoperable patients. Metyrapone, an 11-hydroxylase inhibitor, has been used with some success, but ACTH levels will soon increase and overwhelm the block in cortisol production, leading to renewed symptoms of hypercortisolism. Radiotherapy has been used in some series, but the risk of hypopituitarism developing after radiotherapy has led most clinicians to use other methods of treatment. Bilateral adrenalectomy will cure the hypercortisolism but leave the pituitary tumor. After a period, the hypersecretory pituitary tumor, released from the suppressive effects of hypercortisolism, may grow and secrete increasing amounts of ACTH: hyperpigmentation and an enlarging pituitary tumor of Nelson syndrome results.

The aim of treatment of autonomous adrenal tumors and ectopic ACTH-secreting tumors is to eradicate the offending neoplasm. If the ectopic ACTH-secreting tumor is inoperable, an adrenal blocking agent or bilateral adrenalectomy is used to control the hypercortisolism.

The goal of medical treatment of Cushing syndrome after the correction of the hypercortisolism is the replacement of glucocorticoids in appropriate dose to avoid the suppression of growth. In the months after the removal of the microadenoma of Cushing disease, the remaining corticotropes will not function, and replacement glucocorticoid therapy will be required. The initial dose of cortisol will have to be relatively high, or the patient may experience the malaise and lethargy characteristic of glucocorticoid withdrawal. Although the desired dose of hydrocortisone is approximately 8 mg/m^2, the initial dose may have to be twice or more that level for several weeks, with gradual weaning to the lower dose necessary (see earlier). After 9 to 18 months, normal adrenal function will return in the majority of cases of Cushing disease treated with transsphenoidal microadenomectomy. Of course, if the adrenal glands are removed, both glucocorticoids and mineralocorticoids will have to be replaced for the life span of the patient.

Hypertension due to Adrenal Disease

Idiopathic hyperaldosteronism is usually bilateral but may occur in only one adrenal gland. Serum aldosterone is high, and plasma renin activity is low. Treatment is accomplished by spironolactone and, if necessary, surgery. This condition may be familial (*605635 HYPERALDOSTERONISM, FAMILIAL, TYPE II)

Glucocorticoid-suppressible hyperaldosteronism (#103900 HYPERALDOSTERONISM, FAMILIAL, TYPE I at 8q21) is an autosomal dominant condition due to an abnormality of the 11β-hydroxylase gene whose activity allows the synthesis of DOC but is suppressible by glucocorticoid. This rare condition is treated by glucocorticoid administration. 17α-Hydroxylase deficiency (*202110 ADRENAL HYPERPLASIA, CONGENITAL, DUE TO 17α-HYDROXYLASE DEFICIENCY) and 11β-hydroxylase deficiency (*202010 ADRENAL HYPERPLASIA, CONGENITAL, DUE TO 11β-HYDROXYLASE DEFICIENCY) all produce a hypertensive state (see earlier in chapter). 11-Hydroxysteroid dehydrogenase deficiency interrupts the normal conversion of cortisol to cortisone by 11-hydroxysteroid dehydrogenase (218030 CORTISOL 11β-KETOREDUCTASE DEFICIENCY at 16q22) and leads to apparent mineralocorticoid excess caused by the excess mineralocorticoid effect exerted by cortisol. The condition may be noted at birth and require glucocorticoid administration to decrease cortisol production and mineralocorticoid antagonism by the use of spironolactone. Alternatively, the condition may be acquired by licorice ingestion (true licorice such as found in Europe, not the red candy ropes more prevalent in the United States); the treatment is to discontinue licorice.

Adrenal Medulla
Normal Physiology
The adrenal medulla is derived from neuroectoderm and produces catecholamines in the chromaffin cells. Chromaffin cells also are

located in the sympathetic ganglion and the organ of Zuckerkandl (anterior to the aorta), and although the extraadrenal chromaffin cells mostly disappear in the postnatal period, they remain a potential site of pheochromocytoma formation and must be considered in the diagnostic process.

The catecholamine biosynthetic pathway proceeds from L-tyrosine to L-Dopa (via tyrosine hydroxylase) to dopamine (via aromatic-l-amino acid decarboxylase) to norepinephrine (via dopamine β-hydroxylase) to epinephrine [via phenylethanolamine- N-methyltransferase (PMNT)]. The last step occurs only in specific sympathetic nervous tissue such as the adrenal medulla; the high concentration of cortisol in the blood supply to the adrenal medulla induces PMNT and accounts for the transformation of significant amounts of norepinephrine into epinephrine in this location but not in other chromaffin tissue. Vanillylmandelic acid (VMA) and homovanillic acid (HVA) are deaminated metabolites of catecholamines and are measured when excessive catecholamine production is suspected, but metabolism of catecholamines also is high, such as in neuroblastoma.

Disorders of the Adrenal Medulla

Pheochromocytoma

Pheochromocytomas are derived from the chromaffin cells of the adrenal medulla or the extraadrenal tissue noted earlier. They are rare in childhood but represent a curable cause of hypertension and must be considered in the differential diagnosis of high blood pressure. Familial cases may be inherited in an autosomal dominant pattern (#171300 PHEOCHROMOCYTOMA at 11q23, 1p). They are an integral component of the multiple endocrine neoplasia syndromes (see Chapter 14), neurofibromatosis (*162200 NEUROFIBROMATOSIS, TYPE I; NF1 at 17q11.2), and Von Hippel-Landau disease (*193300 VON HIPPEL-LANDAU SYNDROME; VHL at 3p26-p25) and may develop before or after other components of the syndrome are noted.

Characteristic signs and symptoms of pheochromocytomas include hypertension (more often constant than episodic in children compared with adults), weight loss, headache, vomiting, and, more rarely in childhood than in adults, paroxysmal episodes of tachycardia, flushing, sweating, palpitations, or anxiety. Postural hypotension due to volume depletion may occur. Diagnosis is made by the demonstration of elevated urinary catecholamine, VMA, or total metanephrine excretion in a 24-hour collection. Plasma catecholamine concentrations may not add any information to the urinary collections, which serve as a reflection of the integrated catecholamine production over the previous day. In infants, plasma catecholamine determination may be simpler than urinary collection. Provocative pharmacologic tests are no longer used because of the danger of precipitating a hypertensive crisis and because of the specificity of the plasma and urine collections.

An adrenal pheochromocytoma may be located with abdominal CT scanning or with MRI. To ascertain function, scintiscanning with the synthetic catecholamine precursor, ^{131}I-*meta*-iodoben-zylguanidine, which is concentrated by chromaffin tissue, is used. If imaging techniques fail, selective venous catheterization and analysis of catecholamine efflux may narrow the search for the tumor.

Surgery to remove the tumor is the treatment of choice for pheochromocytoma, but the patient must be prepared for surgery and indeed for invasive radiologic studies by adrenergic block-ade. α-Adrenergic block should be administered before β-adren-ergic blockade. Phenoxybenzamine is given orally (5 to 10 mg every 12 hours, with increasing dosage until high blood pressure is controlled) for long-term therapy; i.v. or i.m. phentolamine (1 mg per dose) is used for hypertensive crises that may occur while the phenoxybenzamine block is being established. β-Blockade by propranolol (5 to 10 mg given 3 to 4 times per day orally for larger children) is added when the heart rate increases as the α-adren-ergic blockade is being established; propranolol may cause para-doxic hypertension if given before the α-adrenergic block is established. If this therapy is ineffective, α-methyltyrosine (a tyrosine hydroxylase inhibitor) can be started at 5 to 10 mg/kg/day, given 4 times per day. Nitroprusside is used as a vasodilator during surgical hypertension. Surgical preparation also includes administration of salt to repair the plasma volume, which is invariably low.

Multiple Endocrine Neoplasia

Pheochromocytomas are part of the multiple endocrine neoplasia (MEN) syndromes (see Chapter 14):

MEN type 1 (Werner syndrome *131100 caused by mutation in the MENEN gene at 11q13) is owing to mutation of the tumor-suppressor gene MEN 1. This condition usually appears in late adolescence and thereafter, rather than in childhood. Affected patients have

Benign pituitary tumors (increased GH secretion causes elevated serum insulin-like growth factor (IGF)-1 and acromegaly; increased prolactin causes galactorrhea).

Benign parathyroid tumors [hyperplasia may affect all glands and increase serum calcium along with inappropriately ele-vated parathyroid hormone (PTH)].

Pancreatic tumors may be malignant or multiple (excess gastrin secretion causes gastric ulcers and Zollinger-Ellison syndrome; increased insulin from beta cells causes hypoglycemia).

MEN type 2 (#171400 MULTIPLE ENDOCRINE NEOPLA-SIA, TYPE II; MEN 2–associated mutations in the RET proto-oncogene with 10q11.2) is due to mutations of the *ret* proto-oncogene, causing constitutive activation of the neural crest cell receptors. Affected patients with MEN 2 have

Medullary carcinoma of the thyroid is usually the first finding of MEN 2 (see Chapters 6 and 14). Those in the family with *ret* mutations may benefit from prophylactic thyroidectomy.

Pheochromocytoma (see earlier): Family members should have annual screening for this tumor, especially if medullary carcinoma of the thyroid (MCT) has occurred.

Parathyroid hyperplasia, possibly in response to the hypocalcemia caused by calcitonin secreted from the MCT.

MEN type 3 (#162300 MULTIPLE ENDOCRINE NEOPLASIA, TYPE IIB; MEN 2B–associated mutations in the RET protooncogene with 10q11.2) (previously MEN 2B) also demonstrate mucosal neuromas, leading to thickened lips and lumps on the tongue and the GI tract, as well as a marfanoid body habitus.

Neuroblastoma

Neuroblastomas are malignant tumors derived from neural crest and are associated with excessive production of catecholamines; in spite of this, they rarely are seen with clinical symptoms of catecholamine excess (probably because of catecholamine catabolism within the tumor), although a minority may have hypertension. They often are diagnosed from their size or the presence of metastases and have a remarkably high incidence of spontaneous regression. Urinary norepinephrine (not epinephrine), VMA, and particularly HVA and dopamine are excreted in increased amounts in neuroblastoma. Ganglioneuromas are benign, mature forms of neuroblastomas derived from sympathetic ganglion cells; usually silent with respect to endocrine function, they may manifest some of the signs of pheochromocytoma.

SUGGESTED READINGS

Bose HS, Sugawara T, Strauss JF III, et al. The pathophysiology and genetics of congenital lipoid adrenal hyperplasia: International Congenital Lipoid Adrenal Hyperplasia Consortium. *N Engl J Med* 1996;335(25):1870–1878.

Chrousos GP. Cushing syndrome and Cushing disease. In: Finberg L, Kleinman RE, eds. *Saunders manual of pediatric practice.* Philadelphia: WB Saunders, 2002:909–911.

Chrousos GP, Linder B. Steroid withdrawal. In: Finberg L, Kleinman RE, eds. *Saunders manual of pediatric practice.* Philadelphia: WB Saunders, 2002:950–952.

Miller WL. The adrenal gland. In: Rudolph CD, Rudolph AM, eds. *Rudolph's pediatrics.* New York: McGraw-Hill, 2002:2028–2055.

Miller WL. The adrenal cortex. In: Sperling MA, ed. *Pediatric endocrinology.* Philadelphia: WB Saunders, 2002:385–438.

Miller WL. 21-Hydroxylase deficiency. In: Finberg L, Kleinman RE, eds. *Saunders manual of pediatric practice.* Philadelphia: WB Saunders, 2000:894–900.

Miller WL. Other congenital adrenal hyperplasia. In: Finberg L, Kleinman RE, eds. *Saunders manual of pediatric practice.* Philadelphia: WB Saunders, 2002:900–905.

Miller WL. Addison disease. In: Finberg L, Kleinman RE, eds. *Saunders manual of pediatric practice.* Philadelphia: WB Saunders, 2002: 905–912.

Oberfield SE, Gallagher MP, Levine LS. Endocrine hypertension. In: Finberg L, Kleinman RE, eds. *Saunders manual of pediatric practice.* Philadelphia: WB Saunders, 2002:912–915.

11 ♣ Diabetes Mellitus

Diabetes mellitus (DM) is a common chronic disease character-ized by elevated blood glucose caused by abnormal insulin pro-duction or abnormal insulin action that leads to disordered car-bohydrate, lipid, and protein metabolism. This may derive from inadequate insulin secretion (in general, the basic defect in type 1 DM), from inadequate insulin action, or both (in general, the description of type 2 DM). Variations are found on these two themes. Until this last decade, type 1 DM was the diagnosis in subjects younger than 18 years with new-onset DM, but now type 2 is becoming more prevalent and is coming closer to matching the incidence of type 1 DM in younger teenagers. The differentiation between the two becomes all the more important in the young patient (Table 11.1).

TYPE 1 DIABETES MELLITUS

Type 1 DM (*222100 DIABETES MELLITUS, INSULIN-DEPENDENT; IDDM) (type 1 DM) is a state of insulin deficiency requiring insulin replacement for therapy; this condition cannot be treated with oral hypoglycemic agents. Absence of insulin causes a catabolic state because of decreased entry of glucose into many cell types such as muscle and adipose tissue (but not brain, which requires no insulin to allow the entry of glucose), and sub-sequent impairment of cellular action occurs. The cells are, in effect, starving, and lipolysis, proteolysis, and glycogenolysis pro-ceed. Counterregulatory hormones (epinephrine, glucagon, growth hormone, and cortisol) stimulate gluconeogenesis, further increas-ing serum glucose. The absence of insulin in the portal circulation eliminates the inhibition of the hepatic acyl carnitine cycle and thereby allows the production of ketone bodies (acetoacetate, ace-tone, and hydroxybutyrate). In the most severe state of DM, diabetic ketoacidosis (DKA) develops, with potentially fatal consequences, as described later.

Type 1 DM is an autoimmune disorder that occurs in an indi-vidual with a genetic susceptibility who encounters an environ-mental stress, causing the development of the clinical disease. Type 1 DM occurs in about 12 to 14 per 100,000 individuals per year, with estimated frequencies from one in 1,430 to 2,500 at age 5 increasing to one in 300 to 360 by age 16 years. Type 1 DM does not have to occur in childhood as half of the cases are diag-nosed in the adult. Type 1 DM is more often found in whites than is type 2 DM (#TYPE 2 DIABETES MELLITUS #125853 DIA-BETES MELLITUS, NON–INSULIN-DEPENDENT; NIDDM at 20q12-q13.1, 20q12-q13.1, 17q25, 13q34, 13q12.1, 12q24.2, 11p12-p11.2, 2q32, 2q24.1), which is more often diagnosed in African Americans, Native Americans, Hispanic Americans and, most recently recognized, Asian Americans. A 50% concordance rate exists of TYPE 1 DIABETES MELLITUS in monozygotic twins, indicating that environmental effects are of importance in addi-tion to genetic factors (or the concordance would be 100%, which is the approximate rate of TYPE 2 DIABETES MELLITUS in monozygotic twins). Relations exist between the likelihood of

Table 11-1. Differential points between various common types of diabetes mellitus

Disorder	Ketosis	Insulin	C peptide	Islet cell antibodies, insulin antibodies, GAD 65 antibody	Inheritance	Defect	Clinical characteristics or habitus
Type 1 diabetes mellitus	Yes	Low	Low	Positive	Usually sporadic	Autoimmune; beta cell failure	Thin with weight loss
Type 2 diabetes mellitus	Sometimes	Normal to high	Normal to high	Negative	Familial	Inherited insulin resistance and beta cell failure worsened with obesity	Overweight, possibly with recent weight loss
Atypical diabetes mellitus	Sometimes	Normal to high	Normal to high	Negative	Autosomal dominant	Beta cell failure	Occurs in African Americans
MODY	No	Normal to high	Normal to high	Negative	Autosomal dominant	Six different genetic mutations in six MODY types	Occurs before age 20 yr

MODY, maturity onset diabetes of the young.

developing type TYPE 1 DIABETES MELLITUS and the human leukocyte antigens (HLAs) coded on chromosome 6, further emphasizing the genetic basis of the condition. Type 1 DM is 10 times more frequently found in individuals that have DR3/DR4 alleles and 100 times more frequent in those with a missing asparatic acid at position 57 in the DQ β chain than when there is an arginine at position 52 of the DQ α chain. The risk of onset of TYPE 1 DIABETES MELLITUS in nonidentical siblings is 1% if they share no HLA D haplotype, 5% to 7% if they share one haplotype, and 12% to 20% if they share both haplotypes. Other HLA alleles also reduce the likelihood of the onset of type 1 DM. For white children, a 6% risk exists for a sibling of an affected proband to develop type 1 DM if the proband is younger than 10 years, and a 3% risk if the proband is older than 10 years. Further, a 2% to 5% risk of type 1 DM is found to an offspring of a diabetic parent, the higher risk occurring if the father is affected.

The onset of type 1 DM is more frequent in fall and winter (suggesting a link to viral infections, which are more prevalent then). Many environmental factors are suggested to play a role in the onset of type 1 DM, but the mechanism of such effects are not always clear. In some cases, similarities are found in the sequence of viruses and those of proteins in the pancreas. This is the case in the glutamic acid decarboxylase 65 (GAD 65) sequence found in the beta cell and in some viruses; type 1 DM is often associated with antibodies directed to GAD 65. Besides viral infections, other factors such as environmental chemical substances are thought to trigger beta cell destruction in susceptible individuals. In most cases, it appears impossible to avoid exposures that are linked to type 1 DM.

A time sequence of beta cell destruction ultimately leads to the clinical picture that we recognize as type 1 DM (Fig. 11-1). Months or longer pass until the beta cell function is reduced to about 20% of normal levels, the degree of impairment that leads to frank clinical disease. An increase in the titer of antibodies to islet cells, insulin, tyrosine phosphatase (usually as a research study), and GAD 65, as well as other antigens, in the serum precedes the onset of clinical type 1 DM by months to years and may be present for as long as 10 years. The increase in such antibodies is implicated in some clinical studies to predict the onset of clinical DM, especially if the antibody titer is combined with a measure of impaired beta cell function. About 90% of individuals with type 1 DM have such positive antibodies concomitant with the discovery of clinical hyperglycemia. An intercurrent infection or other acute stress may precipitate the onset of type 1 DM or even DKA after a period of subclinical impairment of beta cell activity. After the onset of clinical type 1 DM and the start of therapy, there is often a "honeymoon period" of increased beta cell function and decreased insulin requirements, which may, incorrectly, suggest cure of the disease process and may last months to a year or more. Clinical trials of immune-suppressive therapy to lengthen the honeymoon period and other studies have been undertaken to determine how to avoid the development of type 1 DM.

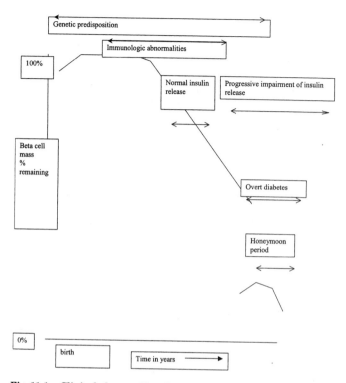

Fig. 11-1. Clinical phases of insulin-dependent diabetes.

The autoimmune basis of type 1 DM also predisposes the affected individual to other autoimmune diseases including Hashimoto thyroiditis, autoimmune Addison disease, autoimmune ovarian disease, and celiac disease. Type 1 DM may be included in auto-immune polyendocrinopathy syndrome 2 (269200 SCHMIDT SYNDROME), which may include candidiasis along with impairment of endocrine glands (see Chapter 10).

Clinical Presentation

Polyuria, polydipsia, and weight loss with dehydration are the classic findings of DM and may be noted, usually in retrospect, for 1 or more weeks before presentation. If the family or physicians are attuned to the findings, the diagnosis might be made before the development of the DKA that is the inevitable consequence of severe untreated insulin deficiency. Thus serum glucose might be moderately elevated at presentation (e.g., 200 to 300 mg/dL) without the presence of substantial serum ketones or decreased mentation, or conversely, the serum glucose might be severely elevated at presentation (700 mg/dL or more) with severe ketoacidosis (pH tending to or even lower than 6.9) and stupor or coma, all depending on when the natural course of the disorder is interrupted with medical evaluation and care. About 25% of subjects are seen in clinically apparent DKA, as described later (Table 11-2).

Laboratory evaluation will reveal elevated serum glucose, and thus rarely is a glucose tolerance test (GTT) required in most affected individuals (Table 11-3 has standards for GTT for completeness). The diagnosis, according to the American Diabetes Association, specifically requires a fasting blood glucose greater than 126 mg/dL or a random (or casual) blood glucose greater than 200 mg/dL, with the presence of the symptoms noted earlier, with repetition of these findings on a second occasion unless frank DKA is found. It must be noted that even a blood sugar (BS) of 126 mg/dL is outside of the normal range that extends only to 120 mg/dL in most laboratories. An elevated titer of antibodies to islet cells, insulin, or GAD 65 is found in the serum in 90% of cases. Urine analysis will be positive for glucose, as the elevation of blood glucose will exceed the renal threshold of 185 mg/dL that allows glucose excretion into the urine; however, glycosuria also can occur in nondiabetic conditions such as a genetic decrease of the renal threshold for glucose or diseases that affect the renal tubule. Positive urine or blood ketone bodies (acetoacetate, acetone, hydroxybutyrate) will develop in the absence of insulin, but ketone bodies also may be found at certain times in some children with type 2 DM, making differentiation between the two types difficult. Because of the elevated serum glucose, the serum sodium will be reported as low, because a 1.6-mEq/L decrease in serum sodium concentration is found for every increase in serum glucose of 100 mg/dL. This "pseudo-hyponatremia" does not itself require sodium administration for treatment, as there is a defect in the measurement of serum sodium rather than a defect in the physiology of sodium at the cellular level in the patient. However, in established DKA, actual sodium loss occurs, so that after correcting the reported sodium for the level of blood glucose, still a decreased serum sodium and total body sodium stores will be found, and administration of exogenous sodium is usually necessary. Insulin deficiency leads to elevation of serum triglyceride, sometimes to a remarkable degree, which may itself factitiously reduce the measurement of blood glucose and cholesterol, and may precipitate pancreatitis. The percentage of hemoglobin A_{1c} (HgbA_{1c}) demonstrates the degree to which glucose is nonreversibly bound to Hgb. Because the half-life of Hgb is 21 days, several half-lives are required to replace the previously formed HgbA_{1c}; thus the HgbA_{1c} value reflects the level of serum glucose on a long-term basis over the preceding 12 weeks or so (Table 11-4).

Diabetic Ketoacidosis

Many patients with type 1 DM have frank DKA caused by the severe insulin deficiency (Table 11-2). Besides the usual symptoms

Table 11-2. Treatment of diabetic ketoacidosis

1. Measure blood sugar (>200 mg/dL for diagnosis), blood ketones (positive or moderate to large ketones in urine for diagnosis), pH (venous <7.25 for diagnosis), bicarbonate (<16 mEq/mL for diagnosis), sodium, potassium, BUN and creatinine, and WBC count (usually elevated in DKA even without infection)
2. Fluid and electrolyte replacement
   a. Evaluate clinical deficit, which will usually be between 5% and 12%; average is 7% dehydration, so extra fluid administration for severe dehydration is not always needed
   b. Fluid administration must be done with care but, if indicated by signs of fluid deficit, an intravenous bolus of 10 mL/kg of "isotonic" fluid (0.9% saline or lactated Ringer's) over 30–60 min is used and repeated if necessary
   c. The remaining fluid deficit is administered over the next 48 hr
   d. Maintenance fluids are added to the deficit replacement
   e. Potassium will be deficient in DKA, so after establishing urine output, add potassium to the infusion at 30–40 mEq/mL. Monitor ECG for abnormalities of potassium, as peaked T waves occur in hyperkalemia and low T waves and the development of U waves occurs in hypokalemia
   f. Low phosphorus is a potentially dangerous complication of DKA, so K Phos is used as at least a portion of the replacement of K
   g. Bicarbonate therapy is associated with a higher risk for cerebral edema, and so should not be used unless there is symptomatic hyperkalemia or the acidosis is severe enough to cause hemodynamic instability not responsive to other therapeutic measures. If pH is 7.0–7.1, some suggest the use of bicarbonate at a dose of 40 mEq/mL/m^2 and if <7.0, the use of 80 mEq/mL/m^2, but because the use of bicarbonate is associated with the development of cerebral edema, this decision must be individualized
   h. Although excessive and rapid fluid administration might cause serious complications, dehydration leading to thrombosis is an alternative risk, so each patient must be individualized for appropriate fluid and electrolyte therapy
3. Insulin management
   a. Intravenous insulin at a rate of 0.075–0.1 unit/kg/hr is infused, and blood sugar monitored frequently. The use of a priming dose of insulin to prepare the tubing or an initial bolus of insulin before the infusion starts is no longer recommended
   b. When blood sugar decreases to 250–300 mg/dL, intravenous dextrose (5%–10%) is added to allow continued administration of insulin to bring about resolution of the ketoacidosis safely; this process may continue until the serum bicarbonate is >17–18 mEq/mL

Continued

Table 11-2.   *Continued*

4. Monitoring
   a. Measure blood sugar by glucometer or laboratory determinations every hour, and aim to decrease blood glucose by 10 mg/dL/hr. This rate may easily be exceeded as renal function and fluid and insulin administration all exert effects on decreasing blood sugar, so careful observation is mandatory
   b. Measure serum electrolytes every 4 hr

Watch for deteriorating mental condition, headaches, vomiting, or unusual behavior, as these might indicated the development of cerebral edema. Physical signs might include changing neurologic examination and papilledema. If necessary, confirm the development of cerebral edema with head MRI. Treatment of cerebral edema is difficult, and generally the methods are unproven, but mannitol 1 mg/kg i.v., or 10–20 g/m²) may be beneficial as long as dehydration is not allowed to develop after the use of a hyperosmolar agent

BUN, blood urea nitrogen; WBC, white blood cell; DKA, diabetic ketoacidosis; MRI, magnetic resonance imaging.

of polydipsia and polyuria, weight loss may accelerate because of fluid losses caused by osmotic diuresis and vomiting. Abdominal pain is common, sometimes suggesting the incorrect diagnosis of acute abdomen. Patients at presentation usually have severe elevation of blood glucose, metabolic acidosis with ketone bodies in blood and urine, and dehydration with sodium and potassium loss. Dehydration causes increased serum creatinine and blood urea nitrogen (BUN; factitious elevation of creatinine may also occur because of cross-reaction of acetoacetate in the creatinine assay). The respiration rate is increased to counteract the metabolic acidosis, and the ketonemia adds a "fruity" aroma to the breath; Kussmaul respiration is the term used to describe the rapid but shallow respirations. A patient with type 1 DM might certainly have intercurrent pneumonia, but Kussmaul respiration does not by itself indicate pneumonia; conversely, the state of dehydration may minimize the signs of pneumonia, so consideration for this possible coexisting condition must occur during evaluation of DKA. Indeed, infection may be present and may have been the precipitating factor to cause worsening of the diabetic condition, so the possibility of infection must be considered in all cases of DKA. Even if no infection is present, the white cell count is often elevated in DKA, with a marked shift to the left and prevalence of band forms of white blood cells (WBCs), probably related to the elevation of glucocorticoids during stress. Metabolic acidosis may be demonstrated if the anion gap {calculated as $[Na^+ - (HCO_3^- + Cl^-)]$} is increased above the normal limit of 14 mEq/L.

**Table 11-3.   Glucose tolerance test after
1.75 g/kg carbohydrate load (75 g maximum)**

Condition	Baseline	1 hr	2 hr	3 hr
Normal*	<110	<200	<140	<130
Insulin (mU/mL)	9	51	37	20
C-peptide (ng/mL)	1.3	3.3	3.0	2.0
Impaired glucose tolerance*	110–125		140–199	
Diabetes mellitus*	≥126	≥200	≥200	≥200

*Blood glucose in mg/dL.

The arterial pH is 7.3 or less, and serum bicarbonate is less than 15 mEq/L. DKA is not limited to the undiagnosed patient, as DKA may develop in any patient who does not adequately care for the condition or misses several insulin injections.

The life-threatening complication, cerebral edema (CE), occurs in about one in 100 cases of DKA, more often in younger patients, and may occur during the hospitalization at which the initial diagnosis of type 1 DM is made. Mortality is reported in 20% to 40% of cases, and neurologic sequelae in survivors are reported to be about 25%. The cause of CE is in dispute, and proven methods of eliminating this condition are not yet certain. However, a study of 6,000 cases of DKA indicated that CE is more common in patients having the lowest serum bicarbonate levels, in patients who received bicarbonate administration, in those with the youngest ages, in those with the longest duration of symptoms

Table 11-4.   Hgb A1C compared with average blood sugar

HgbA1c %	Average blood sugar mg/dL
4	60
5	90
6	120
7	150
8	180
9	210
10	240
11	270
12	300
13	330

and in those with the highest severity of symptoms, in those with higher BUN, and in those without the normal increase in serum Na during therapy. CE may cause a depressed sensorium from about 12 up to 24 hours after presentation of DKA and after initial improvement of symptoms. Many patients with any degree of DKA have some degree of brain swelling [which can be demonstrated on magnetic resonance imaging (MRI)], but the clinical manifestations of CE, including cerebellar tonsillar herniation and subsequent respiratory arrest, are the most extreme presentations. A patient who appears to be improving but deteriorates, who develops a headache during the improvement phase, or younger children who develop uncharacteristic behavior such as crying, blinking, or restlessness may be developing clinically relevant CE. Early signs of increased intracranial pressure in include (a) altered mental status/headache with decreased papillary response to light; (b) bradycardia; (c) hypertension; and (d) irregular respiration, developing later in the course. Treatment must be rapid and may include hyperventilation, mannitol infusion (0.25 to 1 mg/kg, i.v., every 2 to 4 hours) and possibly glucocorticoid administration, although the glucocorticoid may itself increase blood glucose values. Elevation of the head may help. Central nervous system (CNS) imaging is the direct proof of the condition and should be performed if imaging can be carried out while the subject is carefully observed and emergency therapy is available. Neurosurgical consult is mandatory, as cranial decompression may be necessary. Most sources recommend careful attention to the rate and composition of fluid replacement to avoid fatal CE, and, even if there is no clear proof that this approach will eliminate the development of CE, it certainly is prudent.

Other possible complications of DKA include thromboses of various major vessels including the development of pulmonary embolism and renal insufficiency. Thus although the treating physician must endeavor to moderate fluid administration so as not to increase the likelihood of CE, fluid must be adequate to avoid these complications of severe dehydration. Serious infections, including mucormycosis, are most prevalent in patients with long-term poor control. Pancreatitis may lead to diabetes if pancreatic function is severely affected, but conversely, elevated lipid levels caused by DKA may themselves lead to pancreatitis. Neuritis is rare in the initial presentation of DM but may be seen in rare patients.

DKA is a life-threatening emergency that requires that close monitoring be carried out in a pediatric intensive care unit, whenever possible. Patients from smaller communities are often transported to such centers by air or ambulance for this care. Vital signs and mental status are checked hourly in affected patients. Blood glucose is measured hourly; a true laboratory value is best, but a bedside glucometer is frequently used. Glucometers must be tested for accuracy, and the age of the sensor strips used on the device must be checked for expiration dates to make sure they have not expired, which would make them likely to record incorrect values. As BS values descend to the normal range, the glucometer becomes less accurate, and laboratory confirmation of glucose values becomes even more important. Serum electrolytes are measured every 4 hours. Serum osmolality is measured in the laboratory, but in the interim may be roughly estimated as

$$mOsm/L = 2 \times serum\ sodium\ (mEq/L) + [blood\ glucose\ (mg/dL)/18].$$

This equation indicates that an increase in blood glucose of 180 mg/dL causes an increase in osmolality of 10 mOsm/L. Thus DKA is a condition of hypertonic dehydration, and osmolality is elevated at presentation (Table 11.2).

Treatment of DKA involves fluid and electrolyte resuscitation along with insulin administration. Careful attention to laboratory data and fluid administration is accomplished with a flow sheet kept up to date at all times; such a flow chart is not an option! The concern that excess fluid administration may predispose a patient to CE must be balanced by the possibility that the dehydration at the time of presentation may cause ischemia of kidney, brain, or other organs. Thus any recipe for therapy must be modified by the clinical condition of the patient, and we can only offer guidelines.

The amount of fluid loss in DKA is estimated according to customary clinical findings. Severe cases are usually associated with fluid loss equivalent to 10% to 15% of body weight. Clinical signs of 10% to 15% dehydration are as follows: 5%, normal skin turgor, moist buccal mucosa, tears present, pulse regular; 10%, skin dry, and tenting of skin possible, buccal mucosa, dry eyes, deep set, tears decreased, irritability noted, pulse increased a bit; and 15%, clammy skin, parched buccal mucosa, eyes sunken, no tears, lethargy noted, pulse rapid. Because of the osmotic diuresis, urine output is not a reliable indicator of hydration.

Most recommend that normal saline solutions be used in the initial phases of rehydration but half-normal saline may be used when serum osmolality returns to the normal range. This fluid should be replaced slowly, over a 36- to 48-hour period, according to most recommendations, with half given over the first 12 hours, and the rest, over the remaining 24 to 36 hours. Initial resuscitation may be offered as a bolus of normal saline at 5 to 10 ml/kg if significant dehydration is detected by abnormal vital signs [low blood pressure (BP), rapid pulse, and delayed capillary filling], and this bolus may be repeated if indicators suggest the need for more immediate fluid replacement. If the patient is in shock, blood or plasma expanders may be used according to customary intensive care protocols.

$$\begin{aligned} mEq\ of\ sodium\ required = [&concentration\ desired\ (mEq/L) - \\ &concentration\ present\ (mEq/L)] \\ &\times 0.6\text{--}0.7 \times body\ weight\ in\ kilograms \end{aligned}$$

One half of this deficit is given in the first 12 hours, and the rest, in the next 36 hours. An additional 20 to 40 mEq/L of sodium is added for daily maintenance.

Potassium deficit is likely in all presentations of DKA. A serum potassium value that is normal indicates a moderate deficit in total body potassium, whereas a low value indicates a serve deficit, and even an elevated value is associated with a mild potassium deficit. Potassium deficit will increase with saline administration and expansion of extracellular volume. As acidosis is corrected, or if alkalosis develops, the potassium will leave the intracellular space in exchange for hydrogen, a trend that intensifies with the ultimate glucose and insulin administration later in the course of the treatment. Careful attention to potassium balance is essential. Although laboratory evaluation is essential, the electrocardiogram (ECG) offers some information, as peaked T waves are seen in hyperkalemia, whereas U waves are seen in hypokalemia. Potassium can be replaced, once urinary output is established, by 20 to 40 mEq/L given slowly in the replacement fluid. ECG monitoring is essential, as an excessive amount or speed of potassium administration may be fatal because of the development of arrhythmias. Because Cl may itself cause acidosis, potassium is best given half as potassium acetate and half as potassium phosphate, with the proviso that phosphate infusion is best used only when phosphate is low, because in excess, phosphate can reduce calcium.

Acidosis is almost always corrected by fluid and insulin administration in DKA. Thus added bicarbonate is not indicated in most cases, even with significant acidosis (indeed, added bicarbonate is associated with an increased likelihood of the onset of cerebral edema and may cause cerebral acidosis), although some authorities recommend the use of 40 mEq/m^2 of bicarbonate if the pH is 7.1 and 80 mEq/m^2 if the pH is less than 7.0. **This chapter does not advocate routine bicarbonate administration,** but for completeness, the formula to calculate bicarbonate deficit is (12 − observed bicarbonate value) × 0.6 body weight (kg), and the administration is performed as 1 to 2 mg/kg over a 2-hour period or slower.

Insulin therapy for DKA is generally administered as an i.v. infusion at a rate of 0.05 to 0.1 unit/kg/hr, with the lower dose range usually achieving a more desirable slower decrease in blood glucose. In the past, a bolus of i.v. insulin was given initially, but this is likely to decrease blood glucose too rapidly; some authorities still recommend it, but we believe that it is best to bypass this bolus. The goal of insulin therapy is a decrease of blood glucose of about 50 to 100 mg/dL/hr, although that the rate of decrease may often exceed this goal. Correction of blood glucose may precede correction of acid-base balance. In this situation, it is important to continue insulin administration until acidosis is eliminated. Although no dextrose is given in i.v. fluids at first, as the blood glucose is already elevated, when blood glucose decreases to about 300 to 200 mg/dL, dextrose (usually as D5% in saline) is added to allow the safe continued administration of insulin, which will serve to eliminate ketone bodies while minimizing the likelihood of hypoglycemia.

Insulin is now always administered as recombinant DNA–derived human insulin. Regular insulin is used for i.v. administration to control DKA. It is administered via a "Y" connector, piggy-backed onto the other fluid being administered. Insulin is usually mixed as 50 units into a 250-mL bottle of saline, yielding 1 unit/5 mL of saline. The desired hourly units of insulin will be delivered by the number of milliliters determined by multiplying the units by 5 (e.g., 2 U/hr given as 10 mL/hr yields). The insulin infusion is usually continued until urine ketone bodies are absent, which is often past the persistence of hyperglycemia. This stage usually is reached at the time that the child will be able to tolerate oral feedings. This is the time to consider switching to subcutaneous insulin administration.

Close monitoring of mental status, vital signs, peripheral perfusion, and serum sodium and potassium is important, with evaluation of magnesium and phosphorus also indicated initially, and if abnormal, at intervals thereafter (magnesium deficiency may cause potassium loss in the urine). All the abnormal measurements should improve in a continuous pattern; if sodium decreases rather than increases, excess free water administration may be the cause.

Improvement should be continuous. Thus deteriorating status may be owing to increasing or not resolving acidosis, uncorrected or developing hypokalemia, hypoglycemia, hypotension, untreated infection, or CE.

Onset Without DKA

With increased education of the population, many patients are diagnosed at the earlier stages of the disease and do not have DKA. BS might be only in the range from 200 to 300. These patients might be educated in the outpatient environment if adequate and trained staff is available to administer such education. This is appropriate only if ketosis is absent or minimal and if glucose is only moderately elevated. It is important to differentiate this situation from type 2 DM described later.

Transitioning to the Long-term Management of Diabetes Mellitus Type 1

It is essential to involve the patient and family in the process of monitoring BS by glucometer and the measurement and administration of insulin as soon as possible after the resolution of DKA, or a lengthened hospitalization will result. At initial presentation, the family may be distraught over the new diagnosis, and it is necessary to take clues from them as to when they can be receptive to education about this disease. After the resolution of hyperglycemia and ketonemia/acidosis, the major reason for patient to remain in the hospital is lack of ability to carry out BS monitoring, insulin administration, or dietary planning, and this accomplishment rests on family education. Because the patient will be more active at home than in the hospital and glucose values will therefore likely decrease from values seen in the hospital, BS values do not have to be completely normalized before discharge. It is, however, not useful to expect the family and child to have a complete understanding of the biology of diabetes before discharge after the diagnosis of this life-long condition. An understanding of the more complex details of the disorder will develop during the outpatient-management phase.

Home measurement of BS by glucometer has revolutionized the ability of family and patient to control BS closely. Many glucometers are available for measurement of BS from drops of blood from the finger or arm, and all have various advantages and drawbacks. Most have memories, but electronic memories do not replace the maintenance of a meticulous record book, which assists inpatient and physician's review of BS control. Most glucometer memories can be downloaded to a computer for the generation of BS versus time-of-day graphs and other useful analytic information. Nonetheless, all too often, the family brings in a glucometer that was not set to day and time and therefore cannot be interpreted, or they forget the glucometer completely, leading to a wasted visit. If they keep a record book, they are involved in the process of monitoring and have a second source of historical blood glucose data.

In all regimens, BS is monitored at least 4 times per day (before meals and at bedtime, always before eating), and the insulin dose is adjusted according to these values. It is important to wait 2 hours after any preceding meal or snack to obtain a glucometer reading, as it takes about that long to overcome the peak caused by carbohydrate intake. Insulin is not usually given outside of the scheduled time unless the BS is measured very high at alternative times of the day (e.g., greater than 350) and ketone bodies appear in the urine.

A recent advance is continuous glucose monitoring, which can be carried out for a period of 3 days by using a sensor that is temporarily implanted in subcutaneous tissue; this process is evaluated in a doctor's office and is used to analyze problems of glucose control or to determine adjustments to insulin-pump therapy. A watch-like device measures the glucose in a transudate produced over the hours it is worn on the skin; it is now approved for children and may be used to monitor patterns. Although a delay of 20 minutes elapses between the sample and the reading, limiting its ability to signal an emergency, it can predict a low BS value by monitoring the trend of blood glucose and can alert the patient to a likely problem. Unfortunately, the goal of continuous blood glucose monitoring by a miniature device that accurately and quickly reports BS values is still elusive in spite of exceptional research into the area. One might suspect that such a device will be perfected and linked to the subcutaneous insulin infusion pump to form a closed loop that will function as a replacement pancreas. At the same time, much research is ongoing into the transplantation of islet cells into patients with type 1 DM to allow them to produce and secrete insulin in appropriate amounts.

Once BS is brought close to normal values, acidosis is resolved, and the patient is able to tolerate oral feedings, it is time to consider switching to subcutaneous insulin. Many approaches exist to insulin therapy, and more than one type of insulin and type of device are available for administration (Fig. 11-2, Table 11-5). A decision must first be made about the method of switching from

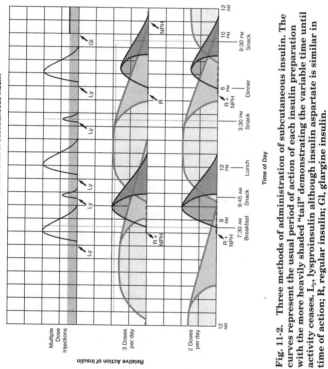

Fig. 11-2. Three methods of administration of subcutaneous insulin. The curves represent the usual period of action of each insulin preparation with the more heavily shaded "tail" demonstrating the variable time until activity ceases. L$_y$, lysproinsulin although insulin aspartate is similar in time of action; R, regular insulin; Gl, glargine insulin.

Table 11-5. Actions of commercially available insulin preparations

Preparation	Onset of action	Peak activity	Duration of action (hr)
Aspart	5 min	30 min to 3 hr	3–5
Lispro	<30 min	30–90 min	2 (<6 hr)
Regular	30–60 min	2–4 hr	5–8
NPH	1–2 hr	6–12 hr	18–24
Glargine	1 hr	None	24

NPH, isophane insulin.

i.v. insulin to subcutaneous insulin. Characteristic management has historically involved two injections per day, each consisting of a moderate-acting and a short-acting insulin preparation. Two injections per day is a compromise, but in some cases must be accepted. In the two-dose-per-day regimen, the child is obliged to eat a meal containing a predictable carbohydrate content to maintain BS as the short- and moderate-acting insulin exert their effects; skipping a meal will cause hypoglycemia, whereas excessive carbohydrate intake will cause hyperglycemia. Some families are not able or willing to give a third noon injection or a fourth bedtime injection of long-acting insulin, and the child may be too young to be independent enough to give the injection, which would be necessary for a multiple-dose injection schedule. However, multiple-dose injection is a better schema for many children (see later).

Insulin is injected subcutaneously, not intramuscularly. The injection sites must change regularly, or lipohypertrophy may develop, a "lump" under the skin that will make the time of absorption vary from injection to injection and lead to unstable control. Insulin is usually injected in the triceps area, the thighs, the abdomen, or the lateral, upper buttocks. Insulin vials are usually kept at room temperature, where they are stable for 30 days. The total daily dose of insulin tends to average about 1 U/kg/day, although significant variations are found to this number as the course of the disease advances.

Assuming that the family will start with two doses of insulin per day, two basic methods may be used to prepare the child for this regimen of insulin administration. When the i.v. insulin is discontinued, the insulin effect will be quickly eliminated. Thus subcutaneous regular insulin must be given at least 30 minutes before discontinuing i.v. insulin to allow it to exert its effect while the i.v. insulin effect wanes. This changeover is best performed before a meal; i.v. glucose is discontinued along with the i.v. insulin, because oral intake is usually tolerated at this stage. If the child has been receiving i.v. insulin for several days and the BS has stabilized on oral intake, the total sum of insulin that was infused over the previous 24 hours is used as an initial estimate of the dose of insulin to be given by subcutaneous injections over the next 24 hours. Without such information, the initial dose of daily insulin is estimated to be 0.5 to 1.0 U/kg/day.

In the first method of insulin therapy after discontinuing i.v. insulin, the total daily dose of insulin is divided into one third given before breakfast, one fourth before lunch, one third before dinner, and one twelfth before bedtime; this adds up to the total daily insulin dosage. If this dosage, or a modification of it, is successful in controlling BS, the next step of therapy proceeds to the use of two doses per day with short- and intermediate-action insulin given before breakfast and before dinner. The insulin dose may be estimated as two thirds of total daily dose before breakfast and one third of the total daily dose of insulin given before dinner, with one third of each dose given as regular and two thirds given as NPH insulin. The amount to be given for a total daily dose is either derived from the i.v. insulin infused the day before, if it was successful in controlling BS or from the formula of the total daily dose equaling 0.5 to 1 U/kg body weight, with a preference to give the lower range at first.

The two dose per day method requires a meal schedule that is rather rigid, or hypoglycemia will occur if no carbohydrate intake occurs at the time of the expected peak of the action of insulin already given.

A technique that is gaining popularity is multiple dose injections (MDIs), which involves the administration of a very long acting insulin (usually glargine insulin, which exerts a stable effect over the 24 hours after an injection) every evening (or more recently, morning) and a dose of very short acting insulin (lispro or Aspartate (not yet approved for children) insulin) given before every substantial meal or snack by using a set ratio of insulin-to-carbohydrate intake (usually 0.5 to 2 units insulin per 15 g of carbohydrate). A dietician is especially helpful in calculating this ratio of insulin-to-carbohydrate intake. The patient or family must count carbohydrates in each meal consumed, so education is more complex for MDI. Someone (if the child is too young, some responsible adult) must be able to calculate insulin doses at midday or at snack time and administer the insulin while the child is away from home. Short-acting insulin may be given by the classic syringe and needle with a bottle of insulin or by a cartridge-and-pen system in which the dose is dialed in and the insulin administered. The short-acting insulin is adjusted both on the basis of the carbohydrates to be consumed (determined by carbohydrate counting) and the BS at the time of injection (determined by glucometer). In this regimen, the child has a more flexible schedule, whereby meals might be delayed, extra snacks might be more easily added, or meals may even be missed (this, of course, is not a recommended action). This MDI regimen may be started just after the insulin infusion ceases during the resolution of DKA in selected patients who appear able to absorb this much information so quickly after diagnosis. In general, the two-dose regimen is begun after the resolution of DKA, and the patient, after a time, chooses to move to MDI after learning carbohydrate counting successfully.

The computerized continuous subcutaneous insulin infusion pump ("insulin pump") has simplified diabetic management to a large degree. In general, a patient must be prepared for the use of an insulin pump, so the patient may not started on the pump while in the hospital for the initial admission. We insist that a patient demonstrate knowledge of carbohydrate counting of a meal, keep records of the four or more BS measurements obtained daily, and accurately calculate the correct dose of rapid-acting insulin according to the amount of carbohydrates ingested and by the serum BS measurement at the time of the injection. We believe that pitfalls exist to the use of the insulin pump that might be avoided by testing the ability of the patient to use it initially.

An insulin pump is computer controlled, small (the size of a pager), and contains enough insulin for at least 3 days of control; the needle (infusion set) is intended to stay in a subcutaneous location for 2 to 3 days but no more, or infection or clogged tubing may occur. One major advantage of a continuous subcutaneous insulin infusion pump is the flexible basal infusion rates. Although a single injection of glargine insulin lasts 24 hours and is rather stable, no way is known to vary its effect during the day for the dawn phenomenon, for example (see later). Insulin pumps vary by manufacturer, but all can change the insulin infusion rate by half-hour intervals, leading to several possible changes per day on a preprogrammed schedule. Most patients use only three to five basal infusion rates per day, but the numerous possible settings may be used to improve control. The patient administers a bolus of short-acting insulin at meal times, depending on blood glucose values and carbohydrate intake, by ordering the dose from a touch-pad keyboard on the pump. The pump has the ability to infuse a peaked bolus or a "square or dual wave" of longer duration based on the amount of fat or protein included in the meal, factors that will change according to the pattern of postprandial glucose values. This method, like MDI, allows a more flexible schedule of meals and may be especially attractive to teenagers. However, the pump cannot sense the BS values and decide on the correct dose of insulin itself (although research is aimed at producing a pump that can do just that). The pump functions completely on the understanding of diabetes by the patient or family.

Some dangers are found in pump therapy, as the user must be able to count CH_2O content of food and scrupulously monitor BS values 4 times or more per day, or control may waver. The infusion set (subcutaneous plastic tubing) must be changed every 2 to 3 days, or it will clog or even become infected, without the patient's becoming aware of this. The pump has alarms but cannot detect all problems. If the tubing is kinked or clogged, the insulin infusion may stop unexpectedly. Short-acting insulin is so quickly cleared from the body that severe insulinopenia and even DKA will develop within hours if the user does not note one of these problems. Thus attention to detail and frequent BS measurement are even more essential in pump therapy. Every insulin-pump company has trainers to teach the patient the important technical, but not medical, points of pump therapy. More details of pump therapy are beyond this chapter.

No matter which schema is followed, careful attention to BS monitoring is essential, at least before breakfast, lunch, and dinner, and before the bedtime snack. A record book of the BS values must be maintained; although glucometers may have memory of the measurements over the previous month or more, observation of the patterns of BS changes is essential if a patient is to learn how to make adjustments of insulin doses and to guard against a dead battery falsifying or emptying the glucometer's memory. Another reason to keep a written record is that some patients use multiple glucometers or may not care for the device correctly: if the glucometer does not have the date or time set (perhaps because of battery change or dropping the device), the memory on the glucometer will be useless, as it will not be possible to determine when any glucose value occurred.

These guidelines are general, and individuals do not follow a simple rule in their response to calculated insulin dosage. For example, once stabilized, when the child resumes the previous daily schedule, the insulin dose might be decreased (10% or more) if the child plans to exercise, as the activity will often decrease the blood glucose value and could possibly precipitate hypoglycemia; this might occur, for example, twice per week, if the child has gym class on a twice-a-week schedule. Alternatively, the family might have to find empirically the amount of carbohydrate needed to maintain the BS during the activity without a change in insulin dose; this might be used to good advantage if unplanned activity occurs. Some children will increase their BS with exercise, so values must be checked before, during, and after exercise. In general, although exercise is a good idea if BS is moderately elevated, if BS is higher than 350 mg/dL, and especially if ketones are present, exercise should be limited or curtailed completely until control is gained by insulin administration.

The patient and family must understand appropriate dietary management of diabetes, although it will take some time before this becomes second nature. A dietician is expert in teaching these skills and should be consulted early in the educational process. An American Diabetes Association (ADA) diet generally consists of 45% to 60% of total calories from carbohydrates, 30% from fat with less than 10% saturated fat, and 10% to 20% calories from protein. Total recommended calories vary by age and size of the child.

The family should learn carbohydrate counting, a skill that will be needed if MDI or insulin pump is considered. In general, carbohydrates are carbohydrates, so that previously "forbidden" foods may be ingested, as long as the insulin administered is appropriate for the carbohydrate load. Birthday cake is not to be a staple of the diet, but on occasion, it can be eaten with insulin coverage, especially in the MDI regimen.

The basic "survival skills" are learned before discharge from the initial hospitalization so that the patient can measure BS by glucometer, measure insulin from the bottle or pen, administer the injection, use emergency measures including intramuscular glucagon injection for hypoglycemia, and choose a reasonable diet. The patient must recognize the signs of hypoglycemia or impending DKA, the steps necessary to reach the doctor for advice (not an easy task in a large medical center), and understand that therapy will change if an intercurrent illness occurs. Although the basics of adjustment of insulin may be taught in the hospital, in this age of mandatory rapid discharges (mandated by funding agencies rather than medical judgment), usually inadequate time is available to teach this all in detail. Thus after discharge, the family/patient will call the physician at the time of scheduled insulin injections for a few days or weeks to discuss the correct dose and explain why it was adjusted as such. This educational process aids the family in achieving independence in understanding the therapy of diabetes. In time the family and patient who have observed the response to therapy will offer suggestions for management that may greatly assist the team in deciding on change in therapy.

Other Aspects of Long-term Therapy

Sick-day management refers to the changes necessary if there is a likelihood that the child's intake will vary from the normal level or if an intercurrent infection itself brings about a tendency to elevated BSs with the stress of the illness; some children will have an increase but some will have a decrease in BS with infections, depending on oral intake, so no hard and fast rule can be made. Intermediate-acting insulin dosage is usually discontinued during the duration of the illness, so that more rapid adjustments in management are possible with the use of more frequent doses of short-acting insulin. Thus four or more injections of regular insulin (or more injections if Humalog is used by the patient) are indicated to achieve control. Frequent BS monitoring is needed during the sickness as well as monitoring for urine ketone bodies. The presence of ketone bodies in the urine will necessitate increased or more frequent doses of insulin or evaluation at the doctor's office or emergency department (ED). Admission to the hospital is a possibility, especially if fluid intake is limited. Telephone contact is necessary at the least during a sick day, if the family has no experience in such management. If the illness involves nausea and vomiting and the patient cannot tolerate fluids, the patient must come to the ED for evaluation; several hours' infusion of fluid (and dextrose if needed) may be all that is required, but hospital admission also may be necessary. It is not appropriate to give an antiemetic [e.g., promethazine (Phenergan)] to a child with diabetes unless careful communication with the family can continue, because the vomiting may be a sign of DKA rather than, for example, a viral illness. Resolution of high BS and moderate ketone bodies may decrease the tendency to vomit, resolving some of the problem. In carefully evaluated situations, the antiemetic may keep a child at home and out of the ED, but it must be emphasized that close communication must eliminate the possibility that the suppositories are simply covering up a worsening situation. In addition, the suppositories might precipitate extrapyramidal effects.

Two phenomena are important in the understanding of DM. The Somogyi phenomenon occurs when hypoglycemia triggers the release of counterregulatory hormones that subsequently increase BS; thus a low BS at 3 a.m. may cause a BS of 300 mg/dL or more in the morning. Nightmares, night sweats, and headaches on awakening may occur in a subject with the Somogyi phenomenon. It would initially seem that more intermediate-acting insulin is indicated at night because the a.m. BS is high, but the opposite is true. Increasing the p.m. dose of intermediate- or long-acting insulin would worsen the situation, because the basic problem is too much insulin, leading to hypoglycemia. The dawn phenomenon is an increase in blood glucose in the early morning hours before waking, due to an elevation of growth hormone. Some children even have an antidawn phenomenon in which the increase in BS occurs just after midnight rather than just before waking. Evaluation of these possibilities requires monitoring BS at intervals during the night, with 2- to 3-a.m. values being quite useful. New 3-day continuous BS-monitoring devices help evaluate these various patterns of blood glucose.

Pattern adjustments are taught to the family and child to allow them to respond to abnormal BS values with a change in insulin administration. Thus they are instructed that the long- or intermediate-acting insulin should remain stable unless a need for changing the dose is demonstrated by an aberrant pattern of BSs at a particular time of the day over at least 3 to 5 days. In contrast, they are taught to change the short-acting insulin at the time the injection is given, based on the concurrent BS. Thus depending on size and insulin sensitivity, one might add 0.5 unit of regular or short-acting insulin to the basal planned dose if BS is greater than 150, 1 unit if BS is greater than 200, 2.5 units if BS is greater than 250, and so on (Table 11-6). Older and larger

Table 11-6.   Typical algorithm for short-term insulin correction (sliding scale)

Blood sugar	Instruction for use of regular insulin
<60 mg/dL	Omit regular, recheck glucose after meal and use rapid acting insulin as needed
60–80 mg/dL	Decrease regular 10%
80–120 mg/dL	Usual dose
120–180 mg/dL	Increase by 10%
180–240 mg/dL	Increase by 15%
240–300 mg/dL	Increase by 20%
>300 mg/dL	Increase by 30% and check urinary ketones

subjects might get twice these doses, and empiric adjustment is used to find the best sliding scale. The rule of 1,500 is useful to determine an appropriate sliding scale: divide the total daily dose of insulin on a normal day into 1,500, and the result is the change in BS that might be expected with the addition of 1 unit of short-acting insulin. Thus if a child uses 50 units per day, the addition of 1 unit as a sliding scale should reduce the blood glucose level by 30. One sliding scale may be developed for one meal, and another sliding scale for another meal.

Time of Insulin Action in Combined Short-acting and Intermediate-acting Insulin

It is important to note when a dose of insulin exerts its effects. The a.m. regular insulin determines the prelunch BS, the a.m. NPH will determine the predinner value, the p.m. regular insulin determines the prebedtime BS, and the p.m. NPH determines the prebreakfast value. However, a dip in BSs might occur in mid-morning if regular insulin is used, because of the long action of the a.m. regular insulin, and at midevening, because of the same effect of the p.m. regular insulin. No such decrease in BS will occur several hours after administration of lispro or Aspartate insulin. The larger a.m. NPH dose can cause a dip in BS at midafternoon. Snacks are therefore given in midmorning, midafternoon, and before bedtime to counteract this tendency in the two-dose-per-day regimen if regular rather than short acting insulin is used. A dip in BS may occur in the middle of the night from the p.m. dose of NPH insulin, so a 3 a.m. BS reading should be obtained on occasion, but not every day, to make sure this is not occurring. If a 3 a.m. decrease in BS if found, the p.m. dose of NPH might be decreased or the Somogyi effect may occur (see later). If the NPH is not lasting until the a.m. BS measurement, or if a 3 a.m. dip is noted, NPH might be given at bedtime, if the child can accept three injections per day. In general, if the BS stays stable between breakfast and lunch or stays stable between dinner and bedtime, the dose of regular or short acting insulin that was given before the first of these times is an appropriate basal dose (Table 11-7). Similarly, if the BSs stay stable between lunch and dinner or bedtime and the next morning, you have found a good basal dose of intermediate-acting insulin. If the BS increases between lunch and dinner (or between bedtime and the next a.m.), you know that the intermediate-acting insulin dose was too low, and you would add one or more units to the inter-mediate dose for the next day (first check that there is no Somo-gyi effect).

Time of Action of Insulin on Multiple-dose-injection Scheme

If the patient is using Lantus insulin and no hypoglycemia is noted during the sleep period (BS should be measured at 3 a.m. on a couple of occasions to be sure), the a.m. BS value will gener-ally determine whether the dose of Lantus is appropriate. If the BS stays stable between a premeal determination and the value

Table 11-7.

	Before breakfast	Before lunch	Before dinner	Bedtime
Blood sugar (mg/dL)	249	250	160	150
Planned regular insulin dose	10	—	5	—
Additional regular insulin on the sliding scale	2	—	—	—
NPH dose	14	—	7	—

In this case, the 10 units of regular insulin plus 2 units on the sliding scale were not able to cover breakfast and bring down the prelunch value, but the sugar stayed stable at ~250 mg/dL, so the 12 total units can hold the sugar values and probably is the correct dose before breakfast with the addition of a sliding scale; if the a.m. blood sugar was normal, the lunch value would likely be as well. Further, because the prebreakfast blood sugar was 249, it appears that the nighttime NPH dose was too low. If the pattern is seen over several days and if the blood sugar tested at 3 a.m. is high, it is safe to add an extra unit or two of NPH insulin to the p.m. NPH dose to bring down the prebreakfast blood sugar. Alternatively, the p.m. NPH dose might be given at bedtime to cause peak action to be delayed, which may bring down the prebreakfast blood sugar; if the breakfast blood sugar is brought down to 100–150 mg/dL, the lunch value may very well follow suit with the a.m. 12-unit dose of regular insulin. Usually it is best to make just one change at a time and evaluate the results of each change. Although the sliding scale of regular insulin is designed to be given for changes in blood sugar encountered on a daily basis, a change in the basal dose of regular or the dose of NPH is usually not invoked unless a pattern is noted over several days. The adjustments of regular insulin as described is usually applicable to adjustments in rapid acting insulin as well.

	Before breakfast	Before lunch	Before dinner	Bedtime
Blood sugar (mg/dL)	165	155	250	240
Planned regular insulin dose	12	—	5	—
Additional regular insulin on the sliding scale	1	—	2	—
NPH dose	14	—	7	—

In this case, the predinner blood morning sugar value was too high. If this occurs over several days, the NPH dose might be increased by 1 or 2 units and the resulting predinner blood sugar evaluated. If the predinner blood sugar value decreases toward normal, the NPH dose is more appropriate. The sum of 5 units of regular insulin before dinner and 2 units of the sliding scale for a total of 7 units regular insulin held the blood sugar relatively constant between dinner and bedtime: thus 7 units is approximately the correct basal dose of regular insulin before dinner. In addition, if the predinner value decreases, the bedtime value might also decrease as an added benefit, so that no extra regular insulin from the sliding scale over the 7 units of regular insulin before dinner is required. The blood sugar before breakfast might be brought down in the same manner as described above.

2 hours later, the short-acting insulin dose per a given serving of carbohydrates is appropriate. If the premeal BS is too high, but the calculated dose of additional short-acting insulin is able to decrease the BS value 2 hours later to a desirable level, the sliding-scale dosage is appropriate.

Hypoglycemia will occur in all individuals with DM at some point, and those with good control or those receiving intensive therapy are more likely to have this complication because their general BS values will be closer to normal and therefore closer to low levels. Sensation of low BS might be lost in those with chronically elevated BS values (hypoglycemic unresponsiveness). Further, more than half of the episodes of hypoglycemia occur at night; some children have night terrors as a sign of this complications, but some have no evidence of hypoglycemia or progress to seizures without warning. Middle-of-the-night BS measurements or a 3-day continuous glucose-monitoring session might help determine if this problem is occurring. Treatment is the administration of glucose (not complex carbohydrates, which will be absorbed too slowly), but overtreatment will lead to hyperglycemia and a seesaw effect of BS values that are too high, leading to another dose of insulin that drives the value down, requiring another dose of glucose. A glass of 4 oz of juice or a few hard candies or a glucose tablet will remedy most mild hypoglycemia; about 15 g of glucose is used. Paste glucose preparations are available as medical agents, but cake frosting might well substitute at lower cost. These oral glucose preparations may be absorbed through the buccal mucosa if the child in not cooperative. In 15 minutes, the BS should increase to more than 100 mg/dL, but if not, the whole process can be repeated. If the patient is not responding to such measures and becomes insensible, injection of glucagon (0.02–0.03 mg/kg or 0.5 to 1.0 mg, subcutaneously) must be given to mobilize the plentiful glycogen stores in diabetic subjects; the BS will increase considerably in a short time but will decrease over the following hours. Unfortunately, a glucagon injection may make the child nauseated, which will further complicate the day's BS and insulin management. All individuals with diabetes must have easily available glucagon emergency kits that contain the medication and a syringe and needle for administration.

Most children with type 1 DM have a period of resumed insulin secretion and improved control known as the "honeymoon period." Some may even not require insulin for months at a time; this period does not define a "cure," but rather a temporary remission, and parents should not develop false hope during this period that the disease process is over. Immune-suppression therapy is under study as a means of prolonging the honeymoon period, and many investigators are attempting truly to "cure" diabetes.

Nationwide study (the diabetes control and complication trial or DCCT) and international studies demonstrate a dramatic decrease in complications of type 1 DM with "tight control," which involves maintaining the HgbA$_{1c}$ and BS values close to normal. Such control cannot be achieved in younger subjects without encountering hypoglycemic reactions, but by the teenage years, this is a noteworthy goal. The American Diabetes Association and all authoritative bodies agree that team management is optimal for close control of diabetes at any age. Thus a nurse educator, a dietician, and a social worker, in the best of situations, join the physician. This team approach may on be available at a larger medical center, which may be at a distance from the patient. Thus initial education and quarterly consultations may be offered, with day-to-day care provided by the patient's local physician. In some remote areas, telemedicine consults are available from major medical centers, so that advice might be dispensed by television hookup if medical personnel are on site with the patient who can supply the necessary physical examinations and provide the needed BS values over the phone, fax, or television. The aim for older patients is achievement of control of BS close to the normal range and achievement of a normal or near-normal value of $HgbA_{1c}$, but this is impossible in younger children and infants. Adolescents and adults are advised by the ADA to have (a) preprandial BS of 80 to 120 mg/dL; (b) 2-hour postprandial BS of less than 180 mg/dL; (c) bedtime BS of 100 to 140 mg/dL; and (d) $HgbA_{1c}$ of less than 1% above the upper limit of normal for the laboratory.

These values are difficult to achieve and are best used as goals rather than expected accomplishments in all young patients. The goal of a preprandial BS close to 150 mg/dL is appropriate at younger ages to lessen the likelihood of hypoglycemia, fully realizing that even this relaxed goal might not be reached. Considerable variation will be found in BS measurements in children of all ages because of the lack of precision of glucose management with present technology, but variations should be minimized as much as possible.

Children are evaluated as needed for insulin adjustments and may receive advice over the phone if they report or fax the BS values to the physician, but these children should be seen in the medical office at least quarterly. Subjects' heights and weights are tracked to see if normal patterns are described. Decreased growth may indicate poor control or the development of hypothyroidism or celiac disease. Decreased BS values and decreased insulin requirements well after the time expected to span the honeymoon period might indicate the development of autoimmune Addison disease. Interphalangeal joints are evaluated for contractures that develop after years of DM. BP is monitored to determine whether hypertension has developed, possibly because of kidney damage. All children should be examined for lipohypertrophy at the sites of insulin injection, as lack of rotation of sites may predispose to this complication and lead to irregular absorption of insulin. Lipoatrophy is rare with the use of human insulin but was seen in the past with the use of animal insulin. Although untreated type 1 DM leads to weight loss due to the loss of calories in the urine and cellular starvation, treatment allows weight regain. However, if a child consumes too many calories and increases insulin dosage to cover the intake, obesity may develop. This is more often encountered with the use of the insulin pump. Dietary counseling and recalculation of insulin dose will help this problem. Some teenagers may skip or decrease insulin dose in a misguided attempt to lose weight, with sometimes tragic consequences. Glycosylated hemoglobin can be measured in minutes by new office-based devices; checking the $HgbA_{1c}$ with the glucose measurements on the glucometer and glucose record book is a good way to evaluate the accuracy of the patient's BS records or recollection of diabetes management. If necessary, an $HgbA_{1c}$ value may lead to a frank discussion of reasons for poorer control than expected. It is important to recall that the $HgbA_{1c}$ is an average, so that near-normal levels are found with excellent control and with a mixture of high and low values of BS; a near-normal value does not always indicate improvement of control, as it may indicate the advent of hypoglycemia. Glucose is nonenzymatically bound to the amino terminus of the β chain of hemoglobin, so that a patient with abnormal hemoglobin (e.g., thalassemia, which increases $HgbA_{1c}$, or sickle cell disease, which decreases it) will have fallacious readings of $HgbA_{1c}$ and will need glucosamine or fructosamine measurements or total glycohemoglobulin by affinity chromatography instead of $HgbA_{1c}$ measurements to determine the long-term status of BS control.

Every year, each child should have determination of thyroid function (autoimmune thyroiditis is common and may occur at presentation of DM) by free T_4 and thyroid-stimulating hormone (TSH), cholesterol and triglycerides (elevated lipid values occur with poor control), and renal function. Yearly ophthalmologic examinations are indicated to check for microvascular disease after the passage of 3–5 years with type 1 DM and at diagnosis for type 2 diabetes in older patients, a celiac panel or evaluation for celiac disease is indicated, especially if gastrointestinal symptoms are found. Neuropathy and gastroparesis are rarely seen in the pediatric population, but history and physical must be directed to evaluating these possibilities and sensation and proprioception should be checked even in the young patient. Microalbumin determinations are carried out as the patient reaches the age of puberty and has had diabetes for 5 years to evaluate the possibility of kidney damage in type 1 diabetes and at diagnosis in older patients with type 2 diabetes: angiotensin-converting enzyme treatment may slow the progression of renal disease, but these agents are teratogenic and cannot be used in pubertal girls without an assurance of abstinence from sexual activity or the use of birth control. Dental care must be offered regularly because of the risk of tooth decay or gum disease interfering with the control of diabetes and nutrition.

Children with diabetes must be identified in case they are separated from their guardians at a time that they may be unresponsive. Although a bracelet or necklace can be obtained from most drugstores, the MedAlert system will keep track of basic medical information and physician's phone number and is preferable as a means of identification.

Summer camps for children with diabetes are available nationally and are a wonderful way for patients to meet others with the same problems and, aside from realizing they are not unusual in their condition, to learn ways of dealing with the disease. Local diabetic groups (lay or medically based) offer support and information for the maintenance of good metabolic control.

Nonautoimmune type 1 DM is described in patients that have no autoantibodies measurable and no evidence of immune etiology; these patients are classified as type 1B or idiopathic DM (here, as elsewhere, the nomenclature of classification of disease varies with the source).

IATROGENIC DIABETES MELLITUS TYPE 1

Various drugs can precipitate DM, particularly drugs used in transplantation (such as FK506) and others used in therapy for cancer (e.g., l-asparaginase or prednisone for acute lymphocytic leukemia), which complicate the management of those serious conditions. The clinical manifestation of DM may wax and wane with the administration and cessation of the medication. In some cases, the condition may become permanent.

Acquired forms of Insulin-dependent DM (IDDM) in children result from pancreatic degeneration, such as found in cystic fibrosis. With longer-term survival in cystic fibrosis, the number of subjects with diabetes is increasing. In this situation, maximal calories are required for nutrition, so the goal is to match the insulin to the diet rather than tailor the diet to an ADA-recommended diabetic diet.

Long-term Complications

Microvascular and macrovascular complications of diabetes in general are related to the duration of disease and degree of control. The DCCT, as noted earlier, demonstrated that tight control with BS close to normal will decrease the development of these complications and even reverse them. Retinopathy develops through changes in the retinal capillaries and may lead to visual impairment or blindness. Improved control will forestall this complication. Thus ophthalmoscopy with dilation is recommended yearly after the disease has continued for 3 years. Nephropathy may develop as puberty progresses in a child with diabetes or with the increased duration of the disease. The glomeruli may become sclerotic after initial thickening of the basal membrane, so urine evaluation for microalbumin must be carried out yearly after the onset of puberty. Improved control will delay or eliminate this complication and even reverse such changes, whereas the use of angiotensin-converting enzyme (ACE) inhibitors may be appropriate therapy if the condition progresses. Neuropathy in the extremities is usually but not always reserved for adults with diabetes and long-term poor control. Macrovascular disease of the cardiac vessels is rare in childhood but will develop with poor control as the patient ages. This also can be forestalled by good control. Lipid values increase with poor control, and this factor, genetic tendencies, and the hypertension of kidney disease all can increase the likelihood of such macrovascular disease.

NEONATAL DIABETES MELLITUS

Rarely DM is found in the neonate without the autoimmune basis of type 1 DM. It has been related to autosomal recessive homozygous deficiency of PDX1, which causes pancreatic agenesis. Transient neonatal DM may be related to paternal isodisomy of chromosome 6 (*601410 DIABETES MELLITUS, TRANSIENT NEONATAL at 6q24).

TYPE 2 DIABETES MELLITUS

Type 2 DM (TYPE 2 DIABETES MELLITUS #125853 DIABETES MELLITUS, NONINSULIN-DEPENDENT; NIDDM variously at 20q12-q13.1, 20q12-q13.1, 17q25, 13q34, 11p12-p11.2, 2q32, 2q24.1) is the preferred term for what was previously called non–insulin dependent DM. This condition has a stronger genetic tendency than type 1 DM and consists of a combination of insulin resistance and of impaired first-phase insulin secretion from the beta cell of the pancreas. Type 2 DM was previously considered a disorder of adults. About 15 years ago, it became clear that Native American children could develop this condition, just as their parents frequently had, but at a younger age than expected, well before age 20 years. Then about a decade ago, it became clear that a tenfold increase in type 2 DM occurred in African-American teenagers and children. Now, with the epidemic of childhood obesity across the United States and the associated insulin resistance, an increase in type 2 DM is found in all ethnic groups but appears highest in Native American, African-American, Hispanic-American, and most recently recognized, Asian-American teenagers and children. It may be found in children as young as 6 years and possibly younger, although it is most prevalent in the teenage years. It is not clear how many new diagnoses of diabetes in children and adolescents represent type 2, but estimates from some approach 50%. The physical finding of acanthosis nigricans, an area of darkened and thickened skin found at the back of the neck or in flexural creases, is physical evidence of insulin resistance, and subjects with this finding should be screened for the clinical features of type 2 DM. The condition is appearing throughout the world in regions where the prevalence of obesity is increasing, and in many areas that also have undernutrition. The recent description of the later development of diseases in the individuals with impaired fetal growth includes type 2 DM. Type 2 DM is found more frequently in those with large birth weights as well as in those with decreased birth weights.

Unlike classic type 2 DM in adults, children can have ketoacidosis, confusing the differential diagnosis between type 1 DM and type 2 DM. Further, the elevated blood glucose may exert glucose toxicity on the beta cells, limiting their ability to secrete insulin to any appreciable degree, making the differential diagnosis even more difficult. Type 2 DM is not an autoimmune condition, so antiislet cell, antiinsulin or anti-GAD antibodies are negative, although they may be negative in some patients with type 1 DM as well. Exogenous insulin is usually administered in the acute hyperglycemic phase; insulin assays may be inaccurate because of interference in the assay by insulin itself or because of antibodies that develop against the administered insulin. Thus serum insulin cannot itself be easily measured after therapy begins). However, patients in the honeymoon phase of type 1 DM also may be able to secrete endogenous insulin and C peptide, further clouding the differential diagnosis between type 1 and type 2 DM. Sometimes observing the course of the patient is necessary before the diagnosis is determined. Measurement of C peptide after a liquid meal (Boost) is used to determine the ability to secrete endogenous insulin.

The mainstay of therapy for type 2 DM should be appropriate diet and exercise, leading to weight loss, but in view of acute metabolic derangements, medical therapies for hyperglycemia are usually needed at first. Insulin is usually the first line of therapy in a patient with significant illness or in whom the differential diagnosis between types 1 and 2 is unclear. If the onset is mild, type 2 DM may be treated with insulin or oral hypoglycemic agents. With weight control, oral hypoglycemic agents and insulin may be decreased or stopped altogether. Only insulin is approved for all ages, whereas metformin, a biguanide, is approved for children older than 10 years. Many potential treatments commonly used in adults are in clinical trials but are not yet approved for use in children, limiting therapeutic possibilities. Metformin is generally considered safe but can precipitate lactic acidosis, and a metabolic panel must be determined to ensure normal function of liver and kidney before initiating therapy. A dose of 500 mg is used at first, and if adequate control is not achieved, the dose may be increased by 500-mg increments at 1- to 2-weekly intervals up to a maximum of 2,000 mg in larger children. Abdominal distress may occur with this therapy but often resolves within a few weeks; the medication should be offered with meals. Insulin dosage is decreased as BS decreases with metformin, as unintended hypoglycemia is a possibility as insulin responsiveness increases. In some patients, insulin therapy will be required for the long term.

It is not yet clear what the prognosis and complications of type 2 DM will be in young subjects, but younger adults in whom type 2 DM develops have serious and early complications if control is poor. Thus, by extension, complications may be more serious in those adolescents and children who do not achieve adequate control.

A group of six disorders called maturity onset diabetes of the young (MODY) are caused by six autosomal dominant inherited genetic mutations, which usually manifest well before adulthood. They are quite different from those of type 2 DM in etiology, genetics, and usually in presentation. Some types of MODY lead to decreased insulin secretion, and others lead to defects in the disposal of glucose. They are generally mild and may be managed with diet rather than insulin or oral hypoglycemic agents (see Table 11-8).

Table 11-8. The MODY conditions

Condition	Gene defect	Inheritance	Clinical features
MODY 1	#125850 MATURITY-ONSET DIABETES OF THE YOUNG, TYPE I; MODY1	(20q12-q13.1) mutation in the gene encoding hepatocyte nuclear factor-4-α (HNF4A; 600281)	Early onset, mild course
MODY 2	#125851 MATURITY-ONSET DIABETES OF THE YOUNG, TYPE II; MODY2	Glucokinase gene defect 7p15-p13	Early onset, mild course common
MODY 3	#600496 MATURITY-ONSET DIABETES OF THE YOUNG, TYPE III; MODY3	(12q22-qter) mutation in the hepatocyte nuclear factor-1-α gene (142410), which maps to chromosome 12q34.	Before age 25 years; severe insulin secretory defect
MODY 4	#606392 MATURITY-ONSET DIABETES OF THE YOUNG, TYPE IV; MODY4	Mutation in the IPF1 gene (600733).	Homozygous infant had pancreatic agenesis; heterozygous individuals had mild presentation; rare
MODY 5	#604284 MATURITY-ONSET DIABETES OF THE YOUNG TYPE V; MODY5	Mutation in the hepatic transcription factor-2 gene (TCF2; 189907), which is located on chromosome 17cen-q21.3. TYPE V; MODY5	May have kidney or uterine defects as well; rare
MODY 6	#606394 MATURITY-ONSET DIABETES OF THE YOUNG, TYPE VI; MODY6	Mutations in the NEUROD1 gene (601724).	Rare

NIDDM can be found in some children with lipodystropic syndromes, ataxia, telangiectasia, myotonic dystrophy, leprechaunism, Mendenhall syndrome, and acanthosis nigricans.

SUGGESTED READINGS

Fiordalisi I, Harris GD. Diabetic ketoacidemia. In: Finberg L, Kleinman RE, eds. *Saunders manual of pediatric practice.* Philadelphia: WB Saunders, 2002:938–945.

Gitelman SE. Diabetes mellitus. In: Rudolph CD, Rudolph AM, eds. *Rudolph's pediatrics.* New York: McGraw-Hill, 2002:2111–2136.

Glaser N. Type 2 diabetes mellitus. In: Finberg L, Kleinman RE, eds. *Saunders manual of pediatrics.* Philadelphia: WB Saunders, 2002: 936–938.

Glaser N, Barnett P, McCaslin I, et al. Risk factors for cerebral edema in children with diabetic ketoacidosis: the Pediatric Emergency Medicine Collaborative Research Committee of the American Academy of Pediatrics. *N Engl J Med* 2001;344(4):264–269.

Glaser N, Enns G, Kuppermann N. *Endocrine and metabolic emergencies: advanced pediatric life support textbook.* 2003 (in press).

Marcin JP, Glaser N, Barnett P, et al. Clinical and therapeutic factors associated with adverse outcomes in children with diabetic ketoacidosis-related cerebral edema. *J Pediatr* 2002;141(6):193–197.

Schatz DA, Winter WE. Autoimmune polyglandular syndromes. In: Sperling MA, ed. *Pediatric endocrinology.* Philadelphia: WB Saunders, 2002:671–689.

Silverstein JH, Rosenbloom AL. Treatment of type 2 diabetes mellitus in children and adolescents. *J Pediatr Endocrinol Metab* 2000;13(suppl 6):1403–1409.

Sperling MA. Etiology of diabetes mellitus. In: Finberg L, Kleinman RE, eds. *Saunders manual of pediatric practice.* Philadelphia: WB Saunders, 2002:926–930.

Sperling MA. Diabetes mellitus. In: Sperling MA, ed. *Pediatric endocrinology.* Philadelphia: WB Saunders, 2002:323–366.

12 ♣ Obesity

DEFINITION

Obesity is the most prevalent nutritional disorder of children in the United States, a remarkable change from the prominent place of malnutrition due to deficient caloric intake in childhood in the past. The surgeon general designated childhood obesity as epidemic in the United States. A 100% increase of the prevalence of a body mass index (BMI) greater than the 95th percentile in children aged 6 to 11 years is recorded between the National Health and Nutrition Evaluation II (1976 to 1980) and NHANES III (1988 to 1994). Presently the prevalence of BMI higher than the 95th percentile is 11.4% in boys and 9.9% in girls; the mathematical impossibility of these figures (how can there be 11.4% of children above the 85th percentile when only 5% should be at that level?) is owing to the present necessity to set normal values by the use of statistics from previous decades. Thus present prevalence figures are derived by comparison with those older standards. A 50% increase in the prevalence of BMI greater than the 85th percentile was found in the same period to a present prevalence of 22.4% in boys and girls. The prevalence of obesity in 6-to 11-year-old African-American girls is higher than that in whites or Mexican-American children, whereas African-American boys of the same age have a greater prevalence than Mexican-American but not than white boys.

Areas of the world previously suffering from malnutrition are now manifesting an increasing prevalence of obesity, with the introduction of a Western (mainly United States style) diet and life style. Type 2 diabetes mellitus is likewise appearing in these same regions of the world. Children figure prominently in these trends.

The definition of obesity is an excess of adipose tissue, not just an increase in weight. The adverse metabolic and psychological effects of this adiposity mandate attention to the condition. Patients and parents may instead be concerned because of esthetic or psychosocial social concerns.

Obesity should be defined by the percentage of the body consisting of fat. Many techniques of measurements are available: measurement of subscapular skin thickness (requires special training and is difficult to reproduce in a clinical office), underwater weighing (requires a tank of water and other rarely available material), bioelectric impedance (easy to perform but sometimes difficult to standardize at a child's age) and DXA (dual x-ray absorptiometry, which is accurate but expensive) or computed tomography (CT) scans (highly accurate but expensive, and require a small exposure to radiation). To simplify the issue, anthropologic methods are used in the office setting to express percentage of body fat. In the past, percentile of weight for age may have been used to indicate the percentage of body fat, but this is not helpful in childhood, as it does not take into consideration height of the child. Percentile weight for height is a better indication, but does not adequately express the relative amount of fat in the individual, because increased muscle tissue will incorrectly increase the weight for height. BMI was adopted as the international standard of adiposity, as it is considered to reflect better the percentage of the body weight that is fat. BMI is known to be more accurate in adults than in children, but it is now the standard in children as well.

BMI is calculated as

BMI in kg/m^2 = weight (kg)/height^2 (in meters).

The percentile of BMI for age changes by age in children, so no simple number defines obesity at all ages, as in adults. A chart of BMI versus age was recently released by the Centers for Disease Control (CDC) and should be used to evaluate the weight of children (Fig. 12-1).

Adults have increased morbidity and mortality when their BMI increases to more than 25 (classified as overweight), which is the 85th percentile of BMI for adults. By extension, a BMI for children that is at the 85th percentile for age is considered "overweight," or to be "at risk for obesity," whereas at the 95th percentile BMI for age, a child is considered to be "overweight." "Overweight is preferred in communication with the family and patient to the term obesity, although "obesity" is used in this chapter as a medical term.

PATHOPHYSIOLOGY

Strong genetic and environmental bases of obesity exist in children, and both types of factors interact. Thus obesity should not simply be considered a condition of overeating and underexercising, although both factors play at least a relative role in the etiology, and both factors must be changed to control obesity. A child with one obese parent has a fivefold increase in the likelihood of becoming an obese adult, and a child with two obese parents has a 12-fold increased risk; these factors appear to be mainly genetic rather than environmental. Further, a macrosomic infant has a high likelihood of becoming an obese 10-year-old. Further, smaller-birth-weight infants owing to a variety of conditions have a tendency to develop insulin resistance later in life, and in some, obesity also develops. Normally an increase in the percentage of body fat is noted at mid-childhood, called the adiposity rebound, but an earlier adiposity rebound at 3 to 4 years or younger increases the likelihood of the development of adult obesity.

A 40% to 60% influence of genetics on obesity is based on numerous studies. Greater similarity is found in the BMIs of monozygotic twins than in those of dizygotic twins. The BMI of an adopted child relates far better to the BMI of the biologic parents than to those of the adoptive parents with whom the child was raised.

However, obesity develops in an individual with a susceptible genetic makeup who is exposed to an unfortunate environment, and the nutritional environment in the United States is particularly unfortunate. Thus in certain ethnic groups who have a genetic tendency toward obesity, particularly African Americans, Hispanic Americans, Native Americans, and Asian Americans,

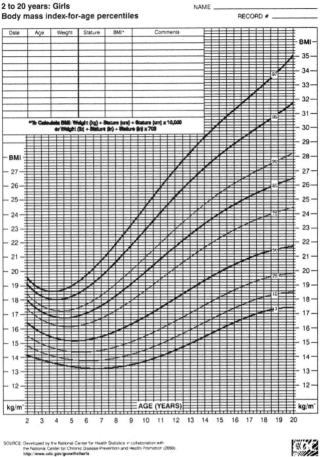

2 to 20 years: Girls
Body mass index-for-age percentiles

NAME _____

RECORD # _____

SOURCE: Developed by the National Center for Health Statistics in collaboration with
the National Center for Chronic Disease Prevention and Health Promotion (2000).
http://www.cdc.gov/growthcharts

Fig. 12-1. A: Body mass index-for-age percentiles for girls aged 2 to 20 years. (From www.cdd)

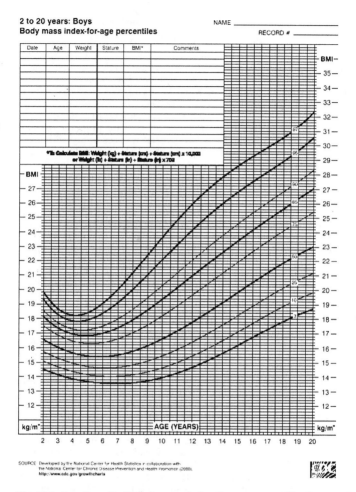

Fig. 12-1. (continued)   B: Body mass index-for-age percentiles for boys aged 2 to 20 years. (From www.cdd)

environmental factors have led to a remarkable increase in the prevalence of obesity. These ethnic groups exhibit a higher prevalence of type 2 diabetes mellitus, and in these same groups, this disease is now found in children as young as 6 years. Whites certainly can develop both obesity and type 2 diabetes in childhood but are at a lower risk, all other things being equal.

An increase in fat tissue must be because of increased caloric intake (by ingestion of food and drink) or decreased total energy expenditure (TEE). TEE consists of the sum of (a) resting energy expenditure (REE), (b) the thermic effect of feeding, and (c) nonresting energy expenditure. However, it is exceedingly difficult to demonstrate that a population of obese children takes in more calories than do matched nonobese children, possibly because of the insensitivity of the methods of observation or recording. An increase of only 25 kcal of intake per day, equivalent to a serving of butter, a change in dietary intake far below the present limit of detection, leads to a 1-kg gain in weight per year; thus obesity is often the result of a subtle but long-term increase in caloric intake.

It also is difficult to demonstrate a difference in energy expenditure in obese compared with lean children, again probably because of inadequate sensitivity of the available methods of evaluation. Likewise, no consistent pattern of decreased basal metabolic rate accounts for the difference between obese and nonobese children in most, but not all, situations. African-American girls appear to have lower basal energy expenditure than that of girls of other ethnic groups, however. It is evident that some individual children and adolescents will be found to have a far greater degree of caloric imbalance, in which the etiology of their obesity will obviously result from overconsumption of calories and decreased physical activity. However, in many cases with a familial tendency to gain weight, it may be appropriate to believe the family if they contend that the child is eating a reasonable diet and is quite active. They may just be fighting a strong genetic tendency toward obesity.

Body weight is regulated by complex and redundant central nervous system (CNS) mechanisms that are revealed by the study of patients and animals with genetic defects. Several hormones act on the brain to regulate appetite. Leptin is a peptide hormone produced by adipocytes that attaches to a receptor in the ventromedial hypothalamus to decrease food intake. Although the rare mutation in genes for leptin or for leptin receptors in human beings (only a handful of cases of mutations are reported) leads to early onset, severe obesity, leptin levels are high in most obese human beings. Because appetite in obese individuals is not suppressed by these values of leptin, a relative leptin resistance may be found in human obesity. Ghrelin is a peptide that can act as a growth-hormone secretagogue, but also is released from the fasting stomach as a signal to the hypothalamus to increase feeding.

A simplified account of the CNS control of appetite includes the following steps: (a) Leptin stimulates production of proopiomelanocortin (POMC), (b) which can be cleaved by enzyme action to

melanocyte-stimulating hormone (MSH), which in turn (c) interacts with melanocortin 4 receptors (MCR4) to reduce food intake;
(d) neuropeptide Y (NPY) is a potent orexogenic (agent to increase
feeding) peptide, and (e) AGRP, produced in the same neuron as
NPY, competes with MSH for the MCR4 and thereby also increases
feeding. Mutations causing obesity are described for each of these
steps, although they are rare. A growing number of other stimu-
lators and inhibitors of appetite are known. Damage to portions
of the hypothalamus may affect these pathways to increase appetite, or in other cases with other locations of lesions, to decrease
appetite.

Norepinephrine (NE) and serotonin exert suppressive effects on
appetite, which led to the development of medications that amplify
or mimic the action of these two neurotransmitters. Phentermine is a NE-reuptake inhibitor that is still in use, but phenyl-
propanolamine was withdrawn from the market when it was
implicated in causing hypertension, stroke, and myocardial infarction. The widespread use of fenfluramine, a 5-HT uptake inhibitor,
and of dexfenfluramine, was halted because of the increased risk
of cardiac valve abnormalities that accompanied the use of these
drugs (a combination of fenfluramine with phentermine was
called Fen-Phen). Presently sibutramine, a serotonin and norepinephrine reuptake inhibitor, is in clinical trials for use in adolescents aged 12 to 16 years; it promotes a feeling of fullness that
decreases appetite, but possible side effects include tachycardia
and hypertension to some degree.

COMORBIDITIES OF CHILDHOOD
AND ADOLESCENT OBESITY

The complications of adult obesity are well known. Visceral fat
surrounds the abdominal organs, and it is an excess of this tissue, rather than the more visible subcutaneous adipose tissue,
that is thought to mediate many of the metabolic derangements
of adult obesity such as insulin resistance and hyperlipidemia.
The influence of this tissue in childhood is less clear but is
suspect.

About 30% of adult obesity has its origin in childhood obesity.
There is tracking of obesity from childhood into adulthood, and
this tendency becomes more likely as the child becomes older and
comes closer to the adult age group. Further, an adult who was
obese as a child has substantially more severe comorbidities of the
obesity during the adult years. BP is higher, and lipid profiles are
more adverse in adults who were overweight or obese as children.
For example, morbidity from all causes is 2-fold higher, and coro-
nary heart disease morbidity is 2.3-fold higher after 50-year follow-
up of British adults who had a BMI at the 75% percentile during
childhood. It is important to note that these children were at the
75th percentile and were not even in what we would now consider
the upper percentiles for BMI for age of 85% or 95%. Studies from
the United States and elsewhere found similar outcomes of childhood obesity in adulthood.

The psychological toll of obesity is significant in childhood and adolescence. Children younger than 10 years demonstrate preference for playmates with a thinner body habitus, and young children are already the target of teasing and ridicule when overweight. The economic well-being, likelihood of advanced education, and ability to marry is decreased with obesity in teenage girls, although no such association is found with overweight boys.

The effects of childhood obesity previously were thought to await the adult years, but more childhood and adolescent comorbidities are now recognized. Type 2 diabetes mellitus, "adult diabetes," was rarely seen in childhood, but now is considered to be a second epidemic, following closely behind the first epidemic of childhood obesity. Pediatric endocrine clinics are now seeing numbers of new-onset type 2 diabetes similar to those of new-onset type 1 diabetes in children, and this tendency may appear as young as 6 years (see Chapter 11).

Comorbidities of Childhood Obesity

Various medical conditions are associated with obesity in childhood and adolescence:

1. Hyperlipidemia manifested as elevated low-density lipoprotein (LDL) cholesterol, decreased HDL cholesterol, and triglycerides when measured after a 14-hour fast (except for water).
2. Insulin resistance or true type 2 diabetes mellitus (see Chapter 11). Increased fasting insulin is a more sensitive indicator of insulin resistance than is the increase in fasting blood sugar or hemoglobin (Hgb)A_{1c}. A glucose tolerance test is rarely if ever indicated, although a boost challenge may be useful. However, diagnosis of type 2 diabetes mellitus rests on particular blood sugar values (see Chapter 11) and not on increased fasting insulin concentrations. Acanthosis nigricans is manifest as dark pigmentation on the back of the neck or other flexural surfaces, with thickening and even papilloma formation in more severe case. This is a physical indication of insulin resistance. Intertrigo and furunculosis may independently develop in skin folds and increase pigmentation as well.
3. Hypertension: BP is increased in many obese children and adolescents, but pitfalls occur in the evaluation. BP measurement in obesity requires larger than normal cuffs, which may not be easily obtained; if the wrong-size cuff is used, the measurement may be fallacious. BP is reactive to emotions and situations, and considerable variation may be found in obese adolescents. BP measurements should be related to height for the greatest accuracy. Standards are found in Tables 12-1 and 12-2.
4. Increased heart rate and cardiac output and possible risk for sudden death because of obstructive sleep apnea. This is associated with CO_2 retention, hypoxia, and right ventricular

hypertrophy and failure. This also is potentially associated with prolongation of the QTc interval and ventricular arrhythmias. The obesity hypoventilation syndrome or pickwickian syndrome, characterized by hypoventilation, somnolence, CO_2 retention, hypoxia, polycythemia, right ventricular hypertrophy and failure, pulmonary embolism, and even sudden death, is an extreme example of this process.

5. Slipped capital femoral epiphysis might occur in obese individuals and also is found in hypothyroidism. Usually hip or even leg pain and waddling develop after the initial presentation. Surgical therapy is the only treatment.

6. Blount disease of the tibia results from increased weight on the proximal tibia.

7. Advanced skeletal development and tall stature is common in most otherwise normal but obese children. A short obese child has a greater likelihood of having a definable endocrine disorder such as hypothyroidism, Cushing syndrome, hypopituitarism or isolated growth hormone deficiency, pseudohypoparathyroidism, or genetic conditions such as Prader-Willi or Bardet-Biedl syndromes (see Chapter 9).

8. Earlier puberty is reported in obese boys and girls. A recent survey confirms this tendency, and a downward revision of the age at onset of puberty may be required as the population becomes heavier. Earlier menarche may occur in obese girls and is worrisome in view of the previously established association of early menarche and breast cancer in girls.

9. Adolescent development of hirsutism and irregular menses, especially in obese girls with precocious adrenarche. This is ovarian hyperandrogenism, previously called Stein-Leventhal syndrome or polycystic ovarian disease.

10. Hepatic steatosis (found in about 50% of obese children after ultrasound examination) and elevated serum transaminases (in about 25%) or other liver-function abnormalities.

11. Cholelithiasis (associated with both obesity and rapid weight loss).

12. Asthma. Asthmatic children may have limited physical activity that fosters the development of obesity, whereas obese children tend to have greater likelihood of reactive airways, which might cause the asthma to worsen.

13. Pseudotumor cerebri, diagnosed by detection of papilledema or with magnetic resonance imaging (MRI). Headaches, as a symptom of the condition, may lead to diagnosis.

Laboratory Evaluation of Childhood Obesity

The degree of investigation is dependent on the BMI and the presence of risk factors.

If the BMI for age is in the 85th to 94th percentile with no risk factors, obtain a fasting lipid profile.

If risk factors are present, obtain a comprehensive chemistry panel with fasting glucose and an alanine aminotransferase (ALT)
(text continues on page 260)

Table 12-1. Blood pressure levels for the 90th and 95th percentiles of blood pressure for boys aged 1 to 17 years by percentiles of height

Age (yr)	% ile	Systolic BP (mm Hg) by percentile of height							Diastolic BP (DBP5) (mm Hg) by percentile of height						
		5%	10%	25%	50%	75%	90%	95%	5%	10%	25%	50%	75%	90%	95%
1	90th	94	95	97	99	101	102	103	49	49	50	51	52	53	54
	95th	98	99	101	103	105	106	107	54	54	55	56	57	58	58
2	90th	98	99	101	103	104	106	107	54	54	55	56	57	58	58
	95th	102	103	105	107	108	110	110	58	59	60	61	62	63	63
3	90th	101	102	103	105	107	109	109	59	59	60	61	62	63	63
	95th	105	106	107	109	111	112	113	63	63	64	65	66	67	68
4	90th	103	104	105	107	109	110	111	63	63	64	65	66	67	67
	95th	107	108	109	111	113	114	115	67	68	68	69	70	71	72
5	90th	104	105	107	109	111	112	113	66	67	68	69	69	70	71
	95th	108	109	111	113	114	116	117	71	71	72	73	74	75	76
6	90th	105	106	108	110	112	113	114	70	70	71	72	73	74	74
	95th	109	110	112	114	116	117	118	74	75	75	76	77	78	79
7	90th	106	107	109	111	113	114	115	72	73	73	74	75	76	77
	95th	110	111	113	115	117	118	119	77	77	78	79	80	81	81
8	90th	108	109	110	112	114	116	116	74	75	75	76	77	78	79
	95th	112	113	114	116	118	119	120	79	79	80	81	82	83	83

Age		1	2	3	4	5	6	7	1	2	3	4	5	6	7
9	90th	109	110	112	114	116	117	118	76	76	77	78	79	80	80
	95th	113	114	116	118	119	121	122	80	81	81	82	83	84	85
10	90th	111	112	113	115	117	119	119	77	77	78	79	80	81	81
	95th	115	116	117	119	121	123	123	81	82	83	83	84	85	86
11	90th	113	114	115	117	119	121	121	77	78	79	80	81	81	82
	95th	117	118	119	121	123	125	125	82	82	83	84	85	86	87
12	90th	115	116	118	120	121	123	124	78	78	79	80	81	82	83
	95th	119	120	122	124	125	127	128	83	83	84	85	86	87	87
13	90th	118	119	120	122	124	125	126	78	79	80	81	81	82	83
	95th	121	122	124	126	128	129	130	83	83	84	85	86	87	88
14	90th	120	121	123	125	127	128	129	79	79	80	81	82	83	83
	95th	124	125	127	129	131	132	133	83	84	85	86	87	87	88
15	90th	123	124	126	128	130	131	132	80	80	81	82	83	84	84
	95th	127	128	130	132	133	135	136	84	85	86	86	87	88	89
16	90th	126	127	129	131	132	134	134	81	82	82	83	84	85	86
	95th	130	131	133	134	136	138	138	86	86	87	88	89	90	90
17	90th	128	129	131	133	135	136	137	83	84	85	86	87	87	88
	95th	132	133	135	137	139	140	141	88	88	89	90	91	92	93

(From: Report of the Second Task Force on Blood Pressure Control in Children—1987. Task force on blood pressure control in children. National Heart, Lung, and Blood Institute, Bethesda, Maryland. *Pediatrics* 1987 79: 1–25.)

Table 12-2. Blood pressure levels for the 90th and 95th percentile of blood pressure for girls aged 1 to 17 years by percentiles of height

Age (yr)	% ile	Systolic BP (mm Hg) by percentile of height							Diastolic BP (DBP5) (mm Hg) by percentile of height						
		5%	10%	25%	50%	75%	90%	95%	5%	10%	25%	50%	75%	90%	95%
1	90th	98	98	99	101	102	103	104	52	52	53	53	54	55	55
	95th	101	102	103	104	106	107	108	56	56	57	58	58	59	60
2	90th	99	99	101	102	103	104	105	57	57	58	58	59	60	60
	95th	103	103	104	106	107	108	109	61	61	62	62	63	64	64
3	90th	100	101	102	103	104	105	106	61	61	61	62	63	64	64
	95th	104	104	106	107	108	109	110	65	65	66	66	67	68	68
4	90th	101	102	103	104	106	107	108	64	64	65	65	66	67	67
	95th	105	106	107	108	109	111	111	68	68	69	69	70	71	71
5	90th	103	103	105	106	107	108	109	66	67	67	68	69	69	70
	95th	107	107	108	110	111	112	113	71	71	71	72	73	74	74
6	90th	104	105	106	107	109	110	111	69	69	69	70	71	72	72
	95th	108	109	110	111	113	114	114	73	73	74	74	75	76	76
7	90th	106	107	108	109	110	112	112	71	71	71	72	73	74	74
	95th	110	111	112	113	114	115	116	75	75	75	76	77	78	78
8	90th	108	109	110	111	112	114	114	72	72	73	74	74	75	76
	95th	112	113	114	115	116	117	118	76	77	77	78	79	79	80

Age		SBP							DBP						
9	90th	110	111	112	113	114	116	116	74	74	74	75	76	77	77
	95th	114	115	116	117	118	119	120	78	78	79	79	80	81	81
10	90th	112	113	114	115	116	118	118	75	75	76	77	77	78	78
	95th	116	117	118	119	120	122	122	79	79	80	81	81	82	83
11	90th	114	115	116	117	119	120	120	76	77	77	78	79	79	80
	95th	118	119	120	121	122	124	124	81	81	81	82	83	83	84
12	90th	116	117	118	119	121	122	123	78	78	78	79	80	81	81
	95th	120	121	122	123	125	126	126	82	82	82	83	84	85	85
13	90th	118	119	120	121	123	124	124	79	79	79	80	81	82	82
	95th	122	123	124	125	126	128	128	83	83	84	84	85	86	86
14	90th	120	121	122	123	124	125	126	80	80	80	81	82	83	83
	95th	124	125	126	127	128	129	130	84	84	85	85	86	87	87
15	90th	121	122	123	124	126	127	128	80	81	81	82	83	83	84
	95th	125	126	127	128	130	131	131	85	85	85	86	87	88	88
16	90th	122	123	124	125	127	128	129	81	81	82	82	83	84	84
	95th	126	127	128	129	130	132	132	85	85	86	87	87	88	88
17	90th	123	123	124	126	127	128	129	81	81	82	83	83	84	85
	95th	127	127	128	130	131	132	133	85	86	86	87	88	88	89

(From: Report of the Second Task Force on Blood Pressure Control in Children—1987. Task force on blood pressure control in children. National Heart, Lung, and Blood Institute, Bethesda, Maryland. *Pediatrics* 1987 79: 1–25.)

measurement. Consider measuring $HgbA_{1c}$ and even a fasting insulin concentration. [An electrocardiogram (ECG) might be considered, depending on family history and symptoms].

If BMI is greater than the 95th percentile, all of the listed tests are recommended.

If appropriate historical features suggest particular problems, perform sleep study, Holter monitor study, or ambulatory BP monitoring, and extremity films. Thyroid-function tests (free T_4 and TSH) are low yield, hypothyroidism should not cause this level of obesity, but parents often insist on thyroid testing.

TREATMENT

Although a history of increased caloric intake and/or decreased activity may be found in some subjects with obesity, some may already be quite active in sports or other activities and may follow a reasonable diet. These children may still require changes in behavior to decrease caloric intake and increase energy expenditure.

The primary treatment for any child requiring weight control is decreased caloric intake (about 500-calorie/day decrease in older children) and increased energy expenditure (mainly by decreased sedentary activity rather than forcing vigorous exercise, which will rarely be maintained); thus life-style changes are in order.

A group program of education and family support is superior to individual sessions for children. Family therapy is used with success in some centers. Group programs may follow the Traffic Light, Shapedown, or our Fit-Kid models. In the youngest children, the parents solely determine the diet and must play an important role in counseling, whereas the message might be more focused on the subjects during in the adolescent years. Unfortunately, only a few programs show long-term success, as constant reinforcement of healthy habits is necessary; obesity should be considered a chronic disease that requires continuous management.

An essential point for anyone caring for obese children is a sense of empathy and a supportive manner that does not further decrease the child's self-esteem; if providers cannot muster such feelings, they should not be involved with affected children or families.

The goals of weight management are based on age, BMI, and complications (Fig. 12-2). If the child can grow into the weight, stopping further weight gain is the goal, but if any weight-based complications are noted, weight loss is needed. Thus in the child younger than 2 years, if the BMI is less than 95%, dietary counseling is recommended, but if the BMI is greater than 95%, specialty consultation is suggested. In a child or early adolescent with a BMI of 85% to 94% and no complications, or in a child younger than 7 years who has a BMI greater than 95% but no complications, weight maintenance is recommended, as the child will grow into the weight if no more is gained. However, if the BMI is greater than 95% at older than

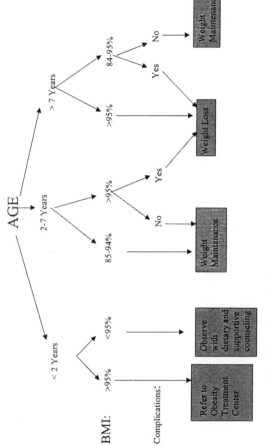

Fig. 12-2. The goals of weight management based on age, body mass index, and complications. (Source is: Barlow SE, Dietz WH. Obesity evaluation and treatment: expert committee recommendations. Maternal and Child Health Bureau, Health Resources and Services Administration and the Department of Health and Human Services. *Pediatrics* 102: E29, 1998.)

7 years or if complications are found, weight loss rather than weight maintenance is required.

A protein-sparing modified fast (PSMF) may be used in children with severe, often life-threatening, consequences of obesity (e.g., sleep apnea) in which rapid weight loss is indicated, if no other method appears applicable, but must be administered only with an experienced practitioner because of inherent dangers. The PSMF is a medically supervised (an experienced clinician must direct the therapy) program of 600 to 800 kcal/day intake, including 1.5 to 2.5 g high-quality protein per kilogram ideal body weight per day (supplied from lean meats, poultry, and fish) but only 20 to 40 g/day of carbohydrate; daily vitamin and mineral supplementation and encouragement to consume more than 1,500 mL free water are additional important features. A PSMF is carried out usually for no more than 12 weeks, with daily monitoring for urinary ketones to demonstrate adherence to the low-caloric plan. The risks of PSMF regimens include cholelithiasis; hyperuricemia; decreases in serum proteins, including transferrin, retinol-binding protein, and complement 1C; orthostatic hypotension; halitosis; and diarrhea. Although long-term weight control may not result, lessening of the initial medical complications may be achieved. If PSMF is not successful, direct treatment of the complication takes precedence, such as BiPAP therapy or adenoidectomy for sleep apnea.

No medication is approved for weight control in children, but sibutramine, discussed earlier, is in clinical trial for 12- to 16-year-olds. Orlistat, an intestinal lipase inhibitor that decreases fat intake and increases the elimination of dietary fat, also is in clinical trials for this age group; side effects include diarrhea and flatus if significant fat remains in the diet, so this becomes a form of aversion therapy if diet is not first modified.

Gastric bypass or other surgery aiming to decrease caloric absorption must be considered an experimental procedure in childhood, as experience and follow-up is extremely limited in this age group.

PREVENTION

It is patently impossible for a nation to mobilize medical resources to treat the more than 22% of the young population who are overweight. Prevention must be the highest priority. Some preventive measures require political or administrative action, whereas some are within the reach of an individual family:

Encourage parental modeling: The parent must model appropriate behaviors in diet and activity. Children are born with a taste for sweet and salt and an aversion to bitter and sour, and demonstrate a tendency to avoid new foods (neophobia); the desire for fat or oil, spice (other than salt), and fat may be learned at an early age. Thus a child will initially spit out green vegetables; if the parent gives up such trials of healthful food, resorting to sugary or salty, initially more palatable substitutes, the child may lose the chance to acquire long-term healthful dietary habits. But just as a lenient approach to diet may be harmful, overly restricting food choices to the point at which the child cannot learn to regulate the intake, conversely, also may lead to obesity.

Encourage breast-feeding for many reasons, not the least because it is associated with a lower likelihood of obesity. Bottle-fed babies may have increased weight. Formula or breast milk may belong in a bottle, but juice and soft drinks do not. Bottles should be used only up to about 1 year, if used at all. Bedtime bottle-feeding is particularly discouraged, as this often leads to formation of dental caries.

Decrease or eliminate the intake of soda and watch the intake of juice: An increase in each soda consumed per day in early teenage years leads to doubling the likelihood of developing obesity. Juice may seem more healthful than sugared drinks, but 8 oz of juice contains 100 calories, just as does 8 oz of soda! Limit juice and encourage water or low fat milk instead.

Increase public safety: If a child cannot leave the house for fear of injury, the child will eliminate vigorous activity and may stay in front of the television set all day.

Decrease television watching: Television viewing is the most proven modifiable factor linked to the development of obesity. The average U.S. child watches 28 hours of television per week. Television viewing decreases beneficial physical activity and socialization. Exposure to television advertising that features highly caloric foods may affect the diet. Some success has occurred with a school-based curriculum aimed to decrease television viewing.

Modify the diet: A small indiscretion in caloric intake adds up. Consistent changes in diet toward decreased calories and increased fruit and vegetables will lead to a beneficial effect. A child cannot exercise off a highly caloric children's fast food meal (contains 750–1,400 calories or more) in the gym or on the exercise bicycle.

Decrease sedentary time: Decreasing the time spent sitting or being driven around by replacement of this time with activities such as walking or playing is beneficial. No child will suddenly change from sedentary habits to vigorous activity, so aim for sustainable small changes. Many children simply watch others participate in gym class, so substitution with fun activities rather than competitive activities may increase participation by all and lead to habits that might be retained.

SUGGESTED READINGS

Arslanian SA, Lewy V, Danadian K, et al. Metformin therapy in obese adolescents with polycystic ovary syndrome and impaired glucose tolerance: amelioration of exaggerated adrenal response to adrenocorticotropin with reduction of insulinemia/insulin resistance. *J Clin Endocrinol Metab* 2002;87(4):1555–1559.

Barlow SE, Dietz WH. Obesity evaluation and treatment: expert committee recommendations: the Maternal and Child Health Bureau, Health Resources and Services Administration and the Department of Health and Human Services. *Pediatrics* 1998; 102(3):E29.

Capriles CC, Levitsky LL. Type 1 diabetes mellitus. In: Finberg L, Kleinman RE, eds. *Saunders manual of pediatric practice.* Philadelphia: WB Saunders, 2002:930–936.

Carrel AL, Myers SE, Whitman BY, et al. Benefits of long-term GH therapy in Prader-Willi syndrome: a 4-year study. *J Clin Endocrinol Metab* 2002;87(4):1581–1585.

Davison KK, Birch LL. Childhood overweight: a contextual model and recommendations for future research. *Obes Rev* 2001;2(3):159–171.

Dietz WH, Robinson TN. Use of the body mass index (BMI) as a measure of overweight in children and adolescents. *J Pediatr* 1998;132:191–193.

Epstein LH, Roemmich JN, Raynor HA. Behavioral therapy in the treatment of pediatric obesity. *Pediatr Clin North Am* 2001;48(4): 981–993.

Farooqi IS, Matarese G, Lord GM, et al. Beneficial effects of leptin on obesity, T cell hyporesponsiveness, and neuroendocrine/metabolic dysfunction of human congenital leptin deficiency. *J Clin Invest* 2002;110(8):1093–1103.

Freemark M, Bursey D. The effects of metformin on body mass index and glucose tolerance in obese adolescents with fasting hyperinsulinemia and a family history of type 2 diabetes. *Pediatrics* 2001;107(4):E55.

Goran MI, Shewchuk R, Gower BA, et al. Longitudinal changes in fatness in white children: no effect of childhood energy expenditure. *Am J Clin Nutr* 1998;67(2):309–316.

Goran MI, Treuth MS. Energy expenditure, physical activity, and obesity in children. *Pediatr Clin North Am* 2001;48(4):931–953.

Gungor N, Arslanian SA. Nutritional disorders. In: Sperling MA, ed. *Pediatric endocrinology.* Philadelphia: WB Saunders, 2002:689–724.

Ibanez L, Valls C, Ferrer A, et al. Sensitization to insulin induces ovulation in nonobese adolescents with anovulatory hyperandrogenism. *J Clin Endocrinol Metab* 2001:86(8):3595–3598.

Jones KL. Treatment of type 2 diabetes mellitus in children. *JAMA* 2002;287(6):716.

Jones KL, Arslanian S, Peterokova VA, et al. Effect of metformin in pediatric patients with type 2 diabetes: a randomized controlled trial. *Diabetes Care* 2002;25(1):89–94.

Robinson TN. Reducing children's television viewing to prevent obesity: a randomized controlled trial. *JAMA* 1999;282:1561–1567.

Styne DM. Childhood and adolescent obesity: prevalence and significance. *Pediatr Clin North Am* 2001;48(4):823–854.

Styne DM, Schoenfeld-Warden N. Obesity. In: Rudolph CD, Rudolph AM, eds. *Rudolph's pediatrics.* New York: McGraw-Hill, 2002: 2136–2142.

Whitaker RC, Wright JA, Pepe MS, et al. Predicting obesity in young adulthood from childhood and parental obesity. *N Engl J Med* 1997;337(13):869–873.

Yanovski JA. Intensive therapies for pediatric obesity. *Pediatr Clin North Am* 2001;48(4):1041–1053.

Yanovski SZ, Yanovski JA. Obesity. *N Engl J Med* 2002;346(8):591–602.

Zadik Z, Wittenberg I, Segal N, et al. Interrelationship between insulin, leptin, and growth hormone in growth hormone-treated children. *Int J Obes Relat Metab Disord* 2001;25(4):538–542.

Zuhri-Yafi MI, Brosnan PG, Hardin DS. Treatment of type 2 diabetes mellitus in children and adolescents. *J Pediatr Endocrinol Metab* 2002;15(suppl 1):541–546.

13 ♣ Hypoglycemia

Hypoglycemia captures the popular imagination, and many fanciful, but nonphysiologic, diagnoses are proposed by the lay public. Hypoglycemia may be devastating, although it is found far more rarely than popular thought would suggest. An etiology cannot always be assigned, but hypoglycemia should always be confirmed by laboratory testing. At the time that glucose decreases, a "critical" blood sample must be obtained or an ideal diagnostic technique is lost, and the diagnostic process may become extremely difficult or expensive.

NORMAL CARBOHYDRATE METABOLISM

The maintenance of normal blood sugar depends on the intake of carbohydrates from the gastrointestinal (GI) tract; the process of gluconeogenesis, or the production of glucose from precursors such as glycerol (derived from fat), amino acids (such as alanine derived from muscle), and factors of anaerobic glycolysis (such as lactate and pyruvate); and glycogenolysis, or the release of glucose from its storage depot, glycogen (Fig. 13-1).

Glucose production and utilization is approximately 5 to 7 mg/kg/min in infants and young children, as compared with 1 to 2 mg/kg/min in the adult; thus an impairment in production of glucose, even with no change in utilization, will reduce serum glucose concentration more quickly in the child than in the adult. Further, as the brain is much larger in relation to body size in the infant than in the adult and consumes relatively more energy, neurologic symptoms and signs of hypoglycemia will be manifest more readily in the child. The muscle mass is smaller in children, and the release of substrates for gluconeogenesis is more limited. Thus for many reasons, the child is more susceptible to hypoglycemia and its symptoms than is the adult. Conversely, if the child has brain damage, resulting in lower metabolic needs for this organ that normally uses so much glucose, hyperglycemia may result.

The fed state: After a meal, in the postprandial state, exogenous glucose is used by, and stored in, tissues whereas the mechanism of glucose production, gluconeogenesis, is decreased. Thus, insulin increases and glucagon decreases with glucose intake in the fed state. Insulin is responsible for the storage of glucose by the production of glycogen, the transport of and incorporation of amino acids into protein and lipids into triglycerides. Insulin suppresses the production of ketone bodies; they are virtually nonexistent in blood in the fed state.

The fasting state: The liver and kidneys are the locations of the enzyme that allows the release of glucose into the circulation during glycogenolysis, glucose-6-phosphate, as are the enzymes necessary for gluconeogenesis. Except for states of severe starvation, the liver plays the major role in gluconeogenesis and glycogenolysis. Glycogenolysis begins first in the fasted state, and when glycogen stores are exhausted (after about 4 hours in infants and after 8 hours in older subjects), gluconeogenesis

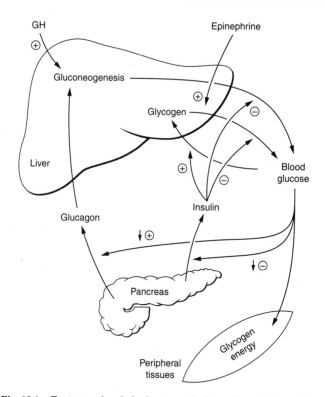

Fig. 13-1. Features of carbohydrate metabolism. (From: Fisher, DA. Pediatric endocrinology. San Juan Capistrano; Quest Diagnostics 2000.)

begins and uses amino acids derived from muscle protein, lactate from blood cell glycolysis, and glycerol from triglycerides. Hepatic fatty acid oxidation provides the energy for gluconeogenesis. Lipolysis breaks triglycerides into glycerol and free fatty acids (FFAs). The liver forms the ketone bodies, acetoacetate (which is converted to acetone), and β-hydroxybutyrate from FFAs during the breakdown of lipids; these ketone bodies can pass the blood–brain barrier and provide energy for brain function. The production of ketone bodies by fatty acid oxidation may be viewed as an adaptive mechanism that spares muscles from breakdown and the release of amino acids that would otherwise be used for gluconeogenesis.

Glucose Can Be Produced by Other Tissues in Various Ways

Anaerobic glycolysis (the Embden-Meyerhof pathway) in muscle will produce pyruvate, which is metabolized to lactate or alanine, which in turn can be used as a gluconeogenic precursor: oxidation of glucose to glycerol-3-phosphate in adipose tissue will esterify fatty acids in the synthesis of triglycerides or alternatively will lead to the production of fatty acids: oxidation through acetyl-coenzyme A (CoA) in the brain will produce carbon dioxide and water.

In states of low glucose availability, the energy needs of some organs can shift to conserve glucose: the liver, adipose tissue, and muscle can use the β-oxidation of fatty acids; the brain can use ketone bodies.

Concentration of Glucose in the Serum of Normal Subjects Is Kept Remarkably Constant by Glucoregulatory Factors

Insulin is secreted from the cells of the pancreatic islets in response to exogenous glucose and, in turn, suppresses endogenous glucose production by inhibiting hepatic glycogenolysis and gluconeogenesis. Insulin is a potent suppressor of ketone body formation, and as a general rule, if ketosis is present in hypoglycemia, abnormally increased insulin is not likely the cause of the hypoglycemia. Further, insulin stimulates the storage of glucose as glycogen and triglycerides and promotes the uptake of glucose in many other tissues, such as skeletal and cardiac muscle and kidney via the GLUT-4 glucose transporter. Thus insulin decreases blood sugar by disposing of glucose into cells and by decreasing the precursors to gluconeogenesis. Glucagon is released from the cells of the pancreas and quickly but transiently stimulates hepatic glycogenolysis and gluconeogenesis. Epinephrine from the adrenal medulla rapidly stimulates hepatic glycogenolysis and gluconeogenesis and acts through adrenergic mechanisms, indirectly affecting insulin and glucagon as well.

Both cortisol and growth hormone (GH) exert antiinsulin effects by limiting glucose utilization and increasing glucose production. GH, however, has an additional transient effect of decreasing serum glucose through the production and action of the insulin-like growth factors, although the ultimate effect of GH is to elevate glucose concentrations (Table 13-1).

HYPOGLYCEMIA

Symptoms of hypoglycemia are due either to effects of adrenergic and cholinergic agents (causing sweating, tremulousness, hunger, weakness, and tachycardia) or to central nervous system (CNS) manifestations (such as headaches or reduced mentation, which may extend on a continuum from drowsiness to coma and seizures). Even if severe and recurrent hypoglycemia is ultimately controlled, the patient may still be left with permanent neurologic impairment such as developmental delay and seizure disorders that manifest even when the blood sugar is normal. Patients taking adrenergic blocking agents may not show the initial symptoms of hypoglycemia in spite of having low blood sugar concentrations, but they still have the potential for neurologic damage. Hypoglycemia is generally diagnosed if serum glucose decreases below 50 mg/dL in a child or older individual (but not a newborn); a normal individual may reach values in the high 50-mg/dL region occasionally but rarely decreases below that limit. Symptoms may begin only when blood sugar decreases below 50 mg/dL, but it is not appropriate to accept values less than 60 mg/dL as normal; careful observation is at the least appropriate when encountering values below that limit.

The timing of hypoglycemia provides an important clue to the diagnosis. Hypoglycemia due to fructose intolerance manifests just after ingesting fructose, glycogen-storage disease, in which there is difficulty in glycogenolysis, in the few hours after eating, and to lipid metabolism abnormalities (acyl-CoA dehydrogenase deficiencies) and hypopituitarism during a prolonged fast.

Hypoglycemia in the Newborn

The definition of hypoglycemia is based on statistical analysis of the normal range of glucose values, and in the newborn, especially, standards change with respect to clinical condition. A prior definition of hypoglycemia in the low-birth-weight infant was a blood glucose less than 20 mg/dL, in the term infant during the first 3 days after birth, less than 30 mg/dL; and thereafter, less than 40 mg/dL (whole-blood glucose is 15% lower than serum or plasma glucose, so adjustment must be made for the method of measurement; for a plasma glucose of 60 mg/dL, the blood glucose could be about 50 mg/dL). However, these lower limits are recommended increased to less than 50 mg/dL at all ages and better yet to less than 60 mg/dL, which is still below the accepted normal of 70 mg/dL. Symptoms of hypoglycemia in the newborn range from grand mal or localized seizures to irritability, hypotonia, lethargy, difficulty in feeding, to other rather nonspecific findings, to no findings at all because of the immaturity of the CNS at birth. Because a hypoglycemic infant may have no symptoms, routine glucose monitoring is performed, especially in certain clinical conditions known to be associated more frequently with hypoglycemia.

The neonate has less tolerance to fasting and stress than does an older individual because of limited glycogen or substrate availability, and hypoglycemia develops faster in the newborn. Disorders causing hypoglycemia in the newborn can be found on a continuum from decreased ability to stabilize metabolically in the postnatal period, continuing to hypoglycemia as a secondary finding associated with other diseases, and ending with disorders in which severe, unremitting hypoglycemia is the immediate and primary problem.

Even a normal newborn who is fasted for 6 hours has a 10% chance of having a blood sugar less than 30 mg/dL and a 30% chance of developing a blood sugar less than 50 mg/dL, so transient hypoglycemia is common. A neonate who is the product of a problem pregnancy or delivery is an even more likely candidate for transient hypoglycemia. Thus infants who are premature or small for gestational age, or who experienced trauma, asphyxia, or cold

(text continues on page 271)

Table 13-1. Causes of hypoglycemia

Condition	Insulin	Ketones	GH	Cortisol	Lactate	Free fatty acids	GIR	Other features
Transient hypoglycemia of the newborn	Low	NI or high	NI	NI	High	High	6–10 mg/kg/min	
Persistent hyperinsulinemic hypoglycemia of infancy	High for glucose value	Low	NI	NI	Low	Low	>12–15 mg/kg/min	Some defects associated with elevated ammonia, IGF BP1 is low
Beckwith-Wiedemann syndrome	High for glucose value	Low	NI	NI	Low	Low	>12–15 mg/kg/min	Organomegaly, elevated IGF-11, IGF BP1 is low
Beta cell adenoma	High for glucose value	Low	NI	NI	Low	Low	>12–15 mg/kg/min	IGF BP1 is low
GH deficiency	NI	High	Peak, <10 ng/mL	NI	High	High	6–10 mg/kg/min	
ACTH or cortisol deficiency	NI	High	NI	Peak, <15 μcg/mL	High	High	6–10 mg/kg/min	

Galactosemia	Low	High	NI	NI	High	High	6–10 mg/kg/min	High galactose
Acyl-CoA dehydrogenase, medium-chain deficiency	NI	Low	NI	NI	High	High	6–10 mg/kg/min	Low carnatine
Glycogen-storage disease types 1, 3, 9, 0	Low	High	NI	NI	High	High	6–10 mg/kg/min	
Ketotic hypoglycemia	Low	High	NI	NI	High	High	6–10 mg/kg/min	Low alanine
Hereditary fructose intolerance	Low	High	NI	NI	High	High	6–10 mg/kg/min	
Fructose 1-6 diphosphatase deficiency	Low	High	NI	NI	High	High	6–10 mg/kg/min	
Muenchhausen's by proxy	High for glucose but C peptide is low	Low	NI	NI	Low	Low	>12–15 mg/kg/min until elimination of exogenous insulin	

GH, growth hormone; NI, normal; ACTH, adrenocorticotropic hormone; GIR, glucose infusion rate. (From Fisher; see Selected Readings.)

exposure at birth should be monitored prospectively for the development of hypoglycemia. Diseases that have other significant manifestations may have hypoglycemia included in the constellation; frequent examples include sepsis, postexchange transfusion or erythroblastosis fetalis, congenital heart disease, or congenital defects of the CNS or elsewhere. The condition of the mother before delivery may affect the neonate as well; e.g., infants of mothers with toxemia, with narcotic addiction, who are taking oral hypoglycemic agents or β-adrenergic blockers are likely candidates for hypoglycemia.

Infants of mothers with permanent or gestational diabetes mellitus (IDMs) have intrauterine hyperglycemia, related to maternal blood sugar concentrations, and develop islet cell hyperplasia because of stimulation by ambient glucose concentrations; after birth, removed from the maternal glucose supply, the increased insulin secretion of the islets will cause minimal to severe hypoglycemia for hours to a few days after delivery. The IDM, unless having intrauterine growth restriction (IUGR), has a characteristic appearance of increased size for gestational age, with extra subcutaneous tissue, a plethoric complexion, and a rather lethargic level of activity. This picture is less frequent if the mother has excellent blood sugar control during pregnancy. Similarly, infants of mothers who were receiving a large amount of intravenous glucose will have increased fetal insulin secretion; because the glucose will abruptly disappear at the time of placental separation, the child also is at risk for transient hyperinsulinemic hypoglycemia.

There is no reason that a child who is a term product of a normal delivery without known complication, fed by 6 hours after birth, should have continued hypoglycemia. Unexplained hypoglycemia in such a situation is worrisome and may result from an abnormality of the hypothalamic pituitary axis or one of the metabolic disorders discussed later.

Newborns with persistent hypoglycemia who require more than 10 to 12 mg/kg/min of intravenous glucose to maintain a normal blood sugar after age 2 days most likely have the hypoglycemia because of hyperinsulinism and will have a more difficult course than most of those with the transient problems mentioned earlier (although some IDMs will require this level of support on a temporary basis). Hyperinsulinism may cause devastating hypoglycemia in the newborn or older child. Diagnosis is suspected if any insulin secretion is detected with hypoglycemia, a state in which normally no insulin should be measurable; even low levels of insulin secretion while the blood sugar is low may suggest hyperinsulinism. Hyperinsulinism is especially likely to cause brain damage, as an absence of glucose as well as lactate and ketone bodies is found, so that all metabolic fuels for the brain are unavailable. Absence of serum ketone bodies and FFAs is a diagnostic clue to hyperinsulinism.

Long-term hyperinsulinism may be caused by the hyperinsulinism of the Beckwith-Wiedemann syndrome (#130650 BECK-

WITH-WIEDEMANN SYNDROME; BWS at 11p15.5), whose features include exomphalos, macroglossia, and gigantism, or in the infant giant syndrome (large body size and microcephaly but no macroglossia or exomphalos). Nesidioblastosis (#256450 NESIDIOBLASTOSIS OF PANCREAS at 11p15.1, 11p15.1) has been classically described as the development of beta-cell islets from pancreatic duct tissue, but more recent histologic studies suggest that this appearance is a normal variant; some of the patients previously diagnosed as having nesidioblastosis have microscopic adenomas that have been missed or a functional defect that cannot be demonstrated histologically but can now be demonstrated by molecular probes.

The most common form of hyperinsulinism results from mutations in the SUR1 or Kir6.2 genes of the short arm of chromosome 11 (#601820 PERSISTENT HYPERINSULINEMIC HYPOGLYCEMIA OF INFANCY) and which code for the adenosine triphosphate (ATP)-sensitive potassium channel, which is a major regulator of insulin secretion by the beta cell. These disorders are called potassium ATP channel hyperinsulinism or KATP-HI. They may be inherited in autosomal recessive (240800 HYPOGLYCEMIA, LEUCINE-INDUCED) or autosomal dominant patterns (#602485 HYPERINSULINISM, AUTOSOMAL DOMINANT at 7p15-p13), with the clinical course determined by the mode of inheritance. Thus autosomal recessive inheritance of mutations of both of these genes may be found, a condition that causes generalized pancreatic disease and hypoglycemia that may not respond to diazoxide therapy. Alternatively a single mutation may exist on the paternal chromosome, with loss of the normal maternal allele, leading to homozygosity for a recessive SUR1 mutation, leading to focal pancreatic disease. This situation may be amenable to surgical correction without the need for total pancreatectomy. Finally, an autosomal dominant pattern of inheritance of a single mutation may cause activating mutations of the glucokinase gene that may be successfully treated with diazoxide and does not require surgery.

Glutamate dehydrogenase hyperinsulinism (GDH #606762 HYPERINSULINISM-HYPERAMMONEMIA SYNDROME at 10q23.3) also is called the hyperinsulinism-hyperammonemia syndrome. This is considered an autosomal dominant condition (although 80% are new mutations and appear to be sporadic). Diagnosis is based on the demonstration of elevated plasma ammonia in addition to low glucose and elevated insulin. Treatment with diazoxide is often successful in this condition, and surgery may not be necessary.

Beta-cell adenomas are extremely rare in infants and newborns and, although more common in later childhood, are still rarer than in adults. Hyperinsulinism of this type may be a part of multiple endocrine neoplasia type 1 but is usually found well after the second decade (see Chapter 14).

Deficiencies of GH and/or adrenocorticotropic hormone (ACTH) may cause neonatal hypoglycemia. In boys, the finding of microphallus (due to gonadotropin and/or GH deficiency) associated with hypoglycemia should strongly suggest this diagnosis; visual impairment and optic hypoplasia also may be found in this constellation (septooptic dysplasia; see Chapter 3). Virilizing congenital adrenal hyperplasia will be indicated by ambiguous genitalia in girls, but boys will appear normal. Adrenal hypoplasia, dysplasia, or atrophy will not necessarily have diagnostic physical findings but will lead to hypoglycemia.

Metabolic abnormalities of branched-chain amino acids, such as maple syrup urine disease (*248600 MAPLE SYRUP URINE DISEASE, TYPE IA at 19q13.1-q13.2), are found in an autosomal recessive pattern and characterized by elevated branched-chain amino acids (leucine, isoleucine, or valine) in serum and urine and causes developmental delay, coma, seizures, vomiting, lethargy, elevated serum ammonia, and metabolic acidosis in the presence of ketotic hypoglycemia. The urine has the odor of maple syrup, as suggested by the name of the disorder. Five different forms and degrees of severity are found, with the basic defect of all being mutations in the branched-chain α-keto acid dehydrogenase, E1α subunit gene (BCKDHA, 248600.0001). Other forms of maple syrup urine disease are termed type 1B (*248611) and type 2 (*448610).

Galactosemia (#230400 GALACTOSEMIA at 9p13) is one of the diseases for which generalized screening is available at birth. Only at the late stages of the disease in which liver failure develops is hypoglycemia apparent. The diagnosis will usually rest on other findings than low blood sugar.

Disorders of organic acid or fatty acid oxidation represent a more common type of disorder (with a prevalence of one in 9,000 to 15,000), leading to fasting hypoglycemia, which may be a life-threatening condition or a mild manifestation. These disorders limit the production of ketone bodies during fasting, so they mimic the hypoglycemic hyperinsulinemic disorders. The conditions are generally the result of defects in the acyl-CoA system, with short-, medium-, or long-chain fatty acids involved in the various classifications. The most common type is medium-chain acyl-CoA dehydrogenase (MCAD) mutations (#201450 ACYL-CoA DEHYDROGENASE, MEDIUM-CHAIN, DEFICIENCY OF at 1p31). Hypoglycemia develops in the newborn or infant period, but sometimes patients are well until several years of age. Hypoglycemia occurs after prolonged fasts that may accompany intercurrent illnesses. Mild hyperammonemia, hyperuricemia, and elevations of liver enzymes may be seen, along with mild hepatomegaly. This may appear in a similar manner to Reye syndrome, with disordered mentation and absent ketone bodies during hypoglycemia. Plasma carnitine is low, and an increased ratio of esterified carnitine to free carnitine is found. Dicarboxylated acids should be measured in the urine to make the specific diagnosis. Diagnosis usually is accomplished through determination of the types of acyl-carnitine present by mass spectroscopy, a technique now becoming more frequently used in newborn screening programs. If screening procedures become more common, life-threatening emergencies may be avoided by early diagnosis. The treatment usually is elimination of fasting for more than a few hours.

Hypoglycemia in Older Children

Some of the same conditions noted under hypoglycemia of the newborn can be diagnosed initially as causes of hypoglycemia in later life, although a change is found in the incidence of the disorders with advancing age. For example, glycogen storage disease (GSD), other than type 1 GSD, becomes more frequently diagnosed at an older age, and beta-cell adenomas replace familial hyperinsulinemic hypoglycemia on the differential diagnosis as children become older.

Hyperinsulinism will be more likely the result of a β-cell adenoma after the newborn period than of a congenital condition, especially after age 3 years. This serious condition requires immediate treatment. In contrast, "reactive hypoglycemia" is all too often diagnosed in children who have unusual behavior or sensations attributed to low serum glucose, but without confirmatory measured glucose values; sometimes pressure is felt from the parents to make the diagnosis because they think that they have hypoglycemia themselves (without laboratory evidence) or because they have read the latest popular book on the subject. Rapid gastric emptying resulting from the dumping syndrome may lead to a sharp increase in serum glucose, causing release of insulin that subsequently causes hypoglycemia, but patients will have a history of GI surgery as an indication of this condition. Reports exist of delayed insulin secretion in rare patients who ultimately develop type 1 diabetes mellitus, but this does not mean that children with unconfirmed episodes only suggested to be hypoglycemia are at risk for diabetes.

Ketotic hypoglycemia classically is seen in a thin (often male) child of age 18 months to 5 years, who has had a longer than average overnight fast (sometimes this is called the Saturday night–Sunday morning syndrome because of the purported late return of parents at night, causing a delay in breakfast the following morning because of late awakening, and therefore a prolonged fast for the child) or has an intercurrent illness that decreases dietary intake. The condition appears to result from a defect in mobilization of alanine for gluconeogenesis or from decreased muscle mass, as muscles are the major source of alanine. Affected patients with ketotic hypoglycemia not related to another diagnosis tolerate an 18-hour fast more poorly than do unaffected patients. This condition may be a more exaggerated intolerance to fasting than normal, as all of the features of ketotic hypoglycemia will develop in a normal child who is fasted for an extended period. Normal children can tolerate a fast of 15 hours by 1 week to 1 year, 24 hours by 1 year, and 36 hours by 5 years.

The term ketotic hypoglycemia is quite general and includes many causes of hypoglycemia, including GH and ACTH deficiency, but does not include conditions involving increased insulin secretion. After reviewing the history of the affected child, it may become clear that the child had neonatal hypoglycemia, which apparently resolved after regular feedings were started. However, the child may still maintain a tendency toward hypoglycemia after prolonged fasting, which could be a clue to a deficiency of GH or ACTH. Maple syrup urine disease is a quite severe defect in the release of alanine from muscle owing to a defect in branched-chain amino acid catabolism (see earlier), which may be first diagnosed after infancy. Thus all ketotic hypoglycemia is not a benign variant, and some forms require medical rather than only dietary management.

Several types of GSDs cause hypoglycemia, but hepatomegaly and poor growth might first bring affected infants to evaluation. GSD type 1 (*232200 GLYCOGEN STORAGE DISEASE I at 17q21) is the result of a hepatic defect in glucose-6-phosphatase, the enzyme that converts glucose-6-phosphate to glucose in the last stage of gluconeogenesis and glycogenolysis. The condition is divided into types 1A and 1B (#232220 GLYCOGEN STORAGE DISEASE IB at 11q23). Deficiency of this enzyme thus eliminates both processes, which leads not only to hypoglycemia but also to hypertriglyceridemia and hypercholesterolemia, lactic acidosis and ketosis, hyperuricemia, hypophosphatemia, and abnormal platelet adhesiveness. Presentation of hypoglycemia with lactic acidosis and ketosis may occur in the neonatal period or later after the development of characteristic growth failure and hepatomegaly that is the result of glycogen and lipid deposition in the liver, although liver function usually remains normal. The spleen is not enlarged, but the kidneys are enlarged because of glycogen deposition, and renal failure may develop, but this is not invariable. Type 1B GSD combines all the features characteristic of type 1A and, in addition, features neutropenia and infections that follow (oral and anal lesions and chronic enteritis). Treatment is frequent or constant administration of glucose, as well as the ingestion of cornstarch to prolong the increase in blood sugar. The aim is to remedy the lack of available glucose and to suppress the counterregulatory hormone secretion that is responsible for many of the complications.

GSD type 3 (*232400 GLYCOGEN STORAGE DISEASE III at 1p21) is the result of a deficiency in amylo-1,6-glucosidase, the debrancher enzyme for glycogenolysis; this is a milder condition than GSD type 1. Because gluconeogenesis is functional, the hypoglycemia is less severe, and many of the complications of GSD 1 are absent. Hepatomegaly does, however, occur because of increased glycogen stores. Frequent feeding of glucose or cornstarch is appropriate therapy for most of these cases. However, some children have absence of amylo-1,6-glucosidase in the muscle as well and have weakness or even cardiac failure because of this defect.

GSD types 6 (*232700 GLYCOGEN STORAGE DISEASE VI at 14q21-q22) and 9 result from a phosphorylase deficiency, leading to diminished glycogen breakdown to free glucose. Affected patients have hepatomegaly and possibly hypoglycemia, but these are usually milder conditions than GSD type 1.

GSD 0 (#240600 GLYCOGEN STORAGE DISEASE 0 at 12p12.2) is a rare condition caused by hepatic glycogen synthetase deficiency, limiting glycogen synthesis in the liver but not in the muscle. Thus ketosis and hypoglycemia occur with fasting, but elevated glucose is found after eating. The liver is of normal size. This condition resembles ketotic hypoglycemia in many ways but has been reported in only a few individuals.

Hereditary fructose intolerance (*229600 FRUCTOSE INTOLERANCE, HEREDITARY at 9q22.3) is the result of a defect in fructose-1-phosphate aldolase, which may precipitate hypoglycemia. Affected patients have severe vomiting, diarrhea, and failure to thrive when exposed to fructose, although they are quite normal if fructose is restricted. The findings may extend to shock and acute liver failure, but the exposure to minimal amounts of fructose may cause failure to thrive and liver and kidney failure without the severe manifestations. Short-term treatment of hypoglycemia is accomplished through the administration of glucose, whereas long-term treatment is the avoidance of all dietary fructose.

The enzyme fructose 1,6-diphosphatase plays an important role in gluconeogenesis by using lactate, alanine, and glycerol and oral fructose intake. Thus children with fructose 1,6-diphosphatase deficiency (*229700 Fructose = 1, b = bisposphatase 1, FBPI) have hypoglycemia when exposed to fructose, alanine, glycerol, sorbitol, and lactate, as well as when they have infections or extended fasting. Lactic acidosis, ketosis, hyperuricemia, and elevated serum FFAs and alanine are found with hypoglycemia. Specific diagnosis is made with liver biopsy and enzyme analysis. The liver is enlarged, as in GSD type 1, in this condition because of hepatic steatosis, and differential diagnosis between the two conditions is through fed glucagon stimulation test. Treatment of hypoglycemia is with glucose treatment, and of acidosis, with bicarbonate. The child is not to be allowed prolonged fasting, and fructose is minimized in the diet.

If a storage disease is strongly suspected, liver biopsy might be performed for definitive diagnosis.

Organic acid or fatty acid oxidation defects (FATTY ACID ACYL-COENZYME A dehydrogenase deficiency; #201450 ACYL-CoA DEHYDROGENASE, MEDIUM-CHAIN, DEFICIENCY OF at 1p31) will demonstrate fasting hypoglycemia, mild hyperammonemia, hyperuricemia, and elevations of liver enzymes along with mild hepatomegaly with low serum ketone values and low serum carnitine but elevated esterified/free carnitine ratio. Dicarboxylated acids should be measured in the urine to make the specific diagnosis.

Other causes of hypoglycemia include malnutrition due to GI disease, diarrhea, or starvation, all of which lead to ketotic hypoglycemia. Alcohol ingestion or even significant skin exposure to alcohol can interfere with gluconeogenesis. Ackee fruit ingestion (Jamaican vomiting disease), Reye syndrome or other causes of hepatic failure, and the use of drugs that cause hypoglycemia as a side effect, such as aspirin or oral hypoglycemic agents, also may precipitate the condition. Propranolol or other β-blocking agents can cause hypoglycemia, especially after a fast (for example, when these agents are used to augment the response to a GH-provocative test after an overnight fast). Subjects who have a Nissen fundoplication and G-tube insertion may have a rapid increase in glucose when fed, leading to insulin secretion, followed by rapid decrease in glucose; this occurs more often if the G-tube infusion is administered in boluses rather than continuously.

An unfortunate condition know as Munchhausen by proxy must always receive consideration; in one possible presentation of this condition, a caregiver injects insulin into a child, which leads to unexplained hypoglycemia. Measurement of elevated serum insulin during hypoglycemia with low C-peptide indicates that the insulin is from exogenous sources rather than the patient's own pancreas (endogenous insulin secretion occurs with C-peptide secretion). Absence of hypoglycemia during scrupulous observation of the child, while eliminating the opportunity for anyone to administer insulin, is suggestive of this diagnosis.

As noted earlier, many adults complain of what they call hypoglycemia and often attribute symptoms in their children to the same condition. Symptoms generally occur a few hours after a meal, but when careful blood glucose measurements are obtained, low values are rarely found and even more rarely match the onset of symptoms. Although a 5-hour glucose tolerance test with measurement of glucose and insulin might be considered, in 25% of individuals, the blood sugar decreases during a oral glucose tolerance test (OGTT) more if CH_2O loading is not provided for 3 days beforehand, thus falsely suggesting the diagnosis of hypoglycemia. Most experts do not support the existence of the condition known as reactive hypoglycemia. Of course, it is harmless to modify the diet of most children to avoid concentrated sweets, a measure often suggested by those who support the diagnosis of reactive hypoglycemia, but it is wrong to suggest that a disease is present. If frequent feedings are advised to avoid factitious hypoglycemia, excessive caloric intake and obesity might be the result. Make sure that a diagnosis can be justified before suggesting such treatment (Tables 13-1 and 13-2).

Diagnosis of Hypoglycemia

Diagnosis of hypoglycemia must involve measuring blood sugar rather than just assuming it is low (Fig. 13-2). Glucometers are designed for the management of diabetes, in whom elevated values are frequent, so they do not reliably measure lower values. Nonetheless, if used appropriately, with reagents or test strips that are not outdated, they can be a useful adjunct to diagnosis, as long as true laboratory values are used as well.

Table 13-2.   The critical blood sample

To be obtained if BS is <50 mg/dL
Glucose
Insulin
Ketones
Growth hormone
Cortisol
Lactate
Pyruvate

If possible:

Free fatty acids
C peptide
IGF-1
IGF-11
IGF BP1
Ammonia
Amino acids
Free and bound carnitine

Save as much serum/plasma as possible for future determinations

IGF, insulin-like growth factor.

Anticipating the possibility that hypoglycemia may occur in a predictable situation will lessen the effort later required for the diagnosis and treatment of the condition. Thus patients with stressful deliveries, with prematurity, with IUGR, or, conversely, infants with large body size suspected to be the product of a mother with diabetes mellitus, should have blood sugar monitoring at frequent intervals during the first 24 hours after birth.

In older patients, the pattern of hypoglycemia is of extreme importance in the differential diagnosis. Fasting hypoglycemia more likely will indicate a defect in glucose production or release, such as a defect in gluconeogenesis or a GSD, whereas postprandial (or true reactive) hypoglycemia suggests a hyperinsulinemic state; overlap occurs, however, as hyperinsulinism will cause fasting hypoglycemia as well. The presence of ketone bodies in the urine or blood at the time of hypoglycemia will reflect the insulin secretory state; ketotic hypoglycemia is virtually incompatible (but not completely incompatible!) with hyperinsulinism, but nonketotic hypoglycemia increases the likelihood that insulin is the etiologic agent in the condition.

When a child has hypoglycemia, a blood sample should be obtained immediately so that determinations crucial to the diagnosis can be ordered; this is the "critical" blood sample (Table 13-2) that is the mainstay of diagnosis. Urine should be obtained for determination of ketonuria at the same time. Hypoglycemia is diagnosed only if a true serum/plasma sugar is low or if a glucometer indicates a low blood sugar that is later confirmed when the

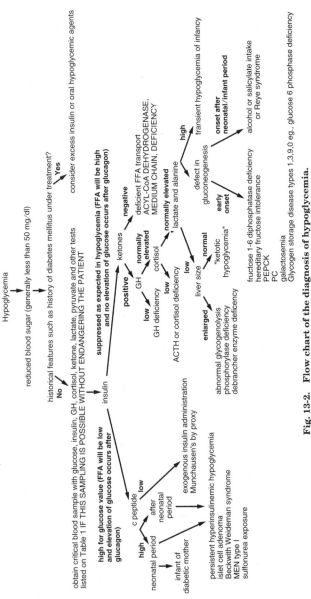

Fig. 13-2. Flow chart of the diagnosis of hypoglycemia.

laboratory determination returns; if only symptoms that suggest hypoglycemia are reported, not yet is a diagnosis of true hypoglycemia appropriate! After the critical blood sample is drawn, glucose is given to increase the blood sugar; the hypoglycemic episode should not be dangerously protracted just to obtain blood for the diagnostic sample, of course. Metabolic derangements (e.g., abnormal serum lactate or pyruvate levels or decreased serum concentration of GH or cortisol) causing hypoglycemia are ideally monitored at the time of the first documented episode. The aim of management of a hypoglycemic child is to prevent the recurrence of hypoglycemia; if the critical blood sample is missed on presentation, it may require long periods of observation before a recurrence allows the diagnostician to have another chance at diagnosis with a critical blood sample during a hypoglycemic event. If no diagnosis is suggested by the history or physical appearance, the blood sample obtained during the hypoglycemic episode should be sent for glucose (a true laboratory glucose rather than a glucometer value), insulin (a value of insulin/glucose greater than 0.3 suggests hyperinsulinism if serum glucose is greater than 60 mg/dL), ketone bodies, cortisol, GH, lactate (elevation suggests a defect in hepatic gluconeogenesis), pyruvate (low pyruvate suggests difficulty in mobilizing substrate for gluconeogenesis) determinations; serum should be frozen for future determinations (such as FFAs, which are elevated in fatty acid oxidation defects) in case another area of diagnostic inquiry seems more likely after the initial results are back (Table 13-1). The critical sample must be analyzed quickly so that glucose is not decreased by the metabolic activity of blood cells in a collection tube without additives; if the glucose determination is separated into a gray top (or other tube with fluoride) tube initially to stop metabolism of glucose, the glucose value is more likely to be accurate if the blood cells are not separated from plasma or serum right away.

If the critical initial sample is not collected, several steps should follow. Frequent measurement of blood glucose is made during a 24-hour period, before each meal, and at 1, 2, and 3 hours after one or more meals and also measured in the middle of the night; this might be called a "nothing tolerance test." If the blood sugar is decreased in any of these samples, as reflected by a finger-stick glucose method by glucometer, the full set of critical value tests noted earlier is performed, if possible, before glucose is given to increase the blood sugar concentration. Of particular importance is an insulin determination, which should be measured contemporaneous with a glucose concentration.

If no episode of spontaneous hypoglycemia occurs, an observed fast should be performed after a high-carbohydrate diet is given for the 3 days before the beginning of the fast. If the child's carbohydrate stores are not repleted by the high-carbohydrate diet, specious hypoglycemia may occur. The fast should start after a usual overnight period of sleep (if the child usually goes without food at night), so that hour 10 to 12 of the routine fast starts at 7:00 to 8:00 a.m., a time when the full hospital staff should be present to handle potential complications. Finger-stick glucose determinations by glucometer are made every 2 hours until a tendency is noted for a decrease in glucose. All urine samples are analyzed for ketone bodies as in ketotic hypoglycemia; the appearance of ketonuria will precede hypoglycemia. At the time that glucose decreases on the glucometer, a true laboratory glucose measurement is made at the same time as the finger-stick sample and the critical sample obtained. If the fast precipitates no decrease in glucose by 5:00 p.m. (after 20 to 22 hours), the test can be continued for a full 24 hours if adequate staff is available to monitor the child safely. If the glucose concentration decreases to less than 60 mg/dL, glucagon is given at a dose of 0.02–0.03 mg/kg to a maximum of 1 mg, and after 10 minutes, blood glucose, insulin, lactate, and pyruvate are measured to see if the child has adequate glycogen stores or if there is an abnormality in mobilization of glucose. Glucagon should not, however, be given if hepatomegaly is present, as it might worsen metabolic acidosis caused by a possible gluconeogenic defect. The fast is usually stopped by 24 hours, and if no hypoglycemia is demonstrated, it is at least apparent that the child can tolerate a 24-hour fast at home; such a long fast is not, of course, recommended, but a good margin of error exists if the child is fed on a reasonable schedule. It should be clear that if the initial critical sample is obtained appropriately, this complex diagnostic plan might often be eliminated altogether.

Various tolerance tests are used in the differential diagnosis of hypoglycemia. The glycogen TT (30 g/kg intravenously or intramuscularly, with blood glucose, FFAs, ketones, insulin, and GH determinations obtained at 0, 5, 15, and 15 minutes thereafter for 2 hours) determines whether glycogen can be broken down to supply glucose; used in the fed or fasting state, no increase in glucose will be seen in GSD type 1 (glucose-6-phosphatase deficiency), whereas in ketotic hypoglycemia or GSD type 3, a normal response will occur in the fed state, and a poor response after a fast. The fructose tolerance test is used to evaluate hereditary fructose intolerance or 1,6-diphosphatase deficiency. Because of GI symptoms after oral fructose, the intravenous test is preferred: 0.25 g/kg/ 5 min is given, with a resulting decrease in glucose (specific glucose measurement by specific laboratory technique must be used so that reducing substances do not interfere with the results) and inorganic phosphorus with an increase in plasma magnesium and uric acid in affected children. The child must be monitored to make sure severe hypoglycemia does not occur. Some tests cannot be recommended without prior experience. They are the leucine (orally, dissolved in a slurry of CO_2-free water administered through a stomach tube, at 150 mg/kg, or intravenously, 75 mg/kg, and blood obtained for glucose and insulin at 5, 10, 20, 30, 45, 60, 90, and 120 minutes or every 10 minutes for an hour, respectively) or the tolbutamide tolerance test (20 to 30 mg/kg up to 1 g intravenously, and blood sampled at 5, 10, 20, 30, 45, 60, 90, and 120 minutes) to determine if insulin secretion is inappropriately high. The tests may be dangerous, as severe hypoglycemia may be precipitated by the insulin secretagogues.

The GTT is rarely indicated, but if performed to rule out reactive hypoglycemia, it is important to carry out several important procedures to ensure that false results do not confuse the issue: 3 days of high-carbohydrate diet must be ingested, or the response to the oral glucose load will be falsely abnormal, even if the patient is normal (this type of preparation also is important for the other tolerance tests listed earlier); an insulin determination should accompany each glucose measurement; the test should extend for 5 hours to look for late hypoglycemia that would be missed on a shorter test; and the dose of glucose is 1.75 g/kg, as a 20% solution. The symptoms manifested by the patient should be recorded during the test so that any low blood sugar determinations can be matched with symptoms of hypoglycemia, making an organic abnormality more likely. Just as important as determining that a low blood sugar is associated with the symptoms is the elimination of the symptoms with an increase in blood sugar.

The method of measurement of glucose also deserves attention. Methods measuring reducing substances, such as Clinitest, will measure other substances, such as galactose, whereas those using a glucose oxidase technique will be specific for glucose. Methods measuring whole blood glucose will report values 15% lower than those with plasma glucose. Finger-stick methods of assessing blood glucose are available by glucometer, but these must be considered a guide and not definitive glucose results. A blood or plasma glucose reading at a licensed laboratory must confirm low blood glucose values. As noted earlier, the method of determining blood glucose depends on the way in which the sample was collected. If an empty tube (red top) is used to collect the blood, metabolic activity in the sample can reduce the concentration of glucose significantly over a period of several hours. Thus any sample collected in an empty tube must be analyzed soon after collection. Tubes containing fluoride (usually grey top), which stops any glucose metabolism and allows the storage of blood for hours without reducing the glucose concentration, are preferable.

Treatment of Hypoglycemia

Treatment of hypoglycemia may be short-term initial treatment to correct the specific event or long-term treatment to ensure continuation of a normal state: prolonged treatment is best aimed to achieve a value greater than 60 mg/dL at all times and normal values of 70 to 120 mg/dL at least most of the time (Table 13-3; see Chapter 15 for discussion of emergency treatment of hypoglycemia). The initial treatment of hypoglycemia must be the administration of glucose sufficient to bring the blood glucose to adequate levels to return neurologic function to normal but not excessive glucose to cause severely increased osmolality. In a child who is only moderately symptomatic, oral glucose is adequate; table sugar, honey (only if the child is older than 1 year and not at risk for infant botulism), or jelly can be administered to the child's buccal mucosa if the child is too disoriented to swallow. For

Table 13-3.   Treatment of hypoglycemia

Acute

If conscious	Oral sugar, cake frosting, 4 oz juice
If unconscious	i.v. Dextrose bolus, 25% at 1 mL/kg
If diabetic or if no evidence of GSD and hepatomegaly	i.m. Glucagon, 30 µg/kg to a maximum of 1 mg

Chronic

Ketotic hypoglycemia	Frequent feedings
GSD 1	Frequent feedings and cornstarch
Hereditary fructose intolerance	Avoidance of fructose
Galactosemia	Avoidance of galactose
Hyperinsulinism	Diazoxide, octreotide, or pancreatectomy
Carnitine deficiency	Carnitine
MCAD	Avoid fasting
Long-chain fatty acid abnormalities	Medium-chain fatty acids

GSD, glycogen-storage disease; MCAD, medium-chain acyl CoA dehydrogenase.

more severe hypoglycemia, intravenous glucose is necessary. Dextrose in water is given in 25% concentration or less as a bolus of 1 mL/kg. If more dextrose in higher concentration (dextrose vials are supplied as 50%) is administered, a risk exists of causing hyperosmolality, and in infants and neonates, D10W is preferable to any more-concentrated preparation. Once the blood sugar increases, the child should be observed; if the sugar again decreases, an infusion of dextrose, 5% to 10%, should be started; appropriate sodium chloride must be present in the infusion to avoid hyponatremia developing as the hypoglycemia is repaired. It is useful to calculate the amount of glucose in terms of milligrams per kilogram per minute to determine the severity of the hypoglycemia. If more than 12 to 15 mg/kg/min of glucose is required and repeatedly needed, the child has severe hypoglycemia, most likely due to hyperinsulinism. Abrupt discontinuation of dextrose support may lead to rebound hypoglycemia after the normal increase in insulin secretion caused by dextrose administration. This rebound condition should not be confused with *bona fide* hyperinsulinism. As transient hypoglycemia resolves, weaning off i.v. dextrose is followed by frequent oral administration of glucose-containing substances, as the child can tolerate under careful observation.

The treatment of several specific diagnoses was presented earlier. Dietary management is possible in some conditions.

Frequent carbohydrate feeding is the management for uncomplicated ketotic hypoglycemia.

GSD type 1, a gluconeogenic defect, is treated with frequent carbohydrate feedings, but overnight blood glucose is supported by uncooked cornstarch preparation or continuous nasogastric feedings.

Hereditary fructose intolerance mandates avoidance of fructose.

Galactosemia mandates avoidance of galactose ingestion.

Fatty oxidation defects, including MCAD, may respond to a low-fat diet and avoidance of fasting that might cause lipid breakdown.

In defects of long-chain fatty acid metabolism, medium-chain triglycerides are administered, and carbohydrates or glucose given during fasting or stress that might lead to lipid breakdown.

Carnitine is administered for *bona fide* carnitine deficiency, either primary or secondary.

Other measures are used for the management of severe hypoglycemia. Diazoxide, a benzothiodiazine hypotensive agent, in doses of 5 to 20 mg/kg/day divided into a dose every 6 hours, will suppress insulin secretion in some cases of hyperinsulinism, as noted earlier, but will not usually be effective in β-cell adenomas. A lack of response to diazoxide is not diagnostic but does suggest the presence of a β-cell adenoma or one of the hyperinsulinemic states discussed earlier that will require surgical removal. Diazoxide has several possible side effects including hirsutism, water and sodium retention (may be opposed by hydrochlorothiazide, which itself is a hypoglycemic agent), mild hyperuricemia, advanced bone age, and decreased immunoglobulin G and neutrophil numbers. Octreotide is a synthetic long-acting somatostatin analogue that will suppress insulin secretion in some cases. Dosing starts at 5 μg/kg subcutaneously, titrating the dose to 40 μg/kg/24 hours, divided into six doses per day. Tachyphylaxis is a possible side effect, as is steatorrhea.

Pancreatectomy is recommended in cases of hyperinsulinism resistant to diet or medications and should not be delayed if no other treatment successfully supports the blood sugar. Glucocorticoids are also used to increase blood sugar but should not be used for long-term replacement, except in cases of cortisol or ACTH deficiency, and then only in replacement doses. GH therapy is offered in cases of GH deficiency. The most important part of therapy is the speedy institution of a treatment designed to increase blood sugar and guard against severe and repetitive hypoglycemia and thereby to salvage mental function.

SUGGESTED READINGS

Enns G, Packman S. Diagnosing inborn errors of metabolism in the newborn: laboratory investigations. *Neoreviews* 2001;2:192–200.

Enns G, Packman S. Diagnosing inborn errors of metabolism in the newborn: clinical features. *Neoreviews* 2001;2:183–191.

Haymond MWSA. Hypoglycemia. In: Rudolph CD, Rudolph AM, eds. *Rudolph's pediatrics.* New York: McGraw-Hill, 2002:2106–2111.

Losek JD. Hypoglycemia and the ABCs (sugar) of pediatric resuscitation. *Ann Emerg Med* 2000;35(1):43–46.

Lovinger RD, Kaplan SL, Grumbach MM. Congenital hypopituitarism associated with neonatal hypoglycemia and microphallus: four cases secondary to hypothalamic hormone deficiency. *J Pediatr* 1975;87:1171.

Lteif AN, Schwenk WF. Hypoglycemia in infants and children. *Endocrinol Metab Clin* 1999;28(3):620–646.

Stanley CA, Thornton PS, Finegold DN, et al. Hypoglycemia in neonates and infants. In: Sperling MA, ed. *Pediatric endocrinology.* Philadelphia: WB Saunders, 2002:135–161.

Thornton PS, Finegold DN, Stanley CA, et al. Hypoglycemia in the infant and child. In: Sperling MA, ed. *Pediatric endocrinology.* Philadelphia: WB Saunders, 2002:367–384.

14 ♣ Endocrine Tumors of Childhood

Endocrine tumors exert influence by their mass or by the secretion of hormones. Hormone-secreting tumors either release hormones normally originating from the tissue encompassing the neoplasm (eutopic hormone-secreting tumors) or secrete increased amounts of hormones not ordinarily produced in the organ in large enough quantities to cause a biologic effect (ectopic hormone-secreting tumors). Some endocrine tumors of childhood are found in groups, often in a familial pattern.

CENTRAL NERVOUS SYSTEM TUMORS

Virtually any tumor of the central nervous system (CNS) can exert pressure effects on the hypothalamic–pituitary area by enlarging or from metastases of tumors arising in other tissues; this mass effect can cause endocrine disorders. Craniopharyngiomas are rare tumors compared with other types of CNS neoplasms, but are those most commonly associated with endocrine deficiencies in children. Other tumors in the area also can lead to pituitary deficiencies if the tumor is located in certain areas. Conversely, tumors may result in increased endocrine activity (e.g., a CNS tumor of the posterior hypothalamus can cause precocious puberty). Last, a human chorionic gonadotropin (hCG)-secreting tumor will exert effects by mass and by endocrine effect. Because of the range of endocrine effects of CNS tumors, they are discussed in general in this chapter; particular endocrine effects are discussed in more details in other appropriate chapters (see Chapter 3).

Craniopharyngiomas are derived from Rathke pouch and therefore arise in the pituitary stalk. They can grow upward into the hypothalamus or down into the sella turcica. Often cystic, they can contain cholesterol-laden fluid, which visually resembles motor oil. They often are calcified, so that 80% show flecks of calcium on lateral skull radiograph, and more will demonstrate calcium on computed tomographic (CT) scans of the hypothalamic–pituitary region. A magnetic resonance imaging (MRI) scan cannot demonstrate calcium, however. In a child of any age, a craniopharyngioma may develop, but the peak incidence is between the ages of 6 and 14 years. Patients will complain of headache and poor vision; they may have the polyuria and polydipsia characteristic of diabetes insipidus, their growth charts will demonstrate decreased growth velocity and, if the patient is old enough, delayed puberty may result. Physical examination may reveal short stature, chubbiness (an appearance characteristic of hypopituitarism), pale atrophic (not dysplastic) optic disks or, alternatively, papilledema, visual field defects on confrontation (usually bitemporal hemianopsia due to impingement on the nearby optic chiasm), and possibly physical findings of hypothyroidism (usually subtle, because this is not primary hypothyroidism); a prepubertal appearance or a cessation of the progression of secondary sexual development may occur, even in an adolescent patient. These historic features and signs and symptoms describe a classic patient; some have been serendipitously diagnosed by the finding of calcium flecks in the sellar area on a lateral skull radiograph taken for head trauma or on a dental radiograph taken for orthodontia. Bone age is often delayed, and in some cases, the bone age can indicate the approximate chronologic age at which the tumor began to exert its effects. Any type of anterior or posterior pituitary deficiency may occur, and even precocious puberty may result. Surgical removal is possible, and if the tumor is small, transsphenoidal microadenomectomy may be used, but a combination of radiation therapy and surgical removal may decrease the risk of recurrence and diminish the likelihood of further CNS damage or visual defects. If radiation is used, a possibility remains of later onset of new pituitary deficiencies. GH deficiency is a possible outcome of radiation to the hypothalamic–pituitary area and may develop in the 6 to 18 months after the therapy.

Germinomas of the hypothalamus are rare tumors as well, but have a peak incidence in the early teenage years. The location of germinomas makes any hypothalamic–pituitary deficiency possible. They may be asymptomatic, except for endocrine effects such as diabetes insipidus, growth failure, and delayed puberty. CNS germinomas may secrete hCG (as can germinomas and teratomas of other locations) and, because hCG acts on the luteinizing hormone (LH) receptor of the testes, cause incomplete precocious puberty in affected boys; a boy with a positive pregnancy test (β-hCG test) has a germ cell tumor until proven otherwise. Because hCG will not affect ovarian function, no effect is seen in girls except for decreased pituitary function caused by the mass of the tumor. These tumors are radiosensitive. Hepatoblastomas and hepatomas can secrete hCG, which also stimulates Leydig cell function. In all hCG-secreting tumors, hCG will cause testicular enlargement from the prepubertal size, but they will not grow so large as seen in the progression of normal puberty because follicle-stimulating hormone (FSH) is not secreted as well. Thus the boy may have a close to adult-size penis and significant pubic and axillary hair with testes of the size found in stage 2 of puberty.

Neurofibromatosis type 1 (*162200 NEUROFIBROMATOSIS, TYPE I; NF1 at 17q11.2) is a dominantly inherited disease characterized by cutaneous freckles, café-au-lait spots, and neurofibromas. The neurofibromas may degenerate into gliomas. Hypothalamic-pituitary disorders, including GH deficiency, hypogonadotropic hypogonadism, and precocious puberty are associated with tumors of the CNS in NF type 1. Pheochromocytomas also are found in this syndrome.

Langerhans cell histiocytosis (Hand-Schüller-Christian disease or histiocytosis X) involves infiltration of the hypothalamus, pituitary, or other organs with lipid-filled histiocytes. Diabetes insipidus is the most common finding, but GH deficiency, hypogonadotropic hypogonadism, and other hypothalamic-pituitary defects are found. Exophthalmos, a radiographic appearance of "floating teeth," and rarification of bones may be found.

HORMONE-SECRETING TUMORS

Childhood neoplasms with endocrine activity may produce an excessive amount of steroids, peptides, or catecholamines that are normally produced in physiologic concentrations in the affected organ or, alternatively, may produce peptide hormones not usually secreted in the same organ. The only sites of steroid biosynthesis in the body are the gonads and the adrenal glands. However, embryonic rests or ectopic adrenal tissue may remain in gonads and enlarge and secrete steroid products under adrenocorticotropic hormone (ACTH) stimulation, thereby simulating an endocrine neoplasm. The disorders listed are discussed in more detail in the chapters devoted to their organ systems.

Tumors Secreting Excessive Amounts of a Hormone That Normally Would Be Produced in the Same Tissue in Physiologic Concentrations: Eutopic Hormone-secreting Tumors

Pituitary tissue rarely forms adenomas during childhood, but prolactinomas, corticotropic adenomas (previously called basophilic adenomas), and, most rarely, somatotroph adenomas (previously eosinophilic adenomas) are reported. Prolactinomas cause amenorrhea or, more rarely, delayed puberty. Galactorrhea may be demonstrated by manual expression of the nipples if is not present spontaneously; serum prolactin is elevated after manipulations of nipples, so if blood sampling is planned, perform it before the examination or a day later. Prolactinomas are treated with surgical removal if possible, bromocriptine suppression if not amenable to surgical extirpation, or a combination of both. If puberty is delayed, progression of spontaneous pubertal development usually occurs after such treatment, assuming that healthy pituitary tissue remains. Psychotropic drugs may increase serum prolactin, so a careful history must be obtained before a diagnosis of a prolactinoma is assigned. Basophilic adenomas are removed by transsphenoidal microadenomectomy if the tumor is intrasellar. Somatotroph adenomas may respond to somatostatin analogues; surgery may be used, but recurrences are possible without medical suppression.

A nodule of the thyroid gland may be medullary carcinoma of the thyroid (MCT), papillary carcinoma, or follicular carcinoma. Family history will be most helpful in the diagnosis of MCT, but rarely a familial form of papillary carcinoma is found. Failing an elevated basal or gastrin-stimulated serum calcitonin value, the diagnosis will have to be confirmed by biopsy, and the local medical expertise may determine whether it will be by ultrasound-guided fine-needle aspiration or open biopsy. Removing as much of the cancer as possible and usually total or near-total thyroidectomy is indicated to decrease the likelihood of recurrence in remaining glandular tissue. Radioactive iodine therapy is sometimes administered to decrease the size of remaining tumor further in papillary and follicular carcinomas. Thyroxine therapy is given to decrease recurrent tumor growth in an amount adequate to suppress serum thyroid-stimulating hormone (TSH).

Parathyroid adenomas may be multiple, so that all four (the usual number of these glands, but more occur on occasion) parathyroid glands must be explored in patients suspected to harbor parathyroid tumors. No malignant tumors of the parathyroid gland have been reported. Hyperplasia of the parathyroid glands can mimic the clinical presentation of parathyroid adenomas; most of the tissue is usually removed surgically to allow relief from hypercalcemia. A parathyroid gland may be implanted in the subcutaneous tissue in the forearm, a site that allows easy access to removal of more tissue if hypercalcemia remains. The goal is to titrate the amount of tissue that remains to the desired normal value of serum calcium.

Islet cell adenomas of the beta cells of the pancreas secrete insulin and can produce symptomatic hypoglycemia. Carcinoma of the pancreas may not secrete sufficient insulin to cause hypoglycemic symptoms, but may secrete ectopic hormones. Other islet cell tumors of the pancreas can secrete gastrin and cause the Zollinger-Ellison syndrome and gastrinomas; somatostatinomas are reported.

Adrenal adenomas or carcinomas can secrete excess cortisol and produce Cushing syndrome, whereas adrenal adenomas can cause virilization because of the secretion of dihydroepiandrosterone (DHEA) or, more rarely, feminization because of the elaboration of estrogens. Carcinomas will usually produce more virilization than found in adenomas. Pheochromocytomas may arise from chromaffin tissue in sympathetic ganglia and the organ of Zuckerkandl, as well as from the adrenal medulla; extraadrenal pheochromocytomas will usually produce more norepinephrine (NE) than will adrenal pheochromocytomas, whereas epinephrine will predominate from tumors developing in the adrenal cortex because the rich supply of cortisol enhances the activity of the enzyme phenylethanolamine-N-methyl transferase, which converts NE to epinephrine. Neuroblastoma and ganglioneuroma also develop from sympathetic ganglia and but have increased formation of dopamine, which is metabolized to a large degree within the tumor, which causes increased urinary excretion of vanillylmandelic acid (VMA), and homovanillic acid (HVA) rather than NE or E.

Testicular Leydig cell tumors secrete testosterone and cause virilization. Adrenal rests may be found in a testes or ovary as the embryologic residua of adrenal cortical formation. With ACTH stimulation such as found in untreated congenital adrenal hyperplasia (CAH), considerable hypertrophy of the tissue can occur, and a false diagnosis of neoplasm may be made. Testicular tumors or masses causing virilization usually can be differentiated from adrenal tumors by the presence of palpable enlargement of the testes.

Tumors Secreting Hormones Not Normally Produced in Physiologic Concentrations from the Organ: Ectopic Hormone-secreting Tumors

hCG is produced in many tissues in small amounts. This suggests that the term ectopic hormone secretion may not be strictly appropriate for a tumor of the liver, for example, that secretes hCG; but for the purposes of this discussion, we retain the term ectopic hormone-secreting tumors.

Ectopic ACTH can be produced from thymomas, lung tumors, Wilms tumors, and islet cell pancreatic tumors. Cushing syndrome will result from intense stimulation of the adrenal cortex, and mineralocorticoid excess (caused by this excessive ACTH) may cause hypokalemic alkalosis in this form of Cushing syndrome; Cushing disease, in which ACTH values are not so far increased, will not lead to hypokalemic alkalosis.

Ovarian thecoma and luteomas and arrhenoblastomas produce virilization from androgen secretion. Granulosa cell tumors of the ovary secrete estrogen and produce feminization. They are usually palpable on bimanual examination. Gonadoblastomas forming in the streak gonads of Turner syndrome or the gonads of patients with other types of gonadal dysgenesis may produce estrogen or testosterone and falsely suggest the presence of normal gonadal function at first. Ovarian and adrenal androgen-secreting tumors may have similar clinical and laboratory features and can be identified from one another by imaging techniques or by selective venous catheterizations. In general, DHEA is the predominant product of adrenal tumors, but androstenedione or testosterone predominate in ovarian tumors.

Multiple Endocrine Neoplasia Syndromes

Multiple endocrine neoplasia syndrome type 1 (MEN 1; Werner syndrome *131100 caused by mutation in the MENEN gene at 11q13) comprises hyperparathyroidism (tumors are often found in all four parathyroid glands), pituitary adenomas (prolactin and GH produced), and pancreatic islet cell tumors (insulin from the beta cells and gastrin from the alpha cells) (all are autosomal dominant; Table 14-1). Thus hypercalcemia, hyperprolactinemia, GH excess, and hypoglycemia (due to hyperinsulinism) may result. Usually pheochromocytomas are not included in MEN type 1, but families rarely are reported with only pheochromocytoma and islet cell pancreatic tumors found in a complex. This disorder usually is first seen in adults, but it may develop in older teenagers.

MEN type 2 (#171400 MULTIPLE ENDOCRINE NEOPLASIA, TYPE II; MEN 2–associated mutations in the *RET* protooncogene at 10q11.2), Sipple syndrome, previously called MEN 2A, includes pheochromocytoma, medullary carcinoma of the thyroid, and parathyroid hyperplasia. The medullary carcinoma of the thyroid often occurs earlier and metastasizes at a younger age than is found in sporadic medullary carcinoma of the thyroid. The

Table 14-1. Features of multiple endocrine neoplasia and hormone values

Condition	Gene defect	Tumors of calcium regulation	Tumors of the pituitary gland	Gastrointestinal tumors	Adrenal tumors	Other features
MEN 1	: MENEN	Hyper-parathyroidism High PTH and Ca	Prolactinomas, growth hormone–secreting adenomas, ACTH-secreting adenomas, chromo-phobe adenomas	Islet cell tumors of the pan-creas: gas-trinomas, insulinomas, glucagono-mas, VIromas, pancreatic polypeptide GHRH and SRIF-secreting tumors	Adrenocorti-cal tumors	Carcinoid, lipomas
MEN 2	RET protooncogene	Parathyroid adenomas High PTH and Ca Medullary carcinoma of the thyroid High calcitonin	—	—	Pheochromo-cytomas High cate-cholamines	—

| MEN 3 | RET protooncogene | — | Rarely parathyroid adenomas
High PTH and Ca
Medullary carcinoma of the thyroid
High calcitonin | — | Pheochromocytomas
High catecholamines | Multiple mucosal neuromas leading to the appearance of lumpy lips, etc. |

MEN, multiple endocrine neoplasia; PTH, parathyroid hormone; ACTH, adrenocorticotropic hormone; VIP, vasoactive intestinal peptide; GHRH, growth hormone–releasing hormone.

pheochromocytomas are usually located in the adrenal gland and may be bilateral or multicentric (see Chapter 15 for a discussion of the emergency management of pheochromocytoma).

MEN type 3 (#162300 MULTIPLE ENDOCRINE NEOPLASIA, TYPE IIB; MEN 2B–associated mutations in the *RET* protooncogene at 10q11.2) includes pheochromocytoma, medullary carcinoma of the thyroid, and multiple mucosal neuromas, and the patient often has a Marfan syndrome–like habitus. The phenotype is quite distinctive; neuromas of the lips and tongue are most common. The physical findings should cause the physician to search for occult pheochromocytomas and medullary carcinomas of the thyroid.

Von Hippel-Lindau disease (retinal cerebellar hemangioblastomatosis (*193300 VON HIPPEL-LINDAU SYNDROME; VHL at 3p26-p25, 11q13) is associated with pheochromocytoma formation.

SCREENING FOR TUMORS

In any of the hereditary conditions that lead to tumor formation, it is essential to screen the family members likely to inherit the tendency (e.g., if a father has the diagnosis of MCT, all offspring must be screened, in view of the autosomal dominant inheritance pattern. See individual disorders for details of diagnosis.

SUGGESTED READINGS

Chernausek SD. Pheochromocytoma and the multiple endocrine neoplasia syndrome. In: Sperling MA, ed. *Pediatric endocrinology.* Philadelphia: WB Saunders, 2002:439–454.

Chernausek SD. Pheochromocytoma. In: Finberg L, Kleinman RE, eds. *Saunders manual of pediatric practice.* Philadelphia: WB Saunders, 2002:915–916.

Chernausek SD. Multiple endocrine neoplasia syndromes. In: Finberg L, Kleinman RE, eds. *Saunders manual of pediatric practice.* Philadelphia: WB Saunders, 2002:917–918.

Iler MA, King DR, Ginn-Pease ME, et al. Multiple endocrine neoplasia type 2A: a 25-year review. *J Pediatr Surg* 1999;34(1):92–96.

15 ♣ Guide to Pediatric Endocrine Emergencies

Much of this information is derived from the previous chapters but is summarized in this format. It is much preferable to read the indicated chapter, which covers the issues in detail.

ACUTE ADRENAL INSUFFICIENCY

1. Signs and symptoms
   a. Adrenal insufficiency should be suspected in children or adolescents who
      i. Have a history of central nervous system (CNS) surgery, trauma, tumors, or congenital defects, as noted in Chapter 3.
      ii. Have a history of ambiguous genitalia.
         1. In this case, investigate possible virilizing or salt-losing congenital adrenal hyperplasia, as described in Chapter 8.
         2. You may assume salt-losing adrenal insufficiency is present if sodium decreases and potassium increases, and treat appropriately while diagnostic measures are pending.
      iii. Have a history of microphallus in boys.
      iv. Have evidence of hyperpigmentation on skin, flexural surfaces, or mucous membranes.
      v. Have a history of previous glucocorticoid maintenance or higher dose therapy because of preexisting conditions of the pituitary gland or adrenal gland.
   b. The patient might exhibit
      i. Weakness, malaise, lethargy increasing to anorexia, nausea, vomiting, and abdominal pain.
      ii. Dehydration with tachypnea, postural hypotension, and decrease skin turgor follows.
      iii. Petechiae and purpura may occur if meningococcemia or Waterson-Fridricksen occurs.
      iv. Hypoglycemia and/or seizures are possible.
      v. Death or coma is possible.
   c. Laboratory evaluation reveals
      i. Low serum cortisol (cortisol should increase in a stressful situation).
      ii. Adrenocorticotropic hormone (ACTH) may be high or low depending on etiology.
      iii. Serum Na is low and K is high if mineralocorticoids are affected, as well as glucocorticoids.
      iv. Serum/blood glucose is low.
      v. Eosinophilia due to decreased cortisol is possible.
2. Glucocorticoid replacement
   a. Immediate administration of hydrocortisone in a dose of 2 mg/kg or 60 mg/m^2 or 2 mg for small children,

up to 100 mg for large teenagers by subcutaneous, intramuscular, or intravenous route is accomplished. An ill effect is not likely from giving too much, so err on the higher dose if necessary.

b.   The maintenance phase is accomplished by the administration of stress doses, which are 3 times maintenance dosage (i.e., 50 mg/m^2 of cortisol or 7.5 mg/m^2 of 6-αmethylprednisolone (Solumedrol) if any stress is present (infection, surgery, severe illness) until the patient is stable, when normal replacement doses of glucocorticoid (6 to 15 mg/m^2/day, divided into four or three doses/day) is instituted. This can be given by mouth if the patient is able to tolerate oral administration or by i.v. or subcutaneous (the oral dose is double the parenteral dose) until maintenance therapy is started.

3.   Hypoglycemia is treated as described later.

4.   Hyponatremia with hyperkalemia is treated as described later.

5.   Volume expansion is accomplished by 20 mL/kg of normal saline as a bolus in the first hour, and maintenance or replacement fluids thereafter in accordance with standard fluid management.

6.   It is imperative if hypothyroidism and glucocorticoid deficiency coexist, that glucocorticoid be administered before or with thyroid hormone, or the minimal glucocorticoid that may be present endogenously will be more rapidly metabolized, leading to acute glucocorticoid deficient crisis.

DIABETIC KETOACIDOSIS

1.   Measure blood sugar (more than 200 mg/dL for diagnosis), blood ketones (positive or moderate to large ketones in urine for diagnosis), pH (venous less than 7.25 for diagnosis), bicarbonate (less than 16 mEq/mL for diagnosis), sodium, potassium, blood urea nitrogen (BUN), creatinine, and white blood cell (WBC) count [usually elevated in diabetic ketoacidosis (DKA) even without infection].

2.   Fluid and electrolyte replacement

a.   Evaluate clinical deficit, which will usually be between 5% and 12% or even 15%; average is 7% dehydration, so extra fluid administration for severe dehydration is not always needed.

b.   Fluid administration must be done with care, but if indicated by signs of fluid deficit, an i.v. bolus of 10 mL/kg of "isotonic" fluid (0.9% saline or lactated Ringers) over a 30- to 60-minute period is used and repeated if necessary.

c.   The remaining fluid deficit is administered over the next 36–48 hours.

d.   Maintenance fluids are added to the deficit replacement.

e. Potassium will be deficient in DKA, so after establishing urine output, add potassium to the infusion at 30 to 40 mEq/mL. Monitor electrocardiogram (ECG) for abnormalities of potassium, as peaked T waves occur in hyperkalemia, and low T waves and the development of U waves occur in hypokalemia.

f. Low phosphorus is a potentially dangerous complication of DKA, so K Phos is used as at least a portion of the replacement of K is Ca is normal.

g. Bicarbonate therapy is associated with a higher risk for cerebral edema, and so should not be used unless symptomatic hyperkalemia is found or the acidosis is severe enough to cause hemodynamic instability not responsive to other therapeutic measures. If pH is 7.0 to 7.1, some suggest the use of bicarbonate at a dose of 40 mEq/mL/m^2, and if Ph is less than 7.0, the use of 80 mEq/mL/m^2, but because the use of bicarbonate is associated with the development of cerebral edema, this decision must be individualized.

h. Although excessive and rapid fluid administration might cause serious complications, dehydration leading to thrombosis is an alternative risk, so each patient must be individualized for appropriate fluid and electrolyte therapy.

3. Insulin management

a. Intravenous insulin at a rate of 0.075 to 0.1 unit/kg/hr is infused, and blood sugar monitored frequently. The use of a priming dose of insulin to prepare the tubing or an initial bolus of insulin before the infusion starts is no longer recommended.

b. When blood sugar decreases to 250 to 300 mg/dL, i.v. dextrose (5% to 10%) is added to allow continued administration of insulin to bring about resolution of the ketoacidosis safely; this process may continue until the serum bicarbonate is above 17 to 18 mEq/mL.

4. Monitoring

a. Measure blood sugar by glucometer or laboratory determinations every hour, and aim to decrease blood glucose by 10 mg/dL per hour. This rate may easily be exceeded, as renal function, fluid, and insulin administration all exert effects on decreasing blood sugar, so careful observation is mandatory. Check extreme values with a laboratory determination of glucose.

b. Measure serum electrolytes every 4 hours.

c. Watch for deteriorating mental condition, headaches, vomiting, or unusual behavior, as these might indicated the development of cerebral edema. Physical signs might include changing neurologic examination and papilledema. If necessary, confirm the development of cerebral edema with head magnetic resonance imaging (MRI). Treatment of cerebral edema is difficult, and generally the methods are unproven, but mannitol (1 mg/kg, i.v., or 10 to 20 g/m^2) may be beneficial as long as dehydration is not allowed to develop after the use of a hyperosmolar agent.

HYPERCALCEMIA

1. Suspect in
   a. Child with history of or hypoparathyroidism with a vitamin D preparation, perhaps with calcium replacement.
   b. Child with family history of multiple endocrine neoplasia type 2 (MEN II).
   c. Child with mucosal neuromas.
   d. Immobilized child.
   e. Child with various malignancies including leukemia.
   f. Child with megavitamin therapy.
   g. Child with physical features of Williams syndrome.
2. Symptoms include
   a. Weakness, listlessness.
   b. Irritability.
   c. Abdominal discomfort and symptoms including nausea and vomiting, abdominal pain, and constipation.
   d. CNS symptoms including depressed consciousness and confusion.
   e. Polyuria and polydipsia.
3. Laboratory values include
   a. Serum Ca more than 11 mg/dL.
   b. If parathyroid hormone (PTH) is present in excess, serum PO$_4$ is low.
4a. Treatment is increased hydration with sodium chloride infusion at twice maintenance if the patient can tolerate increased hydration.
   b. Furosemide, 1 to 2 mg/kg, may be given by i.v. slowly if calcium is not decreasing, to increase urinary calcium excretion. Because the patient may initially have some degree of dehydration, the sodium chloride infusion must be used in concert with the diuretic.
   c. Sodium sulfate and sodium phosphate may be administered during therapy for vitamin D intoxication.
   d. Oral phosphate may be used to bind calcium in the intestine, but may result in diarrhea.
   e. Oral glucocorticoids decrease calcium absorption from the intestines and may be used in severe cases of hypervitaminosis D but are not effective in cases of hyperparathyroidism.
   f. If serum calcium is greater than 14 mg/dL, calcitonin (2 to 4 units/kg/injection s.c., every 6 to 12 hours as needed) or bisphosphonates (pamidronate, 0.5 to 1.0 mg/kg/dose I.V. over 4 to 5 hours, repeated once as necessary up to 2 mg/kg/dose) may be used.
5. If renal failure coexists, renal dialysis might be necessary to decrease serum calcium.

6. If malignancy-derived PTH-releasing protein (PTHRP) is the etiology, mithramycin at 25 mg/kg/day may be used.

HYPERTHYROIDISM IN THE NEONATE

1. This is exceptionally rare in childhood but is seen in infants whose mothers have hyperthyroidism (which might yet not be diagnosed in the mother!). Symptoms including nervousness, diarrhea, shakiness, and tachycardia are indications of hyperthyroidism in the neonate. Congestive heart failure due to supraventricular tachycardia and hepatosplenomegaly may occur in hyperthyroidism.
2. Laboratory findings include
    a. Elevated serum free T_4 (total T_4 might be elevated fallaciously if protein is excessive or patient is taking estrogen).
    b. TSH is usually suppressed as the thyroid gland is stimulated by immunoglobulins in this condition.
3. Digitalis or sedatives might be indicated in this situation in the neonate.
4. Lugol's solution of supersaturated potassium iodine may be used to suppress thyroid hormone output (see later).
5. Propranolol may be used to counter the sympathetic effects of hyperthyroidism (see later).
6. Propylthiouracil (PTU) is given if the condition is severe and is likely to last for several months (see doses later).
7. The child must be watched closely for resolution of hyperthyroidism that usually occurs before 12 weeks and sometimes as soon as 3 weeks; continued treatment with PTU when thyroid function becomes normal would lead to iatrogenic hypothyroidism.

THYROID STORM IN CHILDREN AND ADOLESCENTS

1. This is a rare complication to be suspected in children with
    a. A history of hyperthyroidism with intercurrent
        i.   Infection
        ii. Surgery
        iii. Radioactive iodine therapy.
    b. Alternatively it can occur anew
2. Thyroid storm is indicated by an acute onset of hyperthermia and tachycardia in a patient with underlying hyperthyroidism. Precipitating factors include infection and diabetic ketoacidosis in a patient with hyperthyroidism. It may occur during surgical or radioiodine therapy for hyperthyroidism. Symptoms include high fever, sweating, tachycardia, and reduced mental status, ranging from confusion to coma.
3. Immediate therapy is indicated.
4. Propranolol is used in a starting dose of 2 to 3 mg/kg/day, divided into a dose every 6 hours to control some adrenergic symptoms of thyroid storm. Propranolol may be given i.v. at a dose of 0.01 to 0.1 mg/kg, up to a total of 5 mg over

10 to 15 minutes, but an intraatrial pacing catheter is a necessary precaution: start with the lower range of doses.

5. Dexamethasone in a dose of 1 to 2 mg every 6 hours can decrease conversion of T_4 to T_3 (i.v. dose is 0.2 mg/kg); hydrocortisone at 5 mg/kg i.v. or oral hydrocortisone at triple this dose may be used instead.

6. Intravenous NaI in a dose of 125 to 250 mg/day up to 1 to 2 g/day may decrease the release of thyroid hormone from the thyroid gland; Lugol's solution of concentrated iodine in a dose of 5 drops once every 8 hours by mouth can be given if the patient is conscious.

7. A cooling blanket or tepid bath can help control the hyperpyrexia as can acetaminophen (do not use aspirin in childhood).

8. Propylthiouracil will not take effect for several days, but to plan for the possibly extended course of the disorder, a dose of 6 to 10 mg/kg/day up to a maximum of 200 to 300 mg can be given every 6 hours by slurry, if necessary. Methimazole at a dose of 0.6 to 0.7 mg/kg/day is an alternative.

9. Fluid management must be observed, and if tachycardia causes heart failure, digitalis may be necessary.

HYPOCALCEMIA

1. This is suspected in children or neonates with undiagnosed seizures, a history of hypocalcemia in the family, a tendency to infections, a defect of the great arteries (e.g., truncus arteriosus), cardiac, mucocutaneous candidiasis, papilledema, autoimmune disease, and psychiatric symptoms.

2. Hypocalcemia is defined as serum total Ca less than 7.0 mg/dL or ionized Ca^{2+} less than 3.5 mg/dL, but symptoms might occur if total Ca is less than 8.5 mg/dL.

3. Neonates may require therapy if serum calcium decreases to less than 6 mg/dL or ionized Ca to less than 0.72 mg/mL, but symptoms may occur if total Ca is less than 7.5 mg/dL.

4. ECG may show a prolonged QT interval.

5. For severe symptomatic hypocalcemia, i.v. 10% calcium gluconate in a dose of 0.5 to 1 mL/kg given over 3 to 5 minutes, up to a total of 10 mL given under ECG monitoring (bradycardia and asystole are possible complications, and infusion should stop if pulse decreases to less than 60 beats/min or given extremely carefully if pulse decreases to less than 100 beats/min). During the administration of i.v. calcium, it is important to avoid extravasation that may cause severe sloughing of the skin, possibly requiring plastic surgery. The infusion may be repeated if necessary for the relief of symptoms.

6. The short-term treatment is followed by i.v. 10% calcium gluconate at 100 to 500 mg/kg over 24 hours for neonates and 100 to 200 mg/kg for infants or older subjects. Monitor blood calcium to avoid overtreatment.

7. Prolonged therapy is achieved with 1,25(OH)$_2$ vitamin D (this form eliminates the need for 1-hydroxylation of vitamin D that is impaired in hypoparathyroidism), given at a dose of 20 to 40 ng/kg/day (0.25 to 0.75 μg, calculated as twice daily) with, if necessary, oral calcium supplementation adequate to maintain serum ionized calcium.

8. In the hyperphosphatemic state due to hypoparathyroidism, phosphorus is restricted in the diet until serum phosphorus decreases to near-normal levels, which should occur when serum ionized calcium approaches normal.

9. Serum ionized calcium should be measured regularly until stability is achieved to assure that serum calcium remains in the normal range.

10. If magnesium is low and is a possible etiology for hypoparathyroidism, magnesium sulfate (50% solution) may be given as 0.1 to 0.2 mL/kg i.m. every 12 to 24 hours, as needed.

HYPOGLYCEMIA

1. Hypoglycemia is suspected in a
   a. Child with diabetes mellitus receiving insulin treatment.
   b. Child with error in carbohydrate metabolism.
   c. Child with congenital hypopituitarism.
   d. Boy with microphallus.
   e. Child with midline defect.

2. Diagnosis is made if blood or capillary sugar is less than 40 mg/dL or plasma sugar is less than 45 mg/dL in some texts, but a value of plasma sugar below 60 mg/dL is effectively hypoglycemia.

3. The initial treatment of hypoglycemia must be the administration of glucose sufficient to bring the blood glucose to adequate levels to return neurologic function to normal but not excessive glucose which will cause severe increased osmolality.

4. In a child who is only moderately symptomatic, oral glucose is adequate; table sugar, honey (only if the child is well older than 1 year and not at risk for infant botulism), or jelly can be ingested or administered to the child's buccal mucosa if the child is too disoriented to swallow.

5. For more severe hypoglycemia, i.v. glucose is necessary. Dextrose in water is given in 25% concentration or less as a bolus of 1 mL/kg or 0.25 g of dextrose/kg body weight: this is 2.5 mg/kg of 10% dextrose or 1 mL/kg of 25% dextrose). If more dextrose in higher concentration (dextrose vials are supplied as 50%) is administered, a risk exists of causing hyperosmolality, and in infants and neonates, D10W is far preferable to any more concentrated preparation.

6. Once the blood sugar increases, the child should be observed for improved clinical condition; if the sugar again decreases, an infusion of dextrose, 5% to 10%, should be

started. Sodium chloride must be in the dextrose infusion to avoid hyponatremia developing as the hypoglycemia is repaired. The infusion rate will usually be 6 to 8 mg/kg/min, which is approximately D10W at 1.5 times maintenance.

7. If more than 12 to 15 mg/kg/min of glucose is required and repeatedly needed, the child has severe hypoglycemia, most likely due to hyperinsulinism. Abrupt discontinuation of dextrose support may lead to rebound hypoglycemia due to the normal increase in insulin secretion caused by dextrose administration. This rebound condition should not be confused with *bona fide* hyperinsulinism.

8. As transient hypoglycemia resolves, weaning off i.v. dextrose is followed by frequent oral administration of glucose-containing substances as the child can tolerate under careful observation.

9. Prolonged treatment is best aimed to achieve a value of more than 60 mg/dL at all times and normal values of 70 to 120 mg/dL at least most of the time.

HYPONATREMIA/HYPERKALEMIA DUE TO ADRENAL INSUFFICIENCY

1. This situation is suspected in
   a. Children with ambiguous genitalia.
   b. Children with a history of glucocorticoid deficiency who may also have mineralocorticoid deficiency.
   c. Children in shock (who might have adrenal failure).

2. Laboratory values include serum sodium less than 130 mg/dL.

3. Hypoglycemia: follow the guidelines for hypoglycemia listed earlier.

4. Hyponatremia is treated with the
   a. Intravenous infusion of normal saline in normal replacement volumes.
   b. If the patient is seizing from hyponatremia, 3% NaCl might be infused in doses sufficient to increase the serum Na until seizures stop; 3 ml/kg every 10 to 20 minutes is a useful dose.

5. Hyperkalemia
   a. Replacement i.v. fluid will usually reduce some or all of the hyperkalemia.
   b. If the ECG demonstrates peaked T waves, widening of the P-R interval, first-degree heart block loss of the P wave or ventricular arrhythmia, 10% calcium gluconate at a dose of 0.5 mL/kg i.v., over 2 to 5 minutes, may be administered to stabilize the membranes; if pulse decreases to less than 60 beats/min, calcium infusion should cease, and if the pulse decreases to less than 100 beats/min, calcium infusion can be continued, but only with exceptional care.
   c. Sodium bicarbonate, 7.5%, given as 2 to 3 mL/kg over 30 to 60 minutes, will tend to drive K into the cells, reducing serum K.

      d. 50% Glucose plus 1 unit of insulin for every 5 to 6 g of glucose given over 30 minutes will tend to drive K into the cells, reducing serum K. However, because these children have a tendency toward hypoglycemia, this therapy carries danger and must be used with the utmost caution.

      e. Sodium polystyrene sulfonate (Kayexelate) resin in a dose of 1 g/kg (possibly given in 10% glucose at 1 g/4 mL) may be given every 4 to 6 hours to increase loss of potassium in the gastrointestinal (GI) tract. This is not an emergency treatment.

  6. Oral Florinef is the best treatment for hyponatremia and hyperkalemia of adrenal insufficiency but will take a matter of hours to work. At present, no parenteral treatment exists for mineralocorticoid deficiency.

HYPONATREMIA RESULTING FROM SYNDROME OF INAPPROPRIATE SECRETION OF ANTIDIURETIC HORMONE

  1. Syndrome of inappropriate secretion of antidiuretic hormone (SIADH) should be suspected in a child who

      a. Has had CNS trauma or infection.

      b. Has meningitis or encephalitis.

      c. Has increased intrathoracic pressure due to, for example, pneumonia.

      d. Is receiving positive-pressure ventilation and has decreased serum sodium (laboratory values include serum sodium less than 130 mg/dL), or decreased osmolality in spite of

         i. Urinary concentration to some degree out of proportion for the serum osmolality.

        ii. No hyperlipidemia, hyperproteinemia, or hyperglycemia as a cause of low serum sodium.

       iii. No concomitant hyperkalemia along with hyponatremia.

  2. Sodium loss in the urine will continue until SIADH is resolved, so treatment used to resolve hyponatremic seizures will be effective only temporarily until the cause of SIADH is resolved.

  3. During the episode of hyponatremia, i.v. infusion of normal saline is used in a milliliter-per-milliliter replacement for all urinary loss; this will allow an effective increase in serum sodium without an increase in fluid volume. Alternatively, withholding fluids under close observation until the condition resolves may be tried. This process must consider the state of hydration so that the patient does not become clinically dehydrated and or go into shock while fluids are limited.

  4. If the patient is seizing from hyponatremia, 3% NaCl might be infused in doses sufficient to increase the serum Na until seizures stop; 3 ml/kg given every 10 to 20 minutes until

symptoms of hyponatremia resolve is one recommended therapy.
5. Furosemide (1 mg/kg) might be used, and the volume excreted replaced with 3% NaCl to allow an effective increase of serum sodium to control the seizure; frank dehydration is a possible outcome if fluid volume is not watched carefully.
6. Dilantin, 5 to 10 mg/kg, has been used in patients with seizures due to CNS etiologies of SIADH.
7. For chronic cases, refer to Chapter 4. In addition, democycline is a tetracycline derivative that reduces the ability of the nephron to respond to vasopressin (AVP) and may be used for chronic SIADH in a dose of 10 mg/kg, although this molecule that is a modification of tetracycline might adversely affect tooth development if used for long periods in young children.

HYPERNATREMIA DUE TO DIABETES INSIPIDUS

1. This condition is suspected in a patient who
   a. Has signs of dehydration including sunken eyes, dry mucous membranes, sunken fontanel in infants (because a tendency exists toward hypernatremic dehydration, the loss of skin turgor may not occur, and the skin might feel "doughy" as a result).
   b. Has a history of CNS tumor, surgery or accident, or a bitemporal hemianopsia.
   c. Has a condition causing increased intracranial pressure.
   d. Has an increase serum osmolality and serum sodium while the urine osmolality is low.
2. Laboratory values include serum sodium less than 130 mg/dL with no elevation of serum potassium.
3. This form of hypernatremia is due to loss of free water rather than a condition of excess sodium.
4. The length of time of dehydration is important, as a chronic state will require slower fluid-replacement program than in acute cases.
5. If serum sodium is greater than 160 nM, a bolus of normal saline in a dose of 20 mL/kg may be helpful.
6. Volume deficit is calculated, and fluid replacement is planned for the next 48 hours.
7. The volume of urine output will change remarkably from large volumes before the administration of DDAVP to lower volumes afterward; thus it is best to replace the urine volume lost with an equivalent volume of i.v. fluid for maintenance as the patient is stabilized. Once the volume of urine is controlled, routine maintenance fluid calculations may again be appropriate.
8. DDAVP treatment is established as in Chapter 4, but if the child cannot take oral or nasal DDAVP, i.v. aqueous pitressin, at a dose of 2 to 3 mg/kg/min, or i.m. administration at 1 to 5 units per dose is an alternative.

9. At all times, evaluation of serum sodium and urine osmolality as well as continuous evaluation of the balance of fluid given to fluid excreted is necessary.

HYPERTENSION DUE TO PHEOCHROMOCYTOMA

1. These rare tumors are described in Chapter 14.
2. Symptoms may include headaches of a pounding nature, palpitations with tachycardia and sweating, and possibly flushing.
3. Signs include hypertension, usually of a constant pattern, but episodic hypertension as found in adults may occur in children.
4. Nervousness, tremor, fatigue, and thoracic pain may be present.
5. Patients developing hypertension during the induction of anesthesia, in patients suspected of having MEN II or III, and with malignant hypertension unresponsive to usual methods of therapy.
   a. The hypertension of pheochromocytoma might be treated with
      i. Phentolamine mesylate at 1 mg i.v. or i.m. Usually given 1 hour before surgery. For diagnosis of an untreated hypertensive patient, phentolamine mesylate is given i.v. rapidly after the effects of antihypertensive measures are gone or before they started. BP is monitored for 30 seconds for 3 minutes and thereafter every 60 seconds for 7 minutes. A BP reduction of more than 35 mm Hg systolic and 25 mm Hg diastolic is considered positive for pheochromocytoma. Phentolamine mesylate, i.m., may be used for diagnosis in a dose of 3 mg, and the BP monitored every 5 minutes for 30 to 45 minutes, and the same criteria for change in BP used.
      ii. Sodium nitroprusside, at a done of 0.5 to 8.0 µg/kg/min is an alternative.

SUGGESTED READINGS

Protocols are taken from the other chapters in the book, with specific sources listed.

Hales DE. Endocrine emergencies. In: Fleisher GR, Ludwig S, eds. *Textbook of pediatric emergency medicine.* Philadelphia: Lippincott Williams & Wilkins, 2000:1093–1115.

Hales DE. Endocrine emergencies. In: Fleisher GR, Ludwig S, eds. *Synopsis of pediatric emergencies.* Philadelphia: Lippincott Williams & Wilkins, 2002:439–448.

Wu RHK. Endocrine emergencies. In: Crain EF, Gershel JC, eds. *Clinical manual of emergency pediatrics.* New York: McGraw-Hill, 1997:139–162.

16 ♣ Medications for Pediatric Endocrinology

The following is a list of the most commonly used, but not all, of the mediations for pediatric endocrinology. It is incumbent upon the prescriber to check for allergies, contra indications, side effects and safety in pregnancy as there is too little space here. Also note that some of the medications are used in clinical studies and presented in publications dealing with children without FDA approval: they are presented here for information but the prescriber must take the age of the patient into consideration.

CALCITONIN, HUMAN
Hypercalcemia

CALCITROL (1,25-DIHYDROXYCHOLECALCIFEROL)
0.25 μg/dose, p.o./day initially. Increase by 0.25 μg every 2–4 weeks while observing effects on serum calcium.

Younger than 1 year, 0.04 to 0.08 μg/kg/dose/day
1 to 5 years, 0.25 to 0.75 μg/dose/day
Older than 6 years, 0.5 to 2 μg/dose/day

CALCIUM CARBONATE (TUMS),
40% ELEMENTAL CALCIUM

Neonate: 125 to 325 mg/kg/day, divided into four to six doses/day, not to exceed 2.5 g/day
Children: 112.5 to 162 mg/kg/day, divided into q.i.d.
Adults: 2.5 to 5 g/day, divided into t.i.d. to q.i.d.

CALCIUM GLUBIONATE
Elemental calcium (6%), available as 115 mg/5 mL.

Neonate with hypocalcemia: 1,200 mg/kg/day, divided into q.i.d. to t.i.d.
Maintenance: 600 to 2,000 mg/kg/day, up to 9 g/day, divided q.i.d.

ADULTS: 6 TO 18 G/DAY, DIVIDED INTO Q.I.D.

CALCIUM GLUCONATE
9% elemental calcium; injection is 10% solution.

Maintenance for Hypocalcemia
Neonates: i.v. 200 to 500 mg/kg/day, divided into q.i.d.
Infants: i.v. 200 to 500 mg/kg/day, divided into q.i.d.
Oral: 400 to 800 mg/kg/day, divided into q.i.d.
Child: oral or i.v. is 200 to 500 mg/kg/day, divided into q.i.d.
Adult: oral or i.v. is 5 to 15 g/day, divided into q.i.d.

CALCIUM LACTATE,
13% ELEMENTAL CALCIUM

Infants: 400 to 500 mg/kg/day, divided into q4 to 6 hours
Children: 500 mg/kg/day, divided into q4 to 6 hours

Adults: 1.5 to 3 g/given t.i.d.

DDAVP

1-Deamino-8-ᴅ-arginine vasopressin

Tablets 0.1, 0.2 mg
For diabetes insipidus
Nasal spray: 100 µg/mL or 10 µg/spray
Children: 0.05 mg/dose orally given qd to b.i.d.; 5 to 30 µg/day
  given intranasally divided into qd to b.i.d.
Adults: 0.05 mg/dose orally qd to b.i.d.; 10 to 40 µg/day divided qd
  to t.i.d.

ERGOCALCIFEROL (VITAMIN D2)
Dietary Supplementation

Preterm infant: 400 to 800 IU/day
Infants and children: 400 IU/day

Nutritional Rickets

2,000 to 5,000 IU/day orally, if there is no malabsorption, and
  multiply by 5 if there is.

Vitamin D–resistant Rickets

40,000 to 80,000 IU/day, and increase as necessary

Hypoparathyroidism

Children: 50,000 to 200,000 IU/day
Adults: 25,000 to 200,000 IU/day

FLUDROCORTISONE ACETATE (FLORINEF)

0.5 to 0.1 or even 0.2 mg/day, with added salt to diet, depending
  on degree of salt-losing tendencies and response

FUROSEMIDE

Neonates: 0.5 to 1 mg/kg/dose (maximum, 6 mg/kg/dose) orally
  (p.o.), intramuscularly (i.m.), i.v., with doses q8 to 24 hours
Children: 0.5 to 2 m/kg/day divided into 2–4 doses/day (maximum
  dose, 6 mg/kg)
Adults: 20 to 80 mg/day, divided into b.i.d. or q.i.d. (maximum
  dose, 600 mg/day)

GLUCAGON HCL
Given i.v., i.m., or p.o.

Neonates and children less than 20 kg: give 0.5 mg/dose or 0.02 to
  0.03 mg/kg dose, repeat in 20 minutes as necessary
Children more than 20 kg: 1-mg/doses q20min as needed

Table 16-1.   Glucocorticoid preparations

	Glucocorticoid effect (based on antiinflammatory effect, with cortisol = 1.0)	Mineralocorticoid effect [fludrocortisone (Fluorinef) = 1.0]
Cortisol (hydrocortisone)	1	0.005
Cortisone	0.8	0.005
Prednisone	4	0
Prednisolone	4–5	0
α-Methylprednisolone	5–8	0
Dexamethasone	27–66	0
α-fluorocortisol	15	1

GLUCORTICOID PREPARATIONS
See Table 16-1 and chapters 8 and 10.

HYDROCHLOROTHIAZIDE

Neonates: Younger than 6 months, 2 to 4 mg/kg/day, divided b.i.d.,
  p.o. (maximum dose, 37.5 mg/kg/day)
Older than 6 months: 2 mg/kg/day, divided into b.i.d. (maximum
  dose, 100 mg/day)
Adults: 25 to 100 mg/day, divided into qd, b.i.d. (maximum dose,
  200 mg/day)

INSULIN PREPARATIONS
See Table 16-2.

Table 16-2.   Actions of commercially available insulin preparations

Preparation	Onset of action	Peak activity	Duration of action (hr)
Aspart	5 min	30 min to 3 hr	3–5
Lispro	<30 min	30–90 min	2 (<6 hr)
Regular	30–60 min	2–4 hr	5–8
NPH	1–2 hr	6–12 hr	18–24
Glargine	1 hr	None	24

NPH, neutral protamine Hagedorn.

THYROXINE (LEVO)
Children: p.o. dosing:

0 to 6 months: 8 to 10 µg/kg/dose, qd
6 to 12 months: 6 to 8 µg/kg/dose, qd
1 to 5 years: 5 to 6 µg/kg/dose, qd
6 to 12 years: 4 to 5 µg/kg/dose, qd
Older than 12 years: 2 to 3 µg/kg/dose, qd
Usual adult dose: 100 to 200 µg/24 hours

MAGNESIUM SULFATE
9.9% Elemental Mg

Hypomagnesemia or Hypocalcemia

i.v. / i.m.: 25 to 50 mg/kg/dose, divided into t.i.d. to q.i.d.; repeat as needed.
Maximum single dose: 2 g
Oral: 100 to 200 mg/kg/dose, q.i.d., p.o.

Daily Maintenance

30 to 60 mg/kg/24 hours or 0.25 to 0.5 mEq/kg/24 hours, i.v.
Maximum dose: 1 g/24 hours

MANNITOL (5%, 10%, 15%, 20%, 25%)
Cerebral edema: 0.25 g/kg/dose, i.v., over 20 to 30 minutes. May increase gradually to 1 g/kg/dose if needed. (May give furosemide, 1 mg/kg concurrently or 5 minutes before mannitol.)
Maximum dose: 12.5 g over 3 to 5 minutes.

MEDROXYPROGESTERONE ACETATE
Amenorrhea: 5 to 10 mg, p.o., qd × 5 to 10 days
Abnormal uterine bleeding: 5 to 10 mg, p.o., qd × 5 to 10 days, initiated on day 16 or 21 of the menstrual cycle

METFORMIN
Start with 500 mg p.o., b.i.d., with morning and evening meals; may increase by 500 mg every week, administered in divided doses up to a maximum of 2,500 mg/24 hr. (2000 mg/24 hours in younger teenagers.)

METHIMAZOLE
Hyperthyroidism
Children:

Initial: 0.4 to 0.7 mg/kg/24 hr or 15 to 20 mg/m^2/24 hr, p.o., divided into q8hr
Maintenance: Half to two thirds of initial dose, p.o., q8hr
Maximum dose: 30 mg/24 hr

Adults:

Initial: 15 to 60 mg/24 hr, p.o., divided into t.i.d.
Maintenance: 5 to 15 mg/24 hr, p.o., divided into t.i.d.

NITROPRUSSIDE

Children and adults: i.v., continuous infusion
Dose: Start at 0.3 to 0.5 µg/kg/min, titrate to effect
Usual dose: 3 to 4 µg/kg/min
Maximum dose: 10 µg/kg/min

PAMIDRONATE

Hypercalcemia

Children

Mild hypercalcemia: 0.5 to 1 mg/kg/dose, i.v. × 1
Severe hypercalcemia: 1.5 to 2 mg/kg/dose, i.v. × 1

Adults

Corrected serum Ca^{2+}: 12 to 13.5 mg/dL: 60 mg, i.v., × 1 over 4 hours
   OR 90 mg i.v., × 1 over 24 hours
Corrected serum Ca^{2+}: more than 13.5 mg/dL: 90 mg, i.v. × 1 over
   24 hours
(Dose may be repeated after 7 days.)

Osteogenesis Imperfecta (Limited Data)

Children: 0.5 to 1 mg/kg/dose, i.v., qd × 3 days; may be repeated
   in 4 to 6 months

PHOSPHORUS SUPPLEMENTS

Acute hypophosphatemia: 5 to 10 mg/kg/dose, i.v., over 6 hours

Maintenance/replacement

Children:

i.v.: 15 to 45 mg/kg over 24 hours
p.o.: 30 to 90 mg/kg/24 hr divided into t.i.d. to q.i.d.

Adults:

i.v.: 1.5 to 2 g over 24 hours
p.o.: 3 to 4.5 g/24 hr divided into t.i.d. to q.i.d.
Recommended infusion rate: 3.1 mg/kg/hr (0.1 mM/kg/hr) of phosphate. When potassium salt is used, the rate will be limited by
   the maximum potassium infusion rate. Do not co-infuse with
   calcium-containing products.

POTASSIUM IODIDE

Neonatal Graves disease: 1 drop strong iodine (Lugol's sol) p.o., q8hr
Thyrotoxicosis: Children: 50 to 250 mg, p.o., t.i.d. (about 1 to 5 drops
   of SSKI containing 1g/ml t.i.d.)
Adults: 50–500 mg p.o. t.i.d. (1–10 drops SSKI p.o. t.i.d.)

POTASSIUM SUPPLEMENTS

Hypokalemia

Oral:

Children: 1 to 4 mEq/kg/24 hr divided into b.i.d. to q.i.d. Monitor serum potassium.
Adults: 40 to 100 mEq/24 hr divided into b.i.d. to q.i.d.

Intravenous:
MONITOR SERUM K CLOSELY.

Children: 0.5 to 1 mEq/kg/dose, given as an infusion of 0.5 mEq/kg/hr × 1 to 2 hours.
Maximum infusion rate: 1 mEq/kg/hr. This may be used in critical situations (e.g., hypokalemia with arrhythmia).

Adults:

Serum K ≥ 2.5 mEq/L: Give at rates up to 10 mEq/hr. Total dosage not to exceed 200 mEq/24 hr.
Serum K less than 2 mEq/L: Give at rates up to 40 mEq/hr. Total dosage not to exceed 400 mEq/24 hr.
Maximum peripheral i.v. concentration: 40 mEq/L
Maximum concentration for central line administration: 150 to 200 mEq/L

PROPRANOLOL
Children:
p.o.: Start at 0.5 to 1 mg/kg/24 hr divided into q6 to 8h; increase dosage q3 to 5 days prn.
Usual dosage range: 2 to 4 mg/kg/24 hr divided into q6 to 8h. Maximum dose: 60 mg/24 hr or 16 mg/kg/24 hr.

Adults:

p.o.: 10 to 20 mg/dose t.i.d. to q.i.d. Increase prn. Usual range, 40 to 320 mg/24 hr divided into t.i.d. to q.i.d.

Hypertension
Children:

p.o.: Initial: 0.5 to 1 mg/kg/24 hr divided into q6 to 12h. May increase dose q3 to 5 days prn.
Maximum dose: 8 mg/kg/24 hr

Adults:

p.o.: 40 mg/dose p.o., b.i.d., or 60 to 80 mg/dose (sustained-release capsule) p.o., qd. May increase 10 to 20 mg/dose, q3 to 5 days.
Maximum dose reported: 640 mg/24 hr although lower doses must be tried first

PROPYLTHIOURACIL
Neonates: 5 to 10 mg/kg/24 hr divided into q8h, p.o.
Children:

Initial: 5–7 mg/kg/24 hr divided into q8hr, p.o., or for age:
6 to 10 years: 50 to 150 mg/24 hr divided into q8hr, p.o.
Older than 10 years: 150 to 300 mg/24 hr divided into q8hr, p.o.
Maintenance: Generally begins after 2 months. Usually one third to two thirds the initial dose when the patient is euthyroid.

Adults:

Initial: 300 to 450 mg/24 hr divided into q8hr, p.o.; some may require larger doses of 600 to 1,200 mg/24 hr.
Maintenance: 100 to 150 mg/24 hr divided into q8 to 12 hr, p.o.

SODIUM BICARBONATE
To Correct Metabolic Acidosis
Calculate patient's dose with the following formulas.
Neonates, infants, and children:

$$HCO_3^- \text{ (mEq)} = 0.3 \times \text{weight (kg)} \times \text{base deficit (mEq/L)},$$

Adults:

$$HCO_3^- \text{ (mEq)} = 0.2 \times \text{weight (kg)} \times \text{base deficit (mEq/L)},$$

$$HCO_3^- \text{ (mEq)} = 0.5 \times \text{weight (kg)} \times [24 - \text{serum } HCO_3^- \text{ (mEq/L)}]$$

For either:

$$HCO_3^- \text{ (mEq)} = 0.5 \times \text{weight (kg)} \times [24 - \text{serum } HCO_3^- \text{ (mEq/L)}]$$

SPIRONOLACTONE
Diuretic
Neonates: 1 to 3 mg/kg/24 hr divided into qd to b.i.d., p.o.
Children: 1 to 3.3 mg/kg/24 hr divided into qd to q.i.d., p.o.
Adults: 25 to 200 mg/24 hr divided into qd to q.i.d., p.o.
Maximum dose: 200 mg/24 hr

Diagnosis of Primary Aldosteronism
Children: 125 to 375 mg/m²/24 hr divided into b.i.d. to q.i.d., p.o.
Adults: 400 mg qd, p.o., × 4 days (short test) or 3 to 4 weeks (long test), and then 100 to 400 mg qd maintenance.

Hirsutism in Women
Adults: 50 to 200 mg/24 hr divided into qd to b.i.d., p.o.

VASOPRESSIN
Diabetes Insipidus
Titrate dose to effect

Subcutaneous/intramuscular
Children: 2.5 to 10 U, b.i.d. to q.i.d.
Adults: 5 to 10 U, b.i.d. to q.i.d.
Continuous infusion (adults and children): Start at 0.5 milli-unit/kg/hr (0.0005 U/kg/hr). Double dosage every 30 min prn up to maximum dose of 10 mU/kg/hr (0.01 U/kg/hr).

SUGGESTED READINGS
Dosages as presented in:
Gunn VL, Nechyloa C. *Harriet Lane handbook.* 16th ed. St. Louis: Mosby, 2002.

Dosages from Thomson MICROMEDEX. MICROMEDEX Health-care Series Vol. 114.

Dosages from various textbook chapters noted in the other chapters.

Dosages from manufacturers' information.

Armstrong L. Drugs and hormones used in endocrinology. In: De-Groot LJ, Jameson JL, eds. *Endocrinology*. Philadelphia: WB Saunders, 2001:2601–2621.

17 ♣ Laboratory Values For Pediatric Endocrinology

This list includes the laboratory values of most use in pediatric endocrinology with standards and sample sizes and preparation from Quest Diagnostics/Nichols Institute. Other tests are available from the laboratory and other laboratories perform these tests and a few also have pediatric standards (eg. Esoterix, DSL). However, I do not recommend using a laboratory that does not have pediatric standards established, as the lower detectable limits, or the accurate area of the standard curves of the laboratory, might be well above pediatric values. Laboratories that are set up for pediatric endocrine samples will accept smaller volumes than requested of adult patients. The minimum volumes listed here might yet be decreased in consultation with the laboratory, so I suggest direct communication with the laboratories in such cases. Check your results against the standards of the laboratory you choose.

ADRENOCORTICOTROPIC HORMONE (ACTH)

0.5 mL plasma in ethylenediaminetetraacetic acid (EDTA; lavender-top tube).
Minimum quantity: 0.3 mL.
Transfer the plasma to a plastic transport tube, and ship frozen. Do not thaw.

Drawn at 7–10 a.m.

Adults
9–52 pg/mL
Dexamethasone suppressed, 2–8 pg/mL

Children
Prepubertal: 7–28 pg/mL
Pubertal: 2–49 pg/mL

ALBUMIN (MICROALBUMIN), 24-HOUR URINE

5 mL urine from 24-hr urine container.
Minimum quantity: 0.2 mL.
Record 24-hour urine volume on test-request form and urine vial. Do not use preservatives. Ship refrigerated.

Children and adults: ≤30 mg/24 hr

ALBUMIN (MICROALBUMIN), RANDOM URINE

5 mL urine in sterile screw-cap container
Minimum quantity: 1 mL.
Do not use preservatives. Ship refrigerated.

Children and adults: ≤30 mg/g Cr

ALBUMIN SERUM

1 mL serum.
Minimum quantity: 0.5 mL.

Overnight fasting is preferred. Ship refrigerated.

Children
3–9 yr: 4,120–4,988 mg/dL
10–17 yr: 4,055–5,219 mg/dL

ALDOSTERONE, 24-HOUR URINE

5 mL urine in 24-hr urine container
Minimum quantity: 0.8 mL
Collect urine with 10 g of boric acid to maintain pH <7.5. Record 24-hr urine volume on test-request form and urine vial. Refrigerate during collection and ship refrigerated.

Children
2–7 yr: 0.5–5.7 µg/24 hr
8–11 yr: 0.5–10.2 µg/24 hr
12–16 yr: 0.5–15.6 µg/24 hr

ALDOSTERONE SERUM

2 mL serum in no additive (red-top tube).
Minimum quantity: 0.6 mL.
Draw "upright" samples ≥30 min after patient sits up. Ship refrigerated.

Children (random sodium diet)
Premature infants (31- to 35-wk gestation): ≤144 ng/dL
Term infants, 3 days old: ≤217 ng/dL

After ACTH stimulation

	Baseline	**After ACTH stimulation**
1–12 mo	1–70 ng/dL	5–170 ng/dL
1–5 yr	2–37 ng/dL	13–85 ng/dL
6–12 yr	3–21 ng/dL	14–50 ng/dL
Tanner II–III		
Males	1–13 ng/dL	10–33 ng/dL
Females	2–20 ng/dL	12–31 ng/dL
Tanner IV–V		
Males	3–14 ng/dL	13–30 ng/dL
Females	4–32 ng/dL	10–34 ng/dL

ALKALINE PHOSPHATASE, SERUM

2 mL serum in no additive (red-top tube).
Minimum quantity: 0.5 mL.
Hemolyzed specimens are not acceptable. Ship refrigerated.

Children
1–17 yr: 70–470 IU/L

ALKALINE PHOSPHATASE, BONE SPECIFIC
1 mL serum in no additive (red-top tube).
Minimum quantity: 0.3 mL.
Ship frozen.

Children
2–24 mo: 25.4–124 µg/L
2–9 yr: 24.2–89.5 µg/L
Tanner stages
   I–II: 19.5–87.5 µg/L
   III–IV: 19.5–156 µg/L

ANDROSTENEDIONE
2 mL serum in no additive (red-top tube).
Minimum quantity: 0.5 mL.
An early morning specimen is preferred. Ship refrigerated.

Children
Premature infants (31- to 35-wk gestation): ≤480 ng/dL
Term infants, 3 days old: ≤290 ng/dL
After ACTH stimulation:

	Baseline	**After ACTH stimulation**
1–12 mo	6–78 ng/dL	21–140 ng/dL
1–5 yr	5–51 ng/dL	12–68 ng/dL
6–12 yr	7–68 ng/dL	12–98 ng/dL
Tanner II–III		
Males	17–82 ng/dL	29–88 ng/dL
Females	43–180 ng/dL	58–230 ng/dL
Tanner IV–V		
Males	57–150 ng/dL	78–215 ng/dL
Females	73–220 ng/dL	91–320 ng/dL

ANGIOTENSIN II
1 mL plasma in EDTA (lavender-top tube).
Minimum quantity: 0.3 mL.
Freeze within 1 hr of collection. Ship frozen.

Adults: 10–50 ng/L
Children: No data available

ARGININE VASOPRESSIN
4 mL plasma in EDTA (lavender-top tube).
Minimum quantity: 1.1 mL.

Draw blood in prechilled lavender-top tube. Transport in an ice bath to a refrigerated centrifuge. Separate and freeze immediately. Do not thaw. Ship frozen.

Children and adults: 1.0–13.3 pg/mL (2.5 pg = 1 µU)

ATRIAL NATRIURETIC HORMONE/FACTOR

2 mL plasma in EDTA (lavender-top tube).
Minimum quantity: 0.6 mL.
Do not thaw. Ship frozen.

Children
1 day: 32–60 pg/mL
3 days: 165–185 pg/mL
7 days: 127–153 pg/mL
10 days: 98–122 pg/mL
1–2 mo: 52–72 pg/mL
10–15 yr: ≤54 pg/mL

C PEPTIDE, PLASMA

2 mL plasma in EDTA (lavender-top tube).
Minimum quantity: 0.3 mL.
Overnight fasting is required. Ship frozen.

Children and adults: 0.5–2.0 ng/mL

CALCITONIN

1 mL serum in no additive (red-top tube).
Minimum quantity: 0.3 mL.
Overnight fasting is preferred. Ship frozen.

Children and adults
Females: ≤4 pg/mL
Males: ≤8 pg/mL

CALCIUM, 24-HOUR URINE

10 mL urine from a 24-hr urine container–25 mL 6N HCl.
Minimum quantity: 1 mL.
Collect urine with 25 mL of 6N HCl to maintain a pH <3. Record 24-hr urine volume on test-request form and urine vial. Ship refrigerated.

Adults
Males: 50–300 ng/24 hr
Females: 50–250 ng/24 hr

Children

	African-American	Caucasian
9–17 yr	≤170 mg/24 hr	13–317 mg/24 hr

CALCIUM IONIZED, SERUM

2 mL serum in no additive (red-top tube).
Minimum quantity: 0.6 mL.
Collect in gel-barrier tube, let clot, and spin immediately with cap on. Ship the unopened gel-barrier tube refrigerated, so sample is not exposed to dry ice. Do not open. Ship refrigerated.

Children
8 mo–10 yr: 4.9–5.4 mg/dL
11–17 yr: 4.8–5.3 mg/dL

CALCIUM, SERUM

1 mL serum in no additive (red-top tube).
Minimum quantity: 0.5 mL.
Overnight fasting is preferred. Ship refrigerated.

Children
18 mo–4 yr: 9.3–11.0 mg/dL
7–17 yr: 8.7–10.8 mg/dL

CARNITINE, SERUM

3 mL serum in no additive (red-top tube).
Minimum quantity: 1 mL.
Serum or plasma should be removed from cells immediately after collection. Ship frozen.

Children (M):

	Carnitine total	Carnitine free	Carnitine esters
Premature infants	23–33	13–19	9.4–14.6
Term infants	21–30	12–18	7.7–13.7
Cord blood	17–41	9–26	5.0–17.8
1 wk–12 mo	33–70	28–52	≤22.1
1–17 yr	26–65	18–54	≤19.7

CAROTENE

1 mL serum in no additive (red-top tube).
Minimum quantity: 0.5 mL.
Separate from cells as soon as possible after clotting. Wrap tube in aluminum foil to protect from light. Overnight fasting is preferred. Ship refrigerated.

Children
9 mo–6 yr: ≤47 µg/dL
7–17 yr: ≤94 µg/dL

CATECHOLAMINES, FRACTIONATED, 24-HR URINE

Includes dopamine, epinephrine, and norepinephrine.
10 mL urine from a 24-hr urine container–25 mL 6N HCl.
Minimum quantity: 5 mL.
Collect urine with 15 g of boric acid or 25 mL of 6N HCl to maintain a pH <3. Urine without preservatives is acceptable if pH is <6 and the sample is shipped frozen. Record 24-hr urine volume on test-request form and urine vial. It is preferable for the patient to be off medication for 3 days before collection. Ship refrigerated.

Epinephrine
3–8 yr: 1–7 µg/24 hr
9–12 yr: ≤8 µg/24 hr
13–17 yr: ≤11 µg/24 hr
Adults: 2–24 µg/24 hr

Norepinephrine
3–8 yr: 5–41 µg/24 hr
9–12 yr: 5–50 µg/24 hr
13–17 yr: 12–88 µg/24 hr
Adults: 15–100 µg/24 hr

Dopamine
3–8 yr: 80–378 µg/24 hr
9–12 yr: 51–474 µg/24 hr
13–17 yr: 51–645 µg/24 hr
Adults: 52–480 µg/24 hr

Total (N+E)
3–8 yr: 9–51 µg/24 hr
9–12 yr: 9–71 µg/24 hr
13–17 yr: 13–90 µg/24 hr
Adults: 26–121 µg/24 hr

CATECHOLAMINES, FRACTIONATED, PLASMA

Includes dopamine, epinephrine, and norepinephrine.
4 mL plasma in sodium heparin (green-top tube).
Minimum quantity: 2.5 mL.

Vacutainer is to be chilled before venipuncture. Draw sample as follows: Insert catheter in patient's vein. Instruct patient to lie down for 30 min with catheter in place, and then draw supine specimen in green-top tube. Chill specimen immediately in ice water. Next, instruct patient to sit up for 15 min with catheter still in place. Draw upright specimen in green-top tube. Chill specimen immediately in ice water. Plasma should be separated in a refrigerated centrifuge within 30 min of collection and then frozen immediately at –20°C in plastic vials. Plasma must stay frozen. Thawed samples are unacceptable. Overnight fasting is required. Ship frozen.

Adults

	Supine	**Upright**
Dopamine	<10 pg/mL	<20 pg/mL
Epinephrine	<50 pg/mL	<95 pg/mL
Norepinephrine	12–658 pg/mL	217–1,109 pg/mL
Total (N+E)	123–67s1 pg/mL	242–1,125 pg/mL

Children
  Plasma catecholamine measurements are generally unreliable because of stress in infants and small children. Urinary catecholamine assays are more reliable.

Dopamine:
  3–15 yr: <60 pg/mL
Epinephrine:
  3–15 yr: ≤464 pg/mL
Norepinephrine:
  3–15 yr: ≤1,251 pg/mL

CATECHOLAMINES, RANDOM URINE
Includes epinephrine, norepinephrine, and dopamine.
10 mL urine in sterile screw-cap container.
Minimum quantity: 5 mL.
After urine collection, add 0.5–1.0 g/L boric acid (or 6N HCl) to maintain a pH <3. Urine without preservative is acceptable if pH is <6 and the sample is shipped frozen. It is preferable for the patient to be off medications for 3 days before collection. Ship refrigerated.

Epinephrine
Birth–6 mo: 2–45 µg/g Cr
7–11 mo: 5–45 µg/g Cr
1–2 yr: 1–49 µg/g Cr
3–8 yr: 4–32 µg/g Cr
9–12 yr: 1–15 µg/g Cr
13–17 yr: 1–10 µg/g Cr
Adults: 2–16 µg/g Cr

Norepinephrine
Birth–6 mo: 12–286 µg/g Cr
7–11 mo: 19–250 µg/g Cr
1–2 yr: 25–210 µg/g Cr
3–8 yr: 20–108 µg/g Cr
9–12 yr: 20–73 µg/g Cr
13–17 yr: 15–58 µg/g Cr
Adults: 7–65 µg/g Cr

Total N+NE
Birth–6 mo: 24–322 µg/g Cr
7–11 mo: 10–295 µg/g Cr

1–2 yr: 30–263 µg/g Cr
3–8 yr: 29–134 µg/g Cr
9–12 yr: 22–87 µg/g Cr
13–17 yr: 20–71 µg/g Cr
Adults: 9–74 µg/g Cr

Dopamine
Birth–6 mo: 107–2,180 µg/g Cr
7–11 mo: 96–2,441 µg/g Cr
1–2 yr: 86–1,861 µg/g Cr
3–8 yr: 295–1,123 µg/g Cr
9–12 yr: 164–744 µg/g Cr
13–17 yr: 156–551 µg/g Cr
Adults: 40–390 µg/g Cr

CORTICOSTERONE

1 mL serum in no additive (red-top tube)
Minimum quantity: 0.3 mL.
Ship refrigerated.

Adults
8–10:00 a.m.: 100–700 ng/dL
4–6:00 p.m.: 40–260 ng/dL

Children after ACTH stimulation:

	Baseline	**After ACTH stimulation**
1–12 mo		
Males	78–1,750 ng/dL	2,260–6,540 ng/dL
Females	89–1,200 ng/dL	2,230–4,900 ng/dL
1–5 yr		
Males	120–1,290 ng/dL	2,160–7,565 ng/dL
Females	160–2,040 ng/dL	2,900–5,320 ng/dL
6–12 yr		
Males	235–1,370 ng/dL	3,360–7,565 ng/dL
Females	155–1,100 ng/dL	1,780–4,970 ng/dL
Tanner II–III		
Males	115–1,220 ng/dL	1,475–4,510 ng/dL
Females	110–600 ng/dL	2,260–4,730 ng/dL
Tanner IV–V		
Males	165–840 ng/dL	1,790–5,065 ng/dL
Females	160–390 ng/dL	1,725–5,110 ng/dL

CORTICOTROPIN RELEASING HORMONE

3.1 mL plasma in Parathyroid Hormone–Related Protein and
  Releasing Factors tube.
Minimum quantity: 1.1 mL.

Do not thaw. Ship frozen.

Children and adults: 24–40 pg/mL

Pregnancy
First trimester: 24–40 pg/mL
Second trimester: ≤153 pg/mL
Third trimester: ≤847 pg/mL

CORTISOL-BINDING GLOBULIN

1 mL serum in no additive (red-top tube).
Minimum quantity: 0.2 mL.
Ship refrigerated.
Preterm infants younger than 8 days: 6–26 mg/L
Children and adults: 19–45 mg/L

CORTISOL URINARY FREE 24-HOUR

20 mL urine from a 24-hr urine container.
Minimum quantity: 10 mL.
Collect urine with 10 g of boric acid or keep urine refrigerated
during collection if preservative is not used. Record 24-hr urine
volume on test-request form and urine vial.

Adults
Males and females: ≤50 µg/24 hr

Children
2–7 yr: 1.4–18 µg/24 hr
8–11 yr: 1.6–21 µg/24 hr
12–16 yr: 2.1–38 µg/24 hr

CORTISOL FREE SERUM

2 mL serum in no additive (red-top).
Minimum quantity: 0.7 mL.
Grossly hemolyzed specimens are unacceptable. Ship refrigerated.

Adults
8–10:00 a.m.: 0.6–1.6 µg/dL
4–6:00 p.m.: 0.2–0.9 µg/dL

Children
Term newborns: ≤9.3 µg/dL
Premature newborns (27–36 wk): ≤7.5 µg/dL
Term infants, 3 mo old: ≤3.9 µg/dL
Premature infants, 3 mo old: ≤3.5 µg/dL
6–9 yr: 0.37–1.62 µg/dL
10–11 yr: 0.27–1.12 µg/dL
12–14 yr: 0.23–1.67 µg/dL
15–17 yr: 0.47–1.77 µg/dL

CORTISOL SERUM

1 mL serum in no additive (red-top tube).
Minimum quantity: 0.1 mL.
Specify time of day specimen was collected. Grossly hemolyzed
specimens are unacceptable. Ship refrigerated.

Adults
8–10:00 a.m.: 8–24 µg/dL
4–6:00 p.m.: 2–17 µg/dL
After ACTH stimulation: 14–41 µg/dL

Children
Premature infants (31- to 35-wk gestation): ≤15 µg/dL
Term infants, 3 days old: ≤14 µg/dL

After ACTH stimulation

	Baseline	**After ACTH stimulation**
1–12 mo	3–23 µg/dL	32–60 µg/dL
1–5 yr	6–25 µg/dL	22–40 µg/dL
6–12 yr	3–15 µg/dL	17–18 µg/dL
Tanner II–III		
Males	4–13 µg/dL	15–45 µg/dL
Females	4–16 µg/dL	16–32 µg/dL
Tanner IV–V		
Males	5–15 µg/dL	18–27 µg/dL
Females	6–15 µg/dL	18–35 µg/dL

CREATININE 24-HOUR URINE

10 mL urine in 24-hr urine container.
Minimum quantity: 2 mL.
Record 24-hr urine volume on test-request form and urine vial.
  Ship refrigerated.

Adults
Males and females: 0.63–2.5 g/24 hr

Children
3–8 yr: 0.11–0.68 g/24 hr
9–12 yr: 0.17–1.41 g/24 hr
13–17 yr: 0.29–1.87 g/24 hr

CREATININE RANDOM URINE

10 mL urine in sterile screw-cap container.
Minimum quantity: 2 mL.
Ship refrigerated.

Adults
Males and females: 0.27–3.00 g/L

Children
0–6 mo: 0.02–0.32 g/L
7–11 mo: 0.02–0.36 g/L
1–2 yr: 0.02–1.28 g/L

3–8 yr: 0.02–1.49 g/L
9–12 yr: 0.02–1.83 g/L

CREATININE CLEARANCE

Includes serum and urine creatinine
10 mL urine from a 24-hr urine container and 2 mL serum in no additive (red-top tube).
Minimum quantity: 2 mL/0.2 mL.
Record patient height, weight, and total 24-hr urine volume on test-request form and urine vial. Serum must be collected within 24 hr of urine collection. Ship refrigerated.

Adults
Males: 85–125 mL/min/1.73 m^2 surface area (SA)
Females: 75–115 mL/min/1.73 m^2 SA

Children
Premature infants: 29–65 mL/min/1.73 m^2 SA
Term infants
    2–8 days: 26–60 mL/min/1.73 m^2 SA
    1–3 wk: 28–68 mL/min/1.73 m^2 SA
    1–5.9 mo: 41–103 mL/min/1.73 m^2 SA
    6–11.9 mo: 49–157 mL/min/1.73 m^2 SA
    12–19 mo: 63–191 mL/min/1.73 m^2 SA
    2–12 yr: 89–165 mL/min/1.73 m^2 SA

CREATININE SERUM

2 mL serum in no additive (red-top tube).
Minimum quantity: 0.2 mL.
Hemolyzed specimens are not acceptable. Ship refrigerated.

Adults
Males and females: 0.6–1.4 mg/dL

Children
0–2 days: 0.7–1.4 mg/dL
3–5 days: 0.4–1.1 mg/dL
6–7 days: 0.3–0.9 mg/dL
1 wk–1 mo: 0.3–0.8 mg/dL
1 mo–1 yr: 0.2–0.7 mg/dL
2–9 yr: 0.3–0.7 mg/dL
10–17 yr: 0.5–1.0 mg/dL

CYCLIC ADENOSINE MONOPHOSPHATE, NEPHROGENOUS RANDOM URINE

Includes urine, plasma, and nephrogenous cyclic adenosine mono-phosphate (AMP)
25 mL urine in a sterile screw cap container and 5 mL plasma in EDTA (lavender-top).
Minimum quantity: 2.5 mL/1.2 mL.
Ship frozen.

Postpubertal males and females
Nephrogenous cAMP: 1.4–5.0 n*M*

Cyclic AMP, urine: 0.6–12.0 μ*M*
Cyclic AMP, plasma: 6.3–13.7 n*M*

CYCLIC ADENOSINE MONOPHOSPHATE, PLASMA

3.1 mL plasma in EDTA (lavender-top tube).
Minimum quantity: 1 mL.
Ship frozen.

Adults
Males and females: 6.3–13.7 n*M*

Children
3–36 mo: ≤37 n*M*
11–17 yr: 4–28 n*M*

CYCLIC ADENOSINE MONOPHOSPHATE, RANDOM URINE

1 mL urine in sterile screw-cap container.
Minimum quantity: 0.2 mL.
Collect urine with 2.0 mL of 6N HCl to maintain pH <3. Ship
    frozen.

Adults
Males and females: 0.6–12.0 μ*M*
2.2–63 μmol/g Cr

Children
2 mo–17 yr: 2.9–25.1 μmol/g Cr

DHEA SERUM

1 mL serum in no additive (red-top tube).
Minimum quantity: 0.1 mL.
Specify age and sex on test-request form. Overnight fasting is pre-
    ferred. Ship refrigerated.

Adults
Males: 180–1,250 ng/dL
Females: 130–980 ng/dL
After ACTH stimulation: 545–1,845 ng/dL

Children
Premature infants (31- to 35-wk gestation): ≤3,343 ng/dL
Term infants, 3 days old: ≤1,250 ng/dL

After ACTH stimulation

	Baseline	**After ACTH stimulation**
1–12 mo	26–505 ng/dL	18–1,455 ng/dL
1–5 yr	9–42 ng/dL	21–98 ng/dL
6–12 yr	11–155 ng/dL	34–320 ng/dL
Tanner II–III		
Males	25–300 ng/dL	62–390 ng/dL
Females	69–605 ng/dL	95–885 ng/dL

Continued

	Baseline	After ACTH stimulation
Tanner IV–V		
Males	100–400 ng/dL	195–510 ng/dL
Females	165–690 ng/dL	325–1,460 ng/dL

DHEA SULFATE, SERUM
1 mL serum in no additive (red-top tube).
Minimum quantity: 0.1 mL.
Specify age and sex on test-request form. Ship refrigerated.

	Male	Female
Premature infants		
(31- to 35-wk gestation)	≤700 µg/dL	≤700 µg/dL
Term infants,		
1st wk of life	≤360 µg/dL	≤360 µg/dL
1–5 mo	≤41 µg/dL	5–55 µg/dL
6–11 mo	5–20 µg/dL	5–30 µg/dL
1–5 yr	≤40 µg/dL	≤20 µg/dL
6–9 yr	≤145 µg/dL	≤140 µg/dL
10–11 yr	15–155 µg/dL	15–260 µg/dL
12–14 yr	20–500 µg/dL	20–535 µg/dL
15–17 yr	30–555 µg/dL	35–535 µg/dL
18–30 yr	125–619 µg/dL	45–380 µg/dL
Tanner stages		
I	5–265 µg/dL	5–125 µg/dL
II	15–380 µg/dL	15–150 µg/dL
III	60–505 µg/dL	20–535 µg/dL
IV	65–560 µg/dL	35–485 µg/dL
V	165–500 µg/dL	75–530 µg/dL

DEOXYCORTICOSTERONE, SERUM
3 mL serum in no additive (red-top tube).
Minimum quantity: 1.1 mL.
Ship refrigerated.

Adults
Males: 3.5–11.5 ng/dL
Females
  Follicular phase: 1.5–8.5 ng/dL
  Luteal phase: 3.5–130 ng/dL

Pregnancy
   1st Trimester: 5–25 ng/dL
   2nd Trimester: 10–75 ng/dL
   3rd Trimester: 30–110 ng/dL
After ACTH stimulation: 14–33 ng/dL

Children after ACTH stimulation

	Baseline	**After ACTH stimulation**
1–12 mo	7–57 ng/dL	20–160 ng/dL
1–5 yr	4–49 ng/dL	26–140 ng/dL
6–12 yr		
Males	9–34 ng/dL	33–140 ng/dL
Females	2–13 ng/dL	19–61 ng/dL
Tanner II–III		
Males	4–30 ng/dL	12–74 ng/dL
Females	2–12 ng/dL	13–63 ng/dL
Tanner IV–V		
Males	5–14 ng/dL	19–46 ng/dL
Females	5–10 ng/dL	23–40 ng/dL

11-DEOXYCORTICOSTERONE, SERUM

1 mL serum in no additive (red-top tube).
Minimum quantity: 0.2 mL.
An early morning specimen is preferred. Ship refrigerated.

Adults
Males and females: 20–130 ng/dL
After ACTH stimulation: 82–290 ng/dL
After metyrapone: >5,000 ng/dL (5 µg/dL)

Children
Premature infants (31- to 35-wk gestation): ≤235 ng/dL
Term infants, 3 days old: ≤170 ng/dL

After ACTH stimulation

	Baseline	**After ACTH stimulation**
1–12 mo	10–200 ng/dL	79–390 ng/dL
1–5 yr	7–210 ng/dL	98–360 ng/dL
6–12 yr	14–140 ng/dL	95–320 ng/dL

Continued

	Baseline	**After ACTH stimulation**
Tanner II–III		
Males	11–150 ng/dL	115–280 ng/dL
Females	15–130 ng/dL	90–250 ng/dL
Tanner IV–V		
Males	14–120 ng/dL	87–120 ng/dL
Females	17–120 ng/dL	78–240 ng/dL

11-DEOXYCORTISOL, 24-HOUR URINE

1 mL urine from a 24-hr urine container.
Minimum quantity: 0.2 mL.
Collect urine with 10 g of boric acid or keep urine refrigerated during collection if preservative is not used. Record urine volume on test-request form and urine vial. Ship refrigerated.
Postpubertal males and females: 3–20 µg/24 hr

DIHYDROTESTOSTERONE

4 mL serum in no additive (red-top tube).
Minimum quantity: 1.1 mL.
Specify age and sex on test-request form. Ship refrigerated.

Adults
Males: 25–75 ng/dL
Females: 5–30 ng/dL

Children

	Male	**Female**
Cord blood	≤8 ng/dL	≤5 ng/dL
1–6 mo	12–85 ng/dL	<5 ng/dL
Prepubertal	<5 ng/dL	<5 ng/dL
Puberty		
Tanner stage II–III	3–33 ng/dL	5–19 ng/dL
Tanner stage IV–V	22–75 ng/dL	3–30 ng/dL

DIHYDROTESTOSTERONE, FREE, SERUM

Includes total, free, and percentage free dihydrotestosterone (DHT)
5 mL serum in no additive (red-top tube).
Minimum quantity: 2.5 mL.
Ship refrigerated.

% Free
Postpubertal males: 0.62%–1.10%
Postpubertal females: 0.47%–0.67%

DHT, free
Postpubertal males: 1.00–6.20 pg/mL
Postpubertal females: 0.30–1.90 pg/mL

EPINEPHRINE PLASMA

4 mL plasma in sodium heparin (green-top tube).
Minimum quantity: 2.5 mL.

Vacutainer is to be chilled before venipuncture. Draw sample as follows: Insert catheter in patient's vein. Instruct patient to lie down for 30 min with catheter in place, and then draw supine specimen in green-top tube. Chill specimen immediately in ice water. Next, instruct patient to sit up for 15 min with catheter still in place. Draw upright specimen in green-top tube. Chill specimen immediately in ice water. Plasma should be separated in a refrigerated centrifuge within 30 min of collection and then frozen immediately at –20°C in plastic vials. Plasma must stay frozen. Thawed samples are unacceptable. Each specimen will be invoiced separately. Ship frozen.

Plasma epinephrine measurements are generally unreliable because of stress. Urinary epinephrine is more reliable.

Supine: <50 pg/mL
Upright: <95 pg/mL

ESTRADIOL, FREE

Includes total, free, and percentage free estradiol
3 mL serum in no additive (red-top tube).
Minimum quantity: 1.2 mL.
Grossly hemolyzed specimens are unacceptable. Ship refrigerated.

Adults

Free estradiol:
  Females
    Follicular phase: 0.60–3.20 pg/mL
    Midcycle peak: 0.49–1.09 pg/mL
    Luteal phase: 0.30–4.10 pg/mL
    Postmenopausal: ≤0.23 pg/mL
  Male adults: 0.30–0.90 pg/mL

% Free:
  Females
    Follicular phase: 1.49%–2.04%
    Midcycle peak: 1.59%–2.13%
    Luteal phase: 1.52%–2.03%
    Postmenopausal: 1.50%–2.85%
  Male adults: 1.66%–2.11%

Children
Prepubertal levels will be similar to or less than adult male values.

ESTRADIOL, SERUM

2.5 mL serum in no additive (red-top tube).
Minimum quantity: 0.06 mL.
Specify age and sex on test-request form. Ship refrigerated.

Adults
Males: 10–50 pg/mL
Females
  Early follicular phase: 20–150 pg/mL
  Late follicular phase: 40–350 pg/mL
  Midcycle peak: 150–750 pg/mL
  Luteal phase: 30–450 pg/mL
  Postmenopausal: ≤20 pg/mL

Children

	Males (pg/mL)	Females (pg/mL)
Cord blood	9,000–34,000	9,000–34,000
1–4 days	25–450	25–450
1–5 yr	3–10	5–10
6–9 yr	3–10	5–60
10–11 yr	5–10	5–300
12–14 yr	5–30	25–410
15–17 yr	5–45	40–410
Tanner stages		
I	3–15	5–10
II	3–10	5–115
III	5–15	5–180
IV	3–40	25–345
V	15–45	25–410

ESTRONE, SERUM

4 mL serum in no additive (red-top tube).
Minimum quantity: 1.1 mL.
Specify age and sex on test-request form. Ship refrigerated.

Adults
Males: 15–65 pg/mL
Females
  Early follicular phase: 15–150 pg/mL
  Late follicular phase: 100–250 pg/mL
  Luteal phase: 15–200 pg/mL
  Postmenopausal: 15–55 pg/mL

Children
Cord blood: 9,000–34,000 pg/mL
1–4 days: 15–300 pg/mL
Prepubertal children: 5–15 pg/mL

Tanner stages

	Males	Females
II	10–22 pg/mL	10–33 pg/mL
III	17–25 pg/mL	15–43 pg/mL
IV	21–35 pg/mL	16–77 pg/mL
V	15–45 pg/mL	29–77 pg/mL

FOLLICLE-STIMULATING HORMONE, THIRD GENERATION, SERUM

1 mL serum in no additive (red-top tube).
Minimum quantity: 0.2 mL.
Ship refrigerated.

Adults
Males: 1.48–14.26 IU/L
Females
  Follicular phase: 1.37–9.90 IU/L
  Midcycle peak: 6.17–17.20 IU/L
  Luteal phase: 1.09–9.20 IU/L

Children

	Male	Female
2 wk	1.22–5.19 IU/L	2.09–30.45 IU/L
1–18 mo	0.19–2.97 IU/L	1.14–14.35 IU/L
19 mo–7 yr	0.25–1.92 IU/L	0.70–3.39 IU/L
8–9 yr	0.30–1.67 IU/L	0.28–5.64 IU/L
10–11 yr	0.20–5.79 IU/L	0.68–7.26 IU/L
12–41 yr	0.23–10.37 IU/L	1.02–9.24 IU/L
15–17 yr	0.81–8.18 IU/L	0.33–10.54 IU/L
Tanner stages		
I	0.22–1.92 IU/L	0.50–2.41 IU/L
II	0.72–4.60 IU/L	1.73–4.68 IU/L
III	1.24–10.37 IU/L	2.53–7.04 IU/L
IV	1.70–10.35 IU/L	1.26–7.37 IU/L

FRUCTOSAMINE, SERUM

2 mL serum in no additive (red-top tube).
Minimum quantity: 0.5 mL.
Ship refrigerated.

Adults
Males and females: 190–270 μ*M*

Children
Newborns and children younger than 5 yr have values less than those of adults.
Children older than 5 yr have values similar to those of adults.

GASTRIN SERUM

2 mL serum.
Minimum quantity: 0.5 mL.
Overnight fasting is required. Ship frozen.

Adults
Males and females: <42 pg/mL

Children
Newborns and infants: 69–190 pg/mL
Prepubertal and pubertal children: 1–130 pg/mL

GLUCAGONS

3 mL plasma in EDTA (lavender-top tube).
Minimum quantity: 1.1 mL.
Do not thaw. Overnight fasting is required. Ship frozen.

Children and Adults: 20–100 pg/mL

GLUCOSE, SERUM

1 mL serum in no additive (red-top tube).
Minimum quantity: 0.2 mL.
Overnight fasting is preferred. Ship refrigerated.

Children and Adults
Fasting: 65–109 mg/dL
Impaired fasting glucose: 110–125 mg/dL (ADA Guidelines)
Provisional diagnosis of diabetes: ≥126 mg/dL fasting or > 200 mg/dL casual, non-fasting (ADA Guidelines)

GLUTAMIC ACID DECARBOXYLASE-65 AUTOANTIBODIES

This test is performed by using a test kit that has not been approved or cleared by the Food and Drug Administration (FDA). The performance characteristics of this test have been determined by Quest Diagnostics, Nichols Institute.

1 mL serum in no additive (red-top tube).
Minimum quantity: 0.2 mL.
Ship frozen.

Children and Adults: Positive result, ≥1.0 U/mL.

GLYCATED ALBUMIN

3 mL plasma in EDTA (lavender-top tube).
Minimum quantity: 2 mL.
Spin and separate plasma immediately. Overnight fasting is required. Ship refrigerated.

Children and Adults: 0.8%–1.4%

GROWTH HORMONE, SERUM

1 mL serum in no additive (red-top tube).
Minimum quantity: 0.2 mL.
Ship refrigerated.

Adults: ≤10.0 ng/mL
Children: ≤20.0 ng/mL

Because of diurnal variability, random human growth hormone (hGH) values are not reliable for diagnosis of GH deficiency or acromegaly. See Chapter 5 for instructions on GH testing.

GROWTH HORMONE, HYBRITECH

2 mL serum in no additive (red-top tube).
Minimum quantity: 0.3 mL.
Ship refrigerated.
0–10.2 ng/mL

This method will return lower results than the method above. Because of diurnal variability, random hGH values are not reliable for diagnosis of GH deficiency or acromegaly. See Chapter 5 for instructions on GH testing.

GROWTH HORMONE ANTIBODY

0.5 mL serum in no additive (red-top tube).
Minimum quantity: 0.2 mL.
Ship refrigerated.

Children and adults: Negative

GROWTH HORMONE–BINDING PROTEIN

1 mL serum in no additive (red-top tube).
Minimum quantity: 0.2 mL.
Ship frozen.

Adults
Males and females: 66–306 p*M*

Children

	Males	**Females**
3–5 yr	57–282 p*M*	62–519 p*M*
6–9 yr	60–619 p*M*	58–572 p*M*
10–15 yr	52–783 p*M*	72–965 p*M*

GROWTH HORMONE–RELEASING HORMONE

4 mL plasma in parathyroid hormone–related protein and releasing factors tube.
Minimum quantity: 1.1 mL.
Use special collection tube labeled Parathyroid Hormone RP and Releasing Factors tube, available from Quest Diagnostics Incorporated, Nichols Institute. Do not thaw. Ship frozen.

Adults
Males and females: ≤49 pg/mL

Children
4–14 yr: ≤19 pg/mL

HEMOGLOBIN A$_{1C}$, BLOOD

2 mL whole blood in EDTA (lavender-top tube).
Minimum quantity: 0.3 mL.
Transfer whole blood to plastic shipping vial to prevent breakage. Avoid freezing and thawing. Ship refrigerated.

Children and adults
  Nondiabetic: 4.3%–6.1%
  Therapeutic goal: <7%
  Reevaluate therapy: >8%

HOMOVANILLIC ACID, 24-HOUR URINE

10 mL urine from 24-hr urine container.
Minimum quantity: 5 mL.
Collect urine with 15 g of boric acid or 25 mL of 6N HCl to maintain a pH <3. Urine without preservative is acceptable if pH is <6 and the sample is shipped frozen. Record 24-hr urine volume on test-request form and urine vial. It is preferable for the patient to be off medications for 3 days before collection. Ship refrigerated.

Adults
Males and females: 1.6–7.5 mg/24 hr

Children
3–8 yr: 0.5–6.7 mg/24 hr
9–12 yr: 1.1–6.8 mg/24 hr
13–17 yr: 1.4–7.2 mg/24 hr

HOMOVANILLIC ACID, RANDOM URINE

10 mL urine in sterile screw-cap container.
Minimum quantity: 5 mL.
Collect urine with 15 g of boric acid or 25 mL of 6N HCl to maintain a pH <3. Urine without preservative is acceptable if pH is <6 and the sample is shipped frozen. It is preferable for the patient to be off medications for 3 days before collection. Ship refrigerated.

Adults
Males and females: 1.4–5.3 mg/g Cr

Children
Birth–6 mo: 9.1–36 mg/g Cr
7–11 mo: 11.2–33 mg/g Cr
1–2 yr: 8.5–38 mg/g Cr
3–8 yr: 2.1–23 mg/g Cr
9–12 yr: 1.1–12 mg/g Cr

17-HYDROXYCORTICOSTEROIDS, 24-HOUR URINE

15 mL urine from 24-hr urine container.
Minimum quantity: 5 mL.
Collect urine with 10 g of boric acid to maintain pH <7.5. Record 24-hr urine volume on test-request form and urine vial. Ship refrigerated.

Adults
Males: 4–11 mg/24 hr
Females: 3–10 mg/24 hr

Children
2–17 yr
   Males: 1.1–7.5 mg/24 hr
   Females: 1.1–7.5 mg/24 hr

18-HYDROXYCORTICOSTERONE, SERUM

3 mL serum in no additive (red-top).
Minimum quantity: 1.1 mL.

Adults (8–10 a.m.):
Supine: 4–37 ng/dL
Upright: 5–80 ng/dL

Children
Premature infants (31- to 35-wk gestation): ≤380 ng/dL
Term infants, 3 days old: ≤942 ng/dL

After ACTH stimulation

	Baseline	**After ACTH stimulation**
1–12 mo	5–310 ng/dL	67–470 ng/dL
1–5 yr	7–155 ng/dL	49–370 ng/dL
6–12 yr	10–74 ng/dL	79–360 ng/dL
Tanner II–III		
Males	5–73 ng/dL	91–1,475 ng/dL
Females	11–82 ng/dL	69–195 ng/dL
Tanner IV–V		
Males	14–62 ng/dL	73–205 ng/dL
Females	11–68 ng/dL	82–320 ng/dL

18-HYDROXYDEOXYCORTICOSTERONE (18-OH-DOC)
5 mL serum in no additive (red-top tube).
Minimum quantity: 1.1 mL.
Ship refrigerated.

Adults
8 a.m.: 3–13 ng/dL
6 p.m.: 3–8 ng/dL

Children
Cord blood: ≤40 ng/dL
1 day: 4–21 ng/dL
6 days: ≤34 ng/dL

5-HYDROXYINDOLEACETIC ACID (5-HIAA), 24-HOUR URINE
10 mL urine from 24-hour urine container–25 mL 6N HCl.
Minimum quantity: 5 mL.
Collect urine with 15 g boric acid or 25 mL of 6N HCl to maintain
  a pH <3. Urine without preservative is acceptable if pH is <6
  and the sample is shipped frozen. Keep urine refrigerated
  during collection if preservative is not used. Record 24-hr volume on test-request form and urine vial.
2–10 yr: ≤8.0 mg/24 hr
<10 yr: ≤6.0 mg/24 hr

5-HYDROXYINDOLEACETIC ACID (5-HIAA), RANDOM URINE
10 mL urine in sterile screw-cap container.
Minimum quantity: 5 mL.

  After urine collection, add 0.5–1.0 g boric acid (or 6N HCl) to
maintain a pH <3. Urine without preservative is acceptable if pH
is <6 and the sample is shipped frozen. Keep urine refrigerated
during collection if preservative is not used. Record patient's age
on test-request form and urine vial. Ship refrigerated.

2–10 yr: ≤12 mg/g Cr
>10 yr: ≤10 mg/g Cr

17-HYDROXYPREGNENOLONE, SERUM
2 mL serum in no additive (red-top).
Minimum quantity: 0.4 mL.

Adults
Males and females: 20–450 ng/dL
After ACTH stimulation: 290–910 ng/dL

Children
Premature infants (31- to 35-wk gestation): ≤2,409 ng/dL
Term infants, 3 days old: ≤830 ng/dL

After ACTH stimulation

	Baseline	**After ACTH stimulation**
1–12 mo	14–830 ng/dL	395–3,290 ng/dL
1–5 yr	10–100 ng/dL	45–740 ng/dL
6–12 yr	11–190 ng/dL	70–660 ng/dL
Tanner II–III		
Males	20–360 ng/dL	88–675 ng/dL
Females	58–450 ng/dL	250–800 ng/dL
Tanner IV–V		
Males	32–300 ng/dL	220–860 ng/dL
Females	53–540 ng/dL	500–1,600 ng/dL

See Chapter 10 for more details regarding baseline levels and response to ACTH stimulation.

17-HYDROXYPROGESTERONE, SERUM

1 mL serum in no additive (red-top).
Minimum quantity: 0.1 mL.
Ship refrigerated.

Adults
Males: 50–250 ng/dL
Females
   Follicular phase: 20–100 ng/dL
   Midcycle peak: 100–250 ng/dL
   Luteal phase: 100–500 ng/dL
   Postmenopausal: ≤70 ng/dL
   After ACTH stimulation: 42–250 ng/dL

Children
Premature infants (31- to 35-wk gestation): ≤2,080 ng/dL
Term infants
   3 days old: ≤63 ng/dL
   5 days old: 80–420 ng/dL

After ACTH stimulation

	Baseline	**After ACTH stimulation**
1–12 mo	11–170 ng/dL	85–465 ng/dL
1–5 yr	4–115 ng/dL	50–350 ng/dL
6–12 yr	7–69 ng/dL	75–220 ng/dL

	Baseline	After ACTH stimulation
Tanner II–III		
Males	12–130 ng/dL	69–310 ng/dL
Females	18–220 ng/dL	80–420 ng/dL
Tanner IV–V		
Males	51–190 ng/dL	105–230 ng/dL
Females	36–200 ng/dL	80–225 ng/dL

INSULIN-LIKE GROWTH FACTOR 1 (IGF-1)
(previously call somatomedin c)
1 mL serum in no additive (red-top tube).
Minimum quantity: 0.4 mL.
Ship refrigerated.

	Males	Females
2 mo–5 yr	17–248 ng/mL	17–248 ng/mL
6–8 yr	88–474 ng/mL	88–474 ng/mL
9–11 yr	110–565 ng/mL	117–771 ng/mL
12–15 yr	202–957 ng/mL	261–1,096 ng/mL
16–24 yr	182–780 ng/mL	182–780 ng/mL
25–39 yr	114–492 ng/mL	114–492 ng/mL
40–54 yr	90–360 ng/mL	90–360 ng/mL
Older than 55 yr	71–290 ng/mL	71–290 ng/mL
Tanner stage		
I	109–485 ng/mL	128–470 ng/mL
II	174–512 ng/mL	186–695 ng/mL
III	230–818 ng/mL	292–883 ng/mL
IV	396–776 ng/mL	394–920 ng/mL
V	402–839 ng/mL	308–138 ng/mL

Insulin-Like Growth Factor II (IGF-II)
IGF-2
1 mL plasma in EDTA (lavender-top tube).
Minimum quantity: 0.3 mL.
Overnight fasting is preferred. Ship frozen.

Adults
18–54 yr: 405–1,085 ng/mL
55–65 yr: 230–970 ng/mL

>65 yr: 210–750 ng/mL

Children
2 mo–5 yr: 300–860 ng/mL
6–9 yr: 520–1,050 ng/mL
10–17 yr: 530–1,140 ng/mL

IGF-BINDING PROTEIN-1 (IGFBP-1)

1 mL serum in no additive (red-top tube).
Minimum quantity: 0.2 mL.
Overnight fasting is preferred. Ship frozen.

Adults
Males and females: 13–73 ng/mL

Children
5–9 yr: 20–105 ng/mL
10–14 yr: 10–70 ng/mL
15–18 yr: 10–40 ng/mL

IGF-BINDING PROTEIN-2 (IGFBP-2)

1 mL serum in no additive (red-top tube).
Minimum quantity: 0.2 mL.
Ship frozen.

Adults
18–49 yr: 55–240 ng/mL
>49 yr: 28–444 ng/mL

Children
1–9 yr: 69–480 ng/mL
10–17 yr: 50–326 ng/mL

IGF-BINDING PROTEIN-3 (IGFBP-3)

1 mL serum in no additive (red-top tube).
Minimum quantity: 0.2 mL.
Ship frozen.

Adults
19–55 yr: 2.0–4.0 mg/L
56–82 yr: 0.9–3.7 mg/L

Children
2–23 mo: 0.7–2.3 mg/L
2–7 yr: 0.9–4.1 mg/L
8–11 yr: 1.5–4.3 mg/L
12–18 yr: 2.2–4.2 mg/L

INSULIN ANTIBODIES

For use in patients receiving insulin therapy.
0.5 mL serum in no additive (red-top tube).
Minimum quantity: 0.2 mL.
Ship refrigerated.

Children and adults: Negative

INSULIN ANTIBODIES, HIGHLY SENSITIVE

For detection of insulin autoantibody in patients not receiving
insulin therapy.
1 mL serum in no additive (red-top tube).
Minimum quantity: 0.3 mL.
Ship refrigerated.

Children and adults: ≤1.1%.

INSULIN, FREE

The free (bioactive) insulin test is recommended for patients who
have detectable levels of insulin autoantibodies.
3 mL serum in no additive (red-top tube).
Minimum quantity: 0.6 mL.
Overnight fasting is required. Ship refrigerated.

Children and adults: 4.0–20.0 U/mL
Insulin levels may vary widely in specimens taken from nonfasting individuals.

INSULIN, SERUM

2 mL serum in no additive (red-top tube).
Minimum quantity: 0.3 mL.
  Ship refrigerated. Overnight fasting is required. This assay is
not recommended for patients with positive insulin autoantibody.
Please use the Free Insulin Assay in those cases. Insulin levels
vary widely in specimens taken nonfasting individuals.

Adults
Males and females: ≤20 µU/mL

Children
Cord blood: ≤57 µU/mL
Infants, 2 hr–3 days: 2.7–11.9 µU/L
2–17 yr: ≤33 µU/L
Tanner stage I
   Males: ≤17 µU/L
   Females: ≤21 µU/L
Tanner stage II
   Males: ≤18 µU/L
   Females: ≤19 µU/L
Tanner stage III
   Males: ≤20 µU/L
   Females ≤33 µU/L
Tanner stage IV–V
   Males: ≤28 µU/L
   Females: ≤22 µU/L

ISLET CELL ANTIBODY

2 mL serum in no additive (red-top tube).
Minimum quantity: 0.5 mL.
Ship refrigerated.

Children and Adults: Negative

Note: End-point titers are compared with a single international reference standard, and values are reported in JDF (Juvenile Diabetes Foundation) units.

17-KETOSTEROIDS, 24-HOUR URINE

15 mL urine from 24-hr urine container.
Minimum quantity: 5 mL.
Collect urine with 10 g of boric acid or keep urine refrigerated during collection if preservative is not used. Record 24-hr urine volume on test-request form and urine vial. Ship refrigerated.

Adults
Males: 7–20 mg/24 hr
Females: 5–15 mg/24 hr

Children
2–17 yr: 0.8–8.1 mg/24 hr

LEPTIN, SERUM

1 mL serum in red-top tube.
Minimum quantity: 0.2 mL.
Ship refrigerated.

Adults [lean subjects with body mass index (BMI) of 18–25]
Males: 1.2–9.5 ng/mL
Females: 4.1–25.0 ng/mL

Children
Prepubertal males: 1.6–10.8 ng/mL
Prepubertal females: 1.7–10.6 ng/mL
Tanner stage II–III
    Males: 2.1–11.6 ng/mL
    Females: 2.6–11.5 ng/mL
Tanner stage IV–V
    Males: 3.4–10.2 ng/mL
    Females: 3.4–13.0 ng/mL

LUTEINIZING HORMONE (LH), THIRD-GENERATION SERUM

1 mL serum in no additive (red-top tube).
Minimum quantity: 0.2 mL.
Ship refrigerated.

Adults
Males: 0.95–5.60 IU/L
Females
    Follicular phase: 1.68–15.0 IU/L
    Midcycle peak: 21.94–56.6 IU/L
    Luteal phase: 0.61–16.3 IU/L
    Postmenopausal: 9.0–52.3 IU/L

Children

	Males	**Females**
Cord blood	0.04–2.60 IU/L	0.04–2.60 IU/L
2 wk	4.85–10.02 IU/L	0.29–7.91 IU/L
1–18 mo	0.04–3.01 IU/L	0.02–1.77 IU/L
19 mo–7 yr	0.032–1.03 IU/L	0.03–0.55 IU/L
8–9 yr	0.01–0.78 IU/L	0.02–0.24 IU/L
10–11 yr	0.03–4.44 IU/L	0.02–4.12 IU/L
12–14 yr	0.25–4.84 IU/L	0.28–29.38 IU/L
15–18 yr	0.69–7.15 IU/L	0.11–29.38 IU/L
Tanner stages		
I	0.02–0.42 IU/L	0.01–0.21 IU/L
II	0.26–4.84 IU/L	0.27–4.12 IU/L
III	0.64–3.74 IU/L	0.17–4.12 IU/L
IV	0.55–7.15 IU/L	0.72–15.01 IU/L

METANEPHRINE, FRACTIONATED 24-HOUR URINE

Includes metanephrine, normetanephrine, and total metanephrine
10 mL urine from 24-hour urine container,
Minimum quantity: 3 mL.

Collect urine with 15 g of boric acid or 25 mL of 6N HCl to maintain a pH <3. Urine without preservative is acceptable if pH is <6 and the sample is shipped frozen. Record 24-hour urine volume on test-request form and urine vial. Record patient's age on test request form and urine vial. It is preferable for the patient to be off medications for 3 days before collection. Ship refrigerated.

Metanephrine
3–8 yr: 9–86 µg/24 hr
9–12 yr: 26–156 µg/24 hr
13–17 yr: 31–156 µg/24 hr
Adult males: 26–230 µg/24 hr
Adult females: 19–140 µg/24 hr

Normetanephrine
3–8 yr: 20–186 µg/24 hr
9–12 yr: 10–319 µg/24 hr
13–17 yr: 71–395 µg/24 hr
Adult males: 44–540 µg/24 hr
Adult females: 52–310 µg/24 hr

Total Metanephrine
3–8 yr: 47–360 µg/24 hr
9–12 yr: 72–410 µg/24 hr
13–17 yr: 130–520 µg/24 hr
Adult males: 90–690 µg/24 hr
Adult females: 95–475 µg/24 hr

METANEPHRINE, FRACTIONATED RANDOM URINE

Includes metanephrine, normetanephrine and total metanephrine
10 mL urine in sterile screw-cap container.
Minimum quantity: 3 mL.
Collect urine with 15 g of boric acid or 15 mL of 6N HCl to maintain a pH <3. Urine without preservative is acceptable if pH is
   <6 and the sample is shipped frozen. Record patient's age on test-
   request form and urine vial. It is preferable for the patient to be
   off medications for 3 days before collection. Ship refrigerated.

Metanephrine
Birth–6 mo: 83–523 µg/g Cr
7–11 mo: 45–419 µg/g Cr
1–2 yr: 78–509 µg/g Cr
3–8 yr: 57–237 µg/g Cr
9–12 yr: 38–188 µg/g Cr
13–17 yr: 34–126 µg/g Cr
Adult males: 20–150 µg/g Cr
Adult females: 30–165 µg/g Cr

Normetanephrine
Birth–6 mo: 574–3,856 µg/g Cr
7–11 mo: 527–2,730 µg/g Cr
1–2 yr: 233–2,000 µg/g Cr
3–8 yr: 124–516 µg/g Cr
9–12 yr: 46–517 µg/g Cr
13–17 yr: 45–324 µg/g Cr
Adult males: 70–335 µg/g Cr
Adult females: 105–375 µg/g Cr

Total Metanephrine
Birth–6 mo: 865–4,173 µg/g Cr
7–11 mo: 730–2,980 µg/g Cr
1–2 yr: 311–2,509 µg/g Cr
3–8 yr: 202–750 µg/g Cr
9–12 yr: 100–700 µg/g Cr
13–17 yr: 111–427 µg/g Cr
Adult males: 110–480 µg/g Cr
Adult females: 150–510 µg/g Cr

METANEPHRINE, TOTAL, 24-HOUR URINE

10 mL urine in sterile screw-cap container.
Minimum quantity: 3.5 mL.

Collect urine with 15 g boric acid or 25 mL of 6N HCl to maintain a pH <3. Urine without preservative is acceptable if pH is <6 and the sample is shipped frozen. Record 24-hour urine volume on test-request form and urine vial. Record patient's age on test-request form and urine vial. It is preferable for the patient to be off medications for 3 days before collection. Ship refrigerated.

Adults
Males: 90–690 µg/24 hr
Females: 95–475 µg/24 hr

Children
3–8 yr: 47–360 µg/24 hr
9–12 yr: 72–410 µg/24 hr
13–17 yr: 130–520 µg/24 hr

NOREPINEPHRINE, PLASMA

4 mL plasma in sodium heparin (green-top).
Minimum quantity: 2.5 mL.

Vacutainer is to be chilled before venipuncture. Draw sample as follows: Insert catheter in patient's vein. Instruct patient to lie down for 30 min with catheter in place, and then draw supine specimen in green-top tube. Chill specimen immediately in ice water. Next, instruct patient to sit up for 15 min with catheter still in place. Draw upright specimen in green-top tube. Chill specimen immediately in ice water. Plasma should be separated in a refrigerated centrifuge within 30 min of collection and then frozen immediately at –20°C in plastic vials. Plasma must stay frozen. Thawed samples are unacceptable. Each specimen will be invoiced separately. Overnight fasting is required. Ship frozen.

Adults
Supine: 112–658 pg/mL
Upright: 217–1,109 pg/mL

Children
Plasma norepinephrine measurements are generally unreliable because of stress in infants and small children. Urinary norepinephrine is more reliable.

3–15 yr: ≤1,251 pg/mL

OSMOLALITY, RANDOM URINE

1 mL urine in sterile screw-cap container.
Minimum quantity: 0.2 mL.
Do not use preservatives. Ship refrigerated.

Children and Adults: 200–1,192 mOsm/kg

OSMOLALITY, SERUM

1 mL serum in no additive (red-top tube).
Minimum quantity: 0.2 mL.
Ship refrigerated.

Children and Adults: 282–303 mOsm/kg

OSTEOCALCIN, SERUM

This test is performed by using a test kit that has not been approved or cleared by the Food and Drug Administration (FDA). The performance characteristics of this test have been determined by Quest Diagnostics, Nichols Institute.

1 mL serum in no additive (red-top tube).
Minimum quantity: 0.2 mL.
Avoid hemolysis. Avoid lipemia. Overnight fasting is preferred. Ship refrigerated.

Adults
Males: 8.0–52 ng/mL
Females
  Premenopausal: 5.8–41 ng/mL
  Postmenopausal: 8.0–56 ng/mL

Children

	Male	**Female**
2–12 mo	27–149 ng/mL	27–149 ng/mL
1–4 yr	23–105 ng/mL	23–105 ng/mL
5–9 yr	24–123 ng/mL	24–123 ng/mL
Tanner stages		
I	20–89 ng/mL	20–89 ng/mL
II	26–91 ng/mL	44–144 ng/mL
III–IV	48–123 ng/mL	31–90 ng/mL

PARATHYROID HORMONE ANTIBODY, SERUM

1 mL serum in no additive (red-top tube).
Minimum quantity: 0.2 mL.
Ship refrigerated.

Children and Adults: Negative

PARATHYROID HORMONE (PTH), C-TERMINAL (MID-MOLECULE)

Includes total calcium
2 mL serum in no additive (red-top tube).
Minimum quantity: 1 mL.
Overnight fasting is preferred. Ship refrigerated.

Adults
Males and females: 50–330 pg/mL

Children
2–16 yr: 54–230 pg/mL

PARATHYROID HORMONE (PTH), INTACT, SERUM

Includes total calcium. The intact PTH is the recommended initial assay for the differential diagnosis of calcium-related abnormalities.

2 mL serum in no additive (red-top tube).

Minimum quantity: 1 mL.

Spin and separate serum immediately. Ship refrigerated.

Adults
Males and females: 10–65 pg/mL

Children
Cord blood: <10 pg/mL
3 days–1 yr: ≤56 pg/mL
2–17 yr: 9–52 pg/mL

PARATHYROID HORMONE–RELATED PROTEIN (PTH-RP)

This test is performed by using a test kit that has not been approved or cleared by the Food and Drug Administration (FDA). The performance characteristics of this test have been determined by Quest Diagnostics, Nichols Institute.

3 mL plasma in PTH-RP and Releasing Factors tube.

Minimum quantity: 2 mL.

Do not thaw. For plasma, draw blood in the special Quest Diagnostics Nichols Institute collection tube labeled Parathyroid Hormone-RP and Releasing Factors and gently invert the tube twice. Centrifuge refrigerated immediately. Transfer the plasma to a plastic transport tube and ship frozen.

Postpubertal males and females: ≤1.3 p*M*

PHENYLALANINE, PLASMA

2 mL plasma in sodium heparin (green-top tube).

Minimum quantity: 0.5 mL.

Ship frozen.

0–29 days: 42–110 µ*M*
30 days–16 yr: 22–98 µ*M*
>16 yr: 37–88 µM

PREGNENOLONE, SERUM

4 mL serum in no additive (red-top tube).

Minimum quantity: 1.1 mL.

Ship refrigerated.

Adults
Males: 10–200 ng/dL
Females: 10–230 ng/dL

Children

	Baseline	**After ACTH stimulation**
1–12 mo	10–140 ng/dL	49–360 ng/dL
1–5 yr	10–48 ng/dL	34–135 ng/dL
6–12 yr	15–45 ng/dL	39–105 ng/dL
Tanner II–III		
Males	10–45 ng/dL	58–110 ng/dL
Females	15–84 ng/dL	33–140 ng/dL
Tanner IV–V		
Males	1–50 ng/dL	37–150 ng/dL
Females	20–77 ng/dL	91–220 ng/dL

PROGESTERONE, SERUM

2 mL serum in no additive (red-top tube).
Minimum quantity: 0.6 mL.
Specify age, sex, and menopausal status on test-request form.
  Ship refrigerated.

Adults
  Males: 10–50 ng/dL
  Females
  Follicular phase: ≤50 ng/dL
  Luteal phase: 300–2,500 ng/dL
  Postmenopausal: ≤40 ng/dL
  After ACTH stimulation: 21–44 ng/dL

Children

	Baseline	**After ACTH stimulation**
1–12 mo	5–80 ng/dL	74–200 ng/dL
1–5 yr	8–64 ng/dL	51–230 ng/dL
6–12 yr	5–93 ng/dL	38–200 ng/dL
Tanner II–III		
Males	64–115 ng/dL	61–185 ng/dL
Females	6–680 ng/dL	32–575 ng/dL
Tanner IV–V		
Males	17–145 ng/dL	35–225 ng/dL
Females	16–1,290 ng/dL	45–1,080 ng/dL

PROINSULIN, SERUM

3 mL serum in no additive (red-top tube).
Minimum quantity: 1 mL.
Overnight fasting is required. Ship refrigerated.
Children and Adults: ≤0.20 ng/mL

PROLACTIN, SERUM
Chiron-ACS: 180
1 mL serum in no additive (red-top tube).
Minimum quantity: 0.5 mL.
Overnight fasting is preferred. Ship refrigerated.

Adults
Males: 3.0–14.7 ng/mL
Females: 3.8–23.2 ng/mL

Children

Tanner stage	Males	Females
I	≤10 ng/mL	3.6–12.0 ng/mL
II–III	≤6.1 ng/mL	2.6–18.0 ng/mL
IV–V	2.8–11.0 ng/mL	3.2–20.0 ng/mL

RENIN ACTIVITY (PRA), PLASMA
3.1 mL plasma in EDTA (lavender-top tube).
Minimum quantity: 0.4 mL.

Centrifuge and separate blood at room temperature. Avoid refrigerated temperatures. Patient should refrain from taking medications, preferably 3 weeks before draw. Patient should be ambulatory for 30 min before draw. Patient should be on a moderate sodium diet during collection. Ship frozen.

Adults
Supine (a.m. and p.m.): 0.3–3.0 ng/mL/hr
Upright (a.m. and p.m.): 0.4–8.8 ng/mL/hr

Children
1st wk of life: ≤34 ng/mL/hr
2–4 wk: ≤147 ng/mL/hr
Term neonates: ≤26 ng/mL/hr

	Supine (ng/mL/hr)	Upright (ng/mL/hr)
3 mo–1 yr	≤15	NA
1–3 yr	≤10	NA
4–6 yr	≤7.5	≤15
7–9 yr	≤5.9	≤17
10–12 yr	≤5.3	≤16
13–15 yr	≤4.4	≤16

SEX HORMONE–BINDING GLOBULIN (SHBG)
2 mL serum in no additive (red-top tube).
Minimum quantity: 0.2 mL.

Specify age and sex on test-request form. Ship refrigerated.

Adults
Males: 6–44 nM
Females: 8–85 nM

Children

	Males	**Females**
Preterm infants	24–56 nM	14–40 nM
Term infants	24–54 nM	16–44 nM
2–8 yr	29–141 nM	41–137 nM
9–14 yr	32–92 nM	15–123 nM

SOMATOSTATIN

4 mL plasma in EDTA (lavender-top tube).
Minimum quantity: 1.1 mL.
Draw a prechilled lavender-top tube. Separate and freeze plasma
   immediately. Do not thaw. Ship frozen.
10–22 pg/mL

T_3 (TRIIODOTHYRONINE), FREE, NONDIALYSIS

1 mL serum in no additive (red-top tube).
Minimum quantity: 0.5 mL.
Ship at room temperature.

Postpubertal males and females: 230–420 pg/dL

T_3 (TRIIODOTHYRONINE), FREE, TRACER DIALYSIS

T_3, Free is determined by measuring T_3, total, and the dialyzable
fraction of labeled T_3.

1 mL serum in no additive (red-top tube).
Minimum quantity: 0.4 mL.
Ship refrigerated.

Postpubertal males and females: 210–440 pg/dL

T_3 (TRIIODOTHYRONINE), REVERSE

1 mL serum in no additive (red-top tube).
Minimum quantity: 0.2 mL.
Ship refrigerated.

Adults
Males and females: 10–24 ng/dL

Children
Cord blood: 100–340 ng/dL
1 mo–20 yr: 10–35 ng/dL

T_3 (TRIIODOTHYRONINE), TOTAL, RADIOIMMUNOASSAY

1 mL serum in no additive (red-top tube).
Minimum quantity: 0.2 mL.
Ship refrigerated.

Adults
Males and females: 87–180 ng/dL

Children
Cord blood, >37 wk: 43–99 ng/dL
1–3 days: 100–740 ng/dL
1–11 mo: 105–245 ng/dL
1–4 yr: 105–269 ng/dL
5–9 yr: 94–241 ng/dL
10–14 yr: 82–213 ng/dL
15–19 yr: 80–210 ng/dL

T_3 UPTAKE (TBG ASSESSMENT), SERUM

1 mL serum in no additive (red-top tube).
Minimum quantity: 0.2 mL.
Ship refrigerated.

	Males	**Females**
1–9 yr	0.61–1.13	0.68–0.96
10–19 yr	0.67–1.09	0.64–1.00
20–49 yr	0.92–1.14	0.83–1.15
50–90 yr	0.87–1.11	0.80–1.04

T_4 (THYROXINE), BINDING PROTEINS

Includes T_4, total, thyroxine-binding globulin, prealbumin, albumin, thyroxine-binding globulin–bound T_4, prealbumin-bound T_4, albumin-bound T_4.

4 mL serum in no additive (red-top tube).
Minimum quantity: 2 mL.
Ship refrigerated.

For T_4 (thyroxine, total), thyroxine-binding globulin, prealbumin, and albumin, see individual assays.

Thyroxine Binding Globulin–Bound T_4
3–9 yr: 3.5–8.2 µg/dL
10–17 yr: 2.9–8.0 µg/dL
Adults: 2.9–7.1 µg/dL

Prealbumin-Bound T_4
3–9 yr: 0.5–2.9 µg/dL
10–17 yr: 0.7–3.3 µg/dL
Adults: 0.7–3.0 µg/dL

Albumin-Bound T_4
3–9 yr: 0.4–1.3 µg/dL
10–17 yr: 0.4–1.4 µg/dL
Adults: 0.4–1.1 µg/dL

Thyroxine Binding Globulin–Bound
T_4/Thyroxine-Binding Globulin
3–9 yr: 1.3–3.3 µg/mg
10–17 yr: 1.4–3.1 µg/mg
Adults: 0.4–1.1 µg/mg

Prealbumin-Bound T_4/Prealbumin
3–9 yr: 0.03–0.13 µg/mg
10–17 yr: 0.03–0.14 µg/mg
Adults: 1.3–26 µg/mg

Albumin-Bound T_4/Albumin
3–9 yr: 0.08–0.29 µg/g
10–17 yr: 0.07–0.32 µg/g
Adults: 0.08–0.23 µg/g

T_4 (THYROXINE), BINDING PROTEINS, ELECTROPHORESIS

Includes T_4, Total, Thyroxine Binding Globulin–Bound T_4, Albumin-Bound T_4

1 mL serum in no additive (red-top tube).
Minimum quantity: 0.3 mL.
Ship refrigerated.

Thyroxine Binding Globulin–Bound T_4
3–9 yr: 3.5–8.2 µg/dL
10–17 yr: 2.9–8.0 µg/dL
Adults: 2.9–7.1 µg/dL

Prealbumin-Bound T_4
3–9 yr: 0.5–2.9 µg/dL
10–17 yr: 0.7–3.3 µg/dL
Adults: 0.7–3.0 µg/dL

Albumin-Bound T_4
3–9 yr: 0.4–1.3 µg/dL
10–17 yr: 0.4–1.4 µg/dL
Adults: 0.4–1.1 µg/dL

T_4 (THYROXINE), FREE, DIRECT DIALYSIS SERUM

Direct dialysis is the preferred method for determining Free T_4. Free T_4 is measured in undiluted serum by radioimmunoassay of the dialyzable T_4.

2 mL serum in no additive (red-top tube).
Minimum quantity: 0.2 mL.
Ship refrigerated.

Adults 21–87 yr: 0.8–2.7 ng/dL

Children
Prematures, 25–20 wk
   Birth–7 days: 0.5–3.3 ng/dL
Prematures, 31–36 wk
   Birth–7 days: 1.3–4.7 ng/dL
Cord blood, >37 wk: 1.2–2.2 ng/dL
0–4 days: 2.2–5.3 ng/dL
2 wk–20 yr: 0.8–2.7 ng/dL

T₄ (THYROXINE), FREE, NONDIALYSIS, SERUM

Chiron-ACS: 180
1 mL serum in no additive (red-top tube).
Minimum quantity: 0.5 mL.
Ship refrigerated.

Postpubertal males and females: 0.80–1.50 ng/dL

T₄ (THYROXINE), TOTAL, SERUM

1 mL serum in no additive (red-top tube).
Minimum quantity: 0.2 mL.
Ship refrigerated.

Adults
Males and females: 5.6–13.7 µg/dL

Children
Prematures, 28–36 wk, first week of life: 4.0–17.4 µg/dL
Cord blood, >37 wk: 5.9–15.0 µg/dL
0–4 days: 14.0–28.4 µg/dL
2–20 wk: 8.1–15.7 µg/dL
21 wk–20 yr: 5.6–14.9 µg/dL

TESTOSTERONE, TOTAL, SERUM

2 mL serum in no additive (red-top tube).
Minimum quantity: 0.5 mL.
Specify age and sex on test-request form. Ship refrigerated.

Adults
Males: 260–1,000 ng/dL
Females
   Premenopausal: 15–70 ng/dL
   Postmenopausal: 5–51 ng/dL

Children

	Male	**Female**
Cord blood	17–61 ng/dL	16–44 ng/dL
1–10 days	≤187 ng/dL	≤24 ng/dL
1–3 mo	72–344 ng/dL	≤17 ng/dL

Continued

	Male	**Female**
3–5 mo	≤201 ng/dL	≤12 ng/dL
5–7 mo	≤59 ng/dL	≤13 ng/dL
7–12 mo	≤16 ng/dL	≤11 ng/dL
1–5 yr	≤12 ng/dL	≤12 ng/dL
6–9 yr	3–30 ng/dL	2–20 ng/dL
10–11 yr	5–50 ng/dL	5–25 ng/dL
12–14 yr	10–572 ng/dL	10–40 ng/dL
15–17 yr	220–800 ng/dL	5–40 ng/dL
Tanner stages		
I	2–23 ng/dL	2–10 ng/dL
II	5–70 ng/dL	5–30 ng/dL
III	15–280 ng/dL	10–30 ng/dL
IV	105–545 ng/dL	15–40 ng/dL
V	265–800 ng/dL	10–40 ng/dL

TESTOSTERONE, TOTAL AND FREE, SERUM OR PLASMA
Includes total, free, and percentage free testosterone.
3 mL serum in no additive (red-top tube).
Minimum quantity: 0.5 mL

Percentage free
Adults
Males: 1.0%–2.7%
Females
 Premenopausal: 0.5%–1.8%
 Postmenopausal: 0.8%–1.9%

Children

	Male (%)	**Female (%)**
Cord blood:	1.7–4.1	3.1–14.7
1–10 days	0.8–1.7	0.8–1.6
1–3 mo	0.4–0.8	0.4–1.2
3–5 mo	0.3–1.1	0.4–1.2
5–7 mo	0.4–1.2	0.3–1.1
7–12 mo	0.4–1.2	0.3–1.1
1–5 yr	0.3–1.1	0.3–1.1
6–9 yr	0.9–1.7	0.9–1.4
10–11 yr	1.0–1.9	1.0–1.9
12–14 yr	1.3–3.0	1.0–1.9
15–17 yr	1.8–2.7	1.0–1.9

Free Testosterone
Adults
Males: 50–210 pg/mL
Females
   Premenopausal: 1.0–8.5 pg/mL
   Postmenopausal: 0.6–6.7 pg/mL

Children

	Male	**Female**
Cord blood	3–19 pg/mL	2–4 pg/mL
1–10 days	≤24 pg/mL	≤2.5 pg/mL
1–3 mo	5–21 pg/mL	≤1.2 pg/mL
3–5 mo	≤14 pg/mL	≤0.8 pg/mL
5–7 mo	≤4 pg/mL	≤1.1 pg/mL
7–12 mo	≤0.9 pg/mL	≤0.5 pg/mL
1–5 yr	≤0.6 pg/mL	≤0.6 pg/mL
6–9 yr	0.1–3.2 pg/mL	0.1–0.9 pg/mL
10–11 yr	0.6–5.7 pg/mL	1.0–5.2 pg/mL
12–14 yr	1.4–156 pg/mL	1.0–5.2 pg/mL
15–17 yr	80–159 pg/mL	1.0–5.2 pg/mL

THYROGLOBULIN

This test is performed by using a test kit that has not been approved or cleared by the Food and Drug Administration (FDA). The performance characteristics of this test have been determined by Quest Diagnostics, Nichols Institute.

2 mL serum, minimum quantity: 0.3 mL.
Ship refrigerated.

Adults: 3.5–5.6 ng/mL
2–16 years 2.3–4.0 ng/mL

THYROGLOBULIN ANTIBODY, SERUM

1 mL serum in no additive (red-top tube).
Minimum quantity: 0.15 mL.
Ship refrigerated.

Children and adults: ≤2.0 IU/mL

THYROID PEROXIDASE ANTIBODY (ANTI-TPO), SERUM

The Antithyroid Microsomal Antibody test is now replaced with this test.

1 mL serum in no additive (red-top tube).
Minimum quantity: 0.2 mL.
Ship refrigerated.

Children and adults: <2.0 IU/mL

THYROID-STIMULATING HORMONE (TSH), SERUM

2 mL serum in no additive (red-top tube).
Minimum quantity: 0.5 mL.
Ship refrigerated.

Adults
Males and females (non-pregnant): 0.4–4.2 mU/L

Children
Prematures, 28–36 wk (1st wk of life): 0.7–27.0 mU/L
Cord blood, >37 wk: 2.3–13.2 mU/L
Birth–4 days: 1.0–38.9 mU/L
2–20 wk: 1.7–9.1 mU/L
21 wk–20 yr: 0.7–6.4 mU/L

THYROID-STIMULATING IMMUNOGLOBULIN (TSI)

2 mL serum in no additive (red-top tube).
Minimum quantity: 0.4 mL.
Ship refrigerated.

Children and adults: <130% of basal activity

THYROTROPIN-RELEASING HORMONE

2 mL plasma in Parathyroid Hormone–Related Protein and Releasing Factors tube.
Minimum quantity: 0.6 mL.

For plasma, draw blood in the special Quest Diagnostics Nichols
Institute collection tube, labeled Parathyroid Hormone-RP and
Releasing Factors, and gently invert the tube twice. Centrifuge
and refrigerate immediately. Transfer the plasma to a plastic
transport tube, and ship frozen.

Children and adults: <5 pg/mL

THYROXINE-BINDING GLOBULIN (TBG), SERUM

1 mL serum in no additive (red-top tube).
Minimum quantity: 0.2 mL.
Ship refrigerated.

Adults
Males and females: 1.7–3.6 mg/dL

Children

	Males	**Females**
Cord blood, >37 wk	2.1–3.7 mg/dL	2.1–3.7 mg/dL
1–5 days	2.2–4.2 mg/dL	2.2–4.2 mg/dL
1–11 mo	1.6–3.6 mg/dL	1.7–3.7 mg/dL
1–9 yr	1.2–2.8 mg/dL	1.5–2.7 mg/dL
10–19 yr	1.4–2.6 mg/dL	1.4–3.0 mg/dL

VANILLYLMANDELIC ACID (VMA), RANDOM URINE

15 mL urine in sterile screw-cap container.
Minimum quantity: 2 mL.
Collect urine with 15 g of boric acid or 25 mL of 6N HCl to maintain a pH <6, and the sample is shipped frozen. It is preferable for the patient to be off medication for 3 days before collection. Ship refrigerated.

Adults
Males and females: 1.1–4.1 mg/g Cr

Children
Birth–6 mo: 5.5–26 mg/g Cr
7–11 mo: 6.1–20 mg/g Cr
1–2 yr: 2.5–21 mg/g Cr
3–8 yr: 1.7–6.5 mg/g Cr
9–12 yr: 1.5–5.1 mg/g Cr
13–17 yr: 1.5–3.6 mg/g Cr

VANILLYLMANDELIC ACID (VMA), 24-HOUR URINE

15 mL urine from 24-hr urine container.
Minimum quantity: 2 mL.
Collect urine with 15 g of boric acid or 25 mL of 6N HCl to maintain a pH <3. Urine without preservative is acceptable if pH is <6 and the sample is shipped frozen. Record 24-hr urine volume on test-request form and urine vial. It is preferable for the patient to be off medications for 3 days before collection. Ship refrigerated.

Adults
Males and females: ≤6.0 mg/24 hr

Children
3–8 yr: ≤2.3 mg/24 hr
9–12 yr: ≤3.4 mg/24 hr
13–17 yr: ≤3.9 mg/24 hr

VITAMIN D, 1,25-DIHYDROXY, SERUM

3 mL serum in no additive (red-top tube).
Minimum quantity: 1.1 mL.
Ship refrigerated.

Adults
Males and females: 15–60 pg/mL

Children
3–17 yr: 21–71 pg/mL

VITAMIN D, 25-HYDROXY, SERUM OR PLASMA

1 mL serum in no additive (red-top tube).
Minimum quantity: 0.2 mL.
Ship refrigerated.

Adults
Males and females: 9–52 ng/mL

Children
3–17 yr: 13–67 ng/mL

SUGGESTED READINGS

Laboratory values from
Quest Diagnostics. *The Quest Diagnostics manual of pediatric endocrinology.* 1st ed. San Juan Capistrano, CA: Quest Diagnostics, 2000.
Laboratory values are also available from Esoterix Inc.
Fisher DA, Nelson JC. Endocrine testing. In: DeGroot LJ, Jameson JL, eds. *Endocrinology.* Philadelphia: WB Saunders, 2001:2574–2600.
McCabe ER, McCabe LL. State of the art for DNA technology in newborn screening. *Acta Paediatr Suppl* 1999;88(432):58–60.

🔹 Subject Index

Note: Page numbers followed by *f* indicate figures; those followed by *t* indicate tables.

A

Abnormal growth, 44–57
  history and physical examination, 44
Absent septum pellucidum, 24
Acanthosis nigricans, 244
Achalasia-Addisonianism-Alacrima
    syndrome, 203
Achondroplasia, 15, 49
Acidosis
  diabetic ketoacidosis, 228
Ackee fruit, 277
Acquired hypothyroidism, 98–101
  short stature, 98
  thyroxine, 100–101
Acquired nephrogenic diabetes
    insipidus, 33
Acromegaly, 59
ACTH, 1, 5, 26, 92, 145, 201
  elevated, 4
  laboratory values, 314
Acute adrenal crisis, 203
Acute adrenal insufficiency, 295–296
Addison disease, 201–203
Addisonian crisis, 148
Adenomas
  adrenal gland, 290
  beta-cell, 273
  islet cell, 290
  parathyroid, 129
  pituitary, 4–5
  thyroid, 106
Adenosine monophosphate (AMP), 5
  secretion, 9
Adolescence
  constitutional delay in, 62–68, 167–170
Adrenal crisis
  acute, 203
Adrenal gland
  adenomas, 290
  cortex disorders, 201–217
  disease
    hypertension from, 214
  disorders, 196–217
  hyperplasia, 143–147
  insufficiency
    acute, 295–296
  normal physiology, 196–198, 197*f*–200*f*
Adrenal medulla
  disorders, 215–217
  normal physiology, 214–215
Adrenarche, 166–167
  premature, 191
Adrenocorticotropic hormone (ACTH), 1,
    5, 26, 92, 145, 201
  elevated, 4
  laboratory values, 314
Adrenoleukodystrophy, 202
African Americans
  female pubertal age at onset, 164

obesity, 248
  type 2 diabetes mellitus (noninsulin-
    dependent diabetes mellitus), 244
Albright hereditary osteodystrophy, 118
Albumin
  laboratory values
    24-hour urine, 314
    random urine, 314
Albumin serum
  laboratory values, 314
Aldosterone, 201
  laboratory values
    24-hour urine, 315
    serum, 315
Alkaline phosphatase
  laboratory values
    bone specific, 315–316
    serum, 315
9 alpha-fluorohydrocortisone, 207
1 alpha-hydroxylase, 110
17 alpha-hydroxylase deficiency, 151
1 alpha-hydroxylation deficiency rickets,
    124–125, 130
5 alpha-reductase deficiency, 151
Ambiguous genitalia, 140
  diagnosis and treatment, 153–157
    algorithm, 154*f*–155*f*
    hCG, 156
Amenorrhea
  athletic, 174
Amiloride
  nephrogenic diabetes insipidus, 39
AMP, 5
  secretion, 9
Anaerobic glycolysis, 267–268
Androgen
  partial insensitivity
    sex of rearing, 157
Androgen insensitivity syndrome, 152
Androstenedione
  laboratory values, 316
Angiotensin II
  laboratory values, 316
Anorexia nervosa, 174
Anticonvulsant-associated hypocal-
    cemia, 124
Arginine vasopressin (AVP), 26, 29
  central diabetes insipidus, 38
  laboratory values, 316
Arm span, 49
Arrhenoblastomas
  ovaries, 291
Asthma
  childhood obesity, 255
Astrocytomas
  hypothalamic, 21
  optic, 21
Athletic amenorrhea, 174
Atrial natriuretic hormone
  laboratory values, 316–317

Attention deficit/hyperactivity disorder, 95
Autocrine effects, 2f
Autoimmune hypoparathyroidism, 116–117
Autoimmune polyendocrinopathy syndrome, 99, 116–117
Autoimmune polyglandular disease, 99
Autoimmune syndromes, 202
Autoimmune thyroid disease, 99
AVP, 26, 29
  central diabetes insipidus, 38
  laboratory values, 316

B

Bailey-Pinneau tables, 57
Bardet-Biedl syndrome, 173
Baroreceptors, 26
Barr body, 134
Beckwith-Wiedemann syndrome, 80, 272–273
Beta-cell adenomas, 273
17 beta-hydroxysteroid dehydrogenase type 3, 151
Bicarbonate
  diabetic ketoacidosis, 223t, 297
Bilateral adrenal hyperplasia. *See* Cushing disease
Biosynthetic growth hormone (GH), 72
Bipotential gonad, 134
Bisphosphonates
  osteoporosis, 132
Blood pressure
  boys, 256t–257t
  girls, 258t–259t
Blood sample
  critical, 279, 279t
Blood sugar
  glucometer, 229–230
  monitoring, 235
Blount disease
  tibia
    childhood obesity, 255
Body mass index (BMI), 13–14
  boys, 251f
  calculated, 249
  charts, 16, 44
  girls, 250f
Body weight
  regulation, 252
Bone age, 49
Bone mineral density, 132
Bow legs, 119–120
Boys. *See* Males
Breast
  development, 159, 160f
Breast feeding
  obesity, 263
Breech delivery, 69
Bromergocryptine, 22

C

Calcitonin, 108, 110, 112, 306
  laboratory values, 317

Calcitriol, 110, 111, 117, 306
  biosynthesis, 120f
  hypocalcemia, 300–301
Calcium
  deficiency, 119
  feedback loop, 112
  laboratory values
    24-hour urine, 317
    serum, 317–318
  metabolic disorders, 110–132
  metabolism, 110–111
  regulation, 110–111, 120f
Calcium carbonate, 306
  oral
    renal osteodystrophy, 119
Calcium glubionate, 306
Calcium gluconate, 306
  hypocalcemia of infancy, 113–114
  hypoparathyroidism, 117
Calcium lactate, 306
Carbohydrate
  counting, 235
  normal metabolism, 266–268, 267f
Carnitine
  serum
    laboratory values, 318
Carotene
  laboratory values, 318
Catecholamines
  laboratory values
    24-hour urine, 318–319
    plasma, 319–320
    random urine, 320–321
CDC
  growth charts, 15
Cebocephaly, 23–24
Centers for Disease Control (CDC)
  growth charts, 15
Central diabetes insipidus, 29–39
  treatment, 38–39
Central nervous system (CNS)
  abnormalities, 171–178
  congenital defects, 172
  hypothalamus control, 17
  magnetic resonance imaging, 38
  physical examination, 44
  postinfectious disease, 22–23
  precocious puberty, 188
  tumors, 19–22, 171–172, 287–288
Central (complete or true) precocious puberty, 186–189
Cerebral edema
  diabetic ketoacidosis, 225–226
Cerebral gigantism, 78
Cerebral salt wasting, 40
Charts
  for age
    stature, 49
  body mass index (BMI), 16, 44
  growth, 65f
    Centers for Disease Control (CDC), 15
  growth-velocity, 49
    boys, 52f

girls, 53
  sensitivity, 54*f*–56*f*
intrauterine growth, 46*f*
Cholecalciferol, 110
Cholelithiasis
  childhood obesity, 255
Chronic glucocorticoid deficiency, 203
Chronic lymphocytic thyroiditis, 99
Chronic renal disease, 34
Chvostek sign, 113
Clitoromegaly, 144
Clonidine, 71
CNS. *See* Central nervous system (CNS)
Cold nodule, 89
Computerized continuous subcutaneous
  insulin infusion pump, 234
Congenital adrenal hyperplasia, 142,
  202–203
  female pseudohermaphroditism, 149
  lipoid, 150
Congenital growth hormone
  deficiency, 68–70
Congenital hypopituitarism, 23–24
  signs and symptoms, 93
Congenital hypothyroidism
  etiology, 90*t*–91*t*
  thyroxine
    overtreatment with, 97
  treatment, 96
Congestive heart failure, 105
Constitutional precocious puberty, 186
Continuous glucose monitoring, 230
Corticosterone
  laboratory values, 321
Corticotropin
  laboratory values, 321
Corticotropin-releasing factor (CRF), 1,
  26, 196
  Cushing disease, 212
Cortisol, 4, 17
  Cushing disease, 213–214
  laboratory values
    free serum, 322
    serum, 322–323
    urinary free 24-hour, 322
Cortisol-binding globulin
  laboratory values, 322
Cortisone, 204
C peptide
  plasma
    laboratory values, 317
Craniopharyngioma, 19–20, 29,
  171–172, 287–288
  triphasic response after surgery for,
    42–43, 42*f*
Creatinine
  laboratory values
    clearance, 324
    24-hour urine, 323
    random urine, 323
    serum, 324
Cretinism, 94
CRF, 1, 26, 196
  Cushing disease, 212

Critical blood sample, 279, 279*t*
Cryptorchidism, 176–177
Cushing disease, 209–213
  corticotropin-releasing factor (CRF),
    212
  cortisol, 213–214
  dexmethasone-suppression test, 212
  differential diagnosis, 210–212
  evaluation, 211*f*
  glucocorticoids, 213–214
  metyrapone, 213
  transsphenoidal microsurgery, 213
Cushing syndrome, 4, 9, 60, 67, 74,
  208–214
  treatment, 213–214
Cyclic adenosine monophosphate
  laboratory values
    nephrogenous random urine, 324
    plasma, 325
    random urine, 325–326
Cyclopia, 23–24

D
DDAVP (1-deamino-8-D-arginine
  vasopressin), 306–307
  central diabetes insipidus, 38
  diabetes insipidus
    hypernatremia, 304–305
Dehydroepiandrosterone (DHEA),
  166–167, 196
Dehydroepiandrosterone sulfate
  (DHEAS), 166–167
Delayed puberty, 167–186
  causes, 168*t*–169*t*
  classification, 168*t*–169*t*
  differential diagnosis, 178–181
  sex steroids, 181
  temporary *vs.* permanent, 178
  testosterone, 181
  treatment, 181–186
Deoxycorticosterone
  serum
    laboratory values, 326–327
11-deoxycorticosterone
  laboratory values
    24-hours urine, 328
    serum, 327–328
Developmental defects, 23–25
Dexamethasone
  thyroid storm, 300
Dexmethasone-suppression test
  Cushing disease, 212
Dextrose
  hypoglycemia, 284, 301–302
DHEA, 166–167, 196
DHEAS, 166–167
Diabetes insipidus, 22, 29–39
  acquired nephrogenic, 33
  central, 29–39
    treatment, 38–39
  clinical features, 33
  diagnosis, 34
  hypernatremia, 304–305
  nephrogenic, 32–33
    treatment, 39

Diabetes mellitus, 29, 218–246
  differential points between, 219*t*
  neonatal, 243–244
Diabetic ketoacidosis, 218, 222–229,
    296–298
  acidosis, 228
  bicarbonate, 223*t*
  cerebral edema, 225–226
  insulin therapy, 223*t*, 228–229
  monitoring, 297
  potassium deficit, 228
  treatment, 223*t*–224*t*, 227–228
Diazoxide
  hypoglycemia, 285
Diet, 11
  obesity, 263
Dietary
  type 1 diabetes mellitus (insulin-
    dependent diabetes mellitus),
    235–236
DiGeorge syndrome, 116–117
Digitalis
  neonatal hyperthyroidism, 299
Dihydrotestosterone
  laboratory values, 328
  free serum, 329–330
1,25-dihydroxy vitamin D (calcitriol),
    110, 111, 117, 306
  biosynthesis, 120*f*
  hypocalcemia, 300–301
Diiodotyrosine (DIT), 85
Dilantin, 101
Dilantin
  syndrome of inappropriate secretion of
    ADH (SIADH)
    hyponatremia, 304
DIT, 85
DNA
  transcription, 9*f*
Dominican Republic, 152
Donohue's leprechaun syndrome, 60
Dopamine
  laboratory values
    24-hour urine, 319
    plasma, 320
    random urine, 320–321
Drinking habits
  excessive, 37
Drug-induced hypercalcemia, 129–130
Dual-energy x-ray absorptiometry
    (DXA), 132
Dysplasia
  optic, 172

E

Early pubertal development
  variations of, 190–191
Edema
  cerebral
    diabetic ketoacidosis, 225–226
Educational achievement, 11
18-hydroxydeoxycorticosterone
  laboratory values, 336

11-deoxycorticosterone
  serum
    laboratory values, 327–328
Embden-Meyerhof pathway, 267–268
Emergencies, 295–305
Endocrine disease
  evaluation, 11–16
  manifestations, 4–10
  primary *vs.* secondary or tertiary
    differential diagnosis of, 4*t*
Endocrine effects, 2*f*
Endocrine gland
  enlargement, 4
  tumors, 5, 287–294
Endocrine system, 1–10
Epinephrine
  laboratory values
    24-hour urine, 319
    plasma, 320, 329
    random urine, 320
Epiphyseal fusion, 60
Ergocalciferol (vitamin D2), 307
Estradiol
  laboratory values
    free, 329
    serum, 330
Estrone
  laboratory values
    serum, 330–331
Ethnic groups
  obesity, 252
Excessive drinking habits, 37
Exophthalmos, 101
External genitalia, 140
External sex steroid ingestion, 150
Extremities
  examination, 16

F

Failure to thrive, 68
Familial growth hormone deficiency,
    69–70
Familial hyperaldosteronism, 214
Familial hyperthyroidism, 106
Familial hyperthyroxinemia, 95
Familial hypocalciuric hypercalcemia,
    128
Familial thyroglossal duct cyst, 100
Family history, 13
Family therapy
  obesity, 260
Fasting state, 266–267
Fat necrosis, 131
Fed state, 266
Feedback loops, 2*f*–3*f*
Females
  blood pressure, 258*t*–259*t*
  body mass index, 250*f*
  gender identity, 142
  genetic
    virilization, 142–147
  growth-velocity charts, 53
  incomplete precocious puberty, 189
  length-for-age, 51*f*

pseudohermaphroditism, 142–147
  congenital adrenal hyperplasia, 149
pubertal age at onset, 164
  African Americans, 164
pubic hair
  development, 159–160
stature-for-age, 61*f*
weight-for-age, 51*f*
Fertility
  hermaphrodites, 149
Fetal alcohol syndrome, 66
Fetus
  testes, 140
  testosterone, 140
Florinef, 207, 307
  hyponatremia/hyperkalemia, 303
Fludrocortisone acetate, 307
Fluorohydrocortisone, 207
Follicle-stimulating hormone (FSH), 5,
    165, 289
  beta gene
    mutations, 171
  serum
    laboratory values, 331
Follicular thyroid carcinoma (FTC), 107
Fructosamine
  serum
    laboratory values, 332
FSH, 5, 165, 289
  beta gene
    mutations, 171
  serum
    laboratory values, 331
FTC, 107
Furosemide, 307
  hypercalcemia, 131, 298
  syndrome of inappropriate secretion of
    ADH (SIADH)
    hyponatremia, 304

G

Galactorrhea, 22
Galactosemia, 274
Gastric bypass, 262
Gastrin
  serum
    laboratory values, 332
Gender identity, 142
  female, 142
Genetic females
  virilization, 142–147
Genetic history, 12*f*–13*f*
Genetic male
  virilization, 150
Genetics
  short stature, 66
Genitalia
  ambiguous, 140
    diagnosis and treatment, 153–157,
      154*f*–155*f*
    hCG, 156
  development
    boys, 161, 162*f*–163*f*
  external, 140

Genotype, 134
Genu valgum (knock knees), 119–120
Genu varum (bow legs), 119–120
Germinomas, 21, 29, 172, 288
Gestational age
  height, 15
  weight, 15
GH. *See* Growth hormone (GH)
GHBP, 5, 58
GHRH, 5, 71, 118
  laboratory values, 333–334
Gigantism
  cerebral, 78
Girls. *See* Females
Gliomas
  hypothalamic, 21
  optic, 21
Globulin (SHBG)
  laboratory values, 348–349
Glucagon hydrochloride, 307
Glucagons, 5
  laboratory values, 332
Glucocorticoid, 60, 206*t*, 307, 308*t*
  acute adrenal insufficiency, 295–296
  chronic deficiency, 203
  Cushing syndrome, 213–214
  deficiency, 4
  excess, 4
  21-hydroxylase deficiency, 146, 147
  hypercalcemia, 298
Glucometer
  blood sugar, 229–230
Glucose
  continuous monitoring, 230
  hypoglycemia, 283–284
  production, 266, 267–268
  serum
    laboratory values, 332
Glucose tolerance test, 225*t*, 282
Glutamate dehydrogenase hyper-
    insulinism, 273
Glutamic acid decarboxylase-65
    autoantibodies
    laboratory values, 332
Glycated albumin
  laboratory values, 332
Glycogen storage disease, 276–277
GnRH, 5, 165
  agonists, 188
  mutations, 171
GnRH-A, 192–193
Goiter, 87–88
Goitrogen, 89
Gonad
  bipotential, 134
Gonadal conditions, 149–150
Gonadal dysgenesis, 175–176
Gonadal sex, 136
Gonadal steroids, 60
Gonadarche, 164–165
Gonadotropin, 171
  isolated deficiency, 170
  secretion, 166

Gonadotropin-releasing hormone
(GnRH), 5, 165
  agonists, 188
  mutations, 171
Gonadotropin-releasing hormone
analogues (GnRH-A), 192–193
G protein-coupled receptors, 5
Granulomas, 172
Granulomatous disease, 130
Graves disease, 85–86, 101
  neonatal, 105
Growth
  abnormal, 44–57, 62–81
    history and physical examination,
    44
  constitutional delay in, 62–68,
  167–170
  genetic factors, 60
  measurement, 44–45
  postnatal
    endocrine factors, 58–62
Growth charts, 65f
  Centers for Disease Control (CDC), 15
  intrauterine, 46f
Growth factors, 62
Growth hormone (GH), 58, 110
  antibody
    laboratory values, 333
  biosynthetic, 72
  deficiency, 19, 68, 185, 273–274
    congenital, 68–70
    diagnosis, 70–72
    familial, 69–70
    treatment, 72–73
  hybritech
    laboratory values, 333
  hypothalamic, 177
    releasing factor, 58
  idiopathic deficiency, 68
  receptor, 7f
  serum
    laboratory values, 333
Growth hormone-binding protein
(GHBP), 5, 58
Growth hormone-releasing factor
(GHRH), 5, 71
Growth hormone-releasing hormone
(GHRH), 118
  laboratory values, 333–334
Growth rate, 11, 60
Growth suppressors, 60
Growth-velocity charts, 49
  boys, 52f
  girls, 53
  sensitivity, 54f–56f
Gynecomastia, 191–192

H

Hamartomas, 188
Hand-Schuller-Christian disease, 22, 29,
172, 288
Harpenden stadiometer, 45, 48
Harriet Lane Manual, 15
Hashimoto thyroiditis, 86, 99
  clinical characteristics, 99–100

hCG, 21, 140, 291
  ambiguous genitalia, 156
Head
  radiation, 23
Head, eyes, ears, nose, and throat
(HEENT)
  examination, 16
Height
  gestational age, 15
  predicted, 57
Hemangioma
  liver, 100
Hemoglobin
  blood
    laboratory values, 334
Hepatic steatosis
  childhood obesity, 255
Hepatocellular rickets, 121–124
Hereditary fructose intolerance, 277
Hermaphrodites
  fertility, 149
Heuvodoces, 152
Hirsutism
  childhood obesity, 255
Histiocytosis X, 22, 29, 172
History, 11–12
  abnormal growth, 44
Holoprosencephaly, 23–24
Homocystinuria, 79–80
Homovanillic acid (HVA), 290
  laboratory values
    24-hour urine, 334
    random urine, 334–335
Honeymoon period
  type 1 diabetes mellitus (insulin-
  dependent diabetes mellitus), 240
Hormones
  classes, 5–10
Hormone-secreting tumors, 289–294
Human chorionic gonadotropin (hCG),
21, 140, 291
  ambiguous genitalia, 156
HVA, 290
  laboratory values
    24-hour urine, 334
    random urine, 334–335
Hydrocephalus, 22
Hydrochlorothiazide, 307
Hydrocortisone-sodium succinate, 148
17-hydroxycorticosteroids
  24-hours urine
    laboratory values, 335
18-hydroxycorticosterone
  serum
    laboratory values, 335
5-hydroxyindoleacetic acid
  laboratory values
    24-hour urine, 336
    random urine, 336
Hydroxylase, 110
  deficiency, 151
11-hydroxylase deficiency, 149
21-hydroxylase deficiency, 143–147
  electrolyte disturbance, 144

glucocorticoids, 147
late onset
skin pigmentation, 145
mineralocorticoids, 147–148
skin pigmentation, 144–145
treatment, 147–149
virilization, 144
Hydroxylation deficiency rickets,
124–125, 130
17-hydroxypregnenolone
serum
laboratory values, 336–337
17-hydroxyprogesterone
serum
laboratory values, 337
3-hydroxysteroid-dehydrogenase
deficiency, 149
Hydroxysteroid dehydrogenase type 3,
151
Hyperactivity disorder, 95
Hyperadrenal state, 209–214
Hyperaldosteronism
familial, 214
idiopathic, 214
Hypercalcemia, 125–128, 298
causes, 126t–127t
drug-induced, 129–130
furosemide, 131
hyperthyroidism, 129
phosphate, 131
sodium chloride, 131
Hypercalcemia of infancy
idiopathic, 131
Hypercalcemia of malignancy, 129
Hyperglycemia
intrauterine, 272
Hypergonadotropic hypogonadism,
174–175
Hyperinsulinism, 272–273, 275
Hyperkalemia
adrenal insufficiency, 302–303
Hyperlipidemia
childhood obesity, 254
Hypernatremia
diabetes insipidus, 304–305
Hyperosmolality, 28
Hyperparathyroidism
neonatal transient, 129
primary, 128–132
Hyperprolactinemia, 22
Hypertension
from adrenal disease, 214
pheochromocytoma, 305
Hyperthyroidism, 87, 101–106
etiology, 102t
familial, 106
hypercalcemia, 129
iodine, 104
medication, 103–104
methimazole, 103–104
neonate, 299
nuclear medicine, 104–105
propranolol, 104, 105–106
radioactive iodine, 104–105
subtotal thyroidectomy, 104

Hyperthyrotropinemia
transient, 96
Hyperthyroxinemia
familial, 95
Hypervitaminosis D, 130
Hypoadrenal states, 201–204
diagnosis, 204, 205f
treatment, 204–209
Hypocalcemia, 112–113, 300–301
anticonvulsant-associated, 124
causes, 114t–115t
diagnosis, 118–119
etiology, 111f
infant, 113–114
physical examination, 113
Hypocalciuric hypercalcemia
familial, 128
Hypochondroplasia, 15, 49
Hypoglycemia, 266–285, 268–285,
301–302
diagnosis, 278–283, 280f
ketotic, 275
neonate, 269–275
newborn, 269–275
older children, 275–278
treatment, 283–285, 284t
type 1 diabetes mellitus (insulin-
dependent diabetes mellitus), 240
Hypogonadism
hypergonadotropic, 174–175
Hypogonadotrophic hypogonadism, 178
Hyponatremia, 40, 41
adrenal insufficiency, 302–303
syndrome of inappropriate secretion of
ADH (SIADH), 303–304
Hypoosmolality, 28
Hypoparathyroidism, 4, 58, 67–68
autoimmune, 116–117
diagnosis, 117
pathological, 116–117
treatment, 117
Hypophosphatemia
X-linked, 125
Hypopituitarism, 20, 22
congenital, 23–24
signs and symptoms, 93
idiopathic, 172–173
magnetic resonance imaging, 19
Hypopituitary dwarfism
idiopathic, 23–24
Hypospadias, 152
Hypotelorism
orbital, 23–24
Hypothalamic astrocytomas, 21
Hypothalamic gliomas, 21
Hypothalamic growth hormone, 177
releasing factor, 58
Hypothalamic hypogonadism, 170
Hypothalamic-pituitary axis, 84f
disorders, 17–25
central nervous system (CNS)
disorders, 19–25
pathology, 19
physiology, 17–18

Hypothalamic-pituitary tumor, 29
Hypothalamus, 17
  anatomy, 18*f*
  hormones, 1
  releasing or inhibiting factors, 17
Hypothyroidism, 15, 74, 89–106, 95, 174
  acquired, 98–101
    short stature, 98
    thyroxine, 100–101
  congenital
    etiology, 90*t*–91*t*
    thyroxine, 97
    treatment, 96
  neonates, 89–98
    screening, 93–94
  premature sexual development, 99
  secondary *vs.* tertiary, 86

I

Iatrogenic type 1 diabetes mellitus
    (insulin-dependent diabetes
    mellitus), 243
Idiopathic growth hormone
  deficiency, 68
Idiopathic hyperaldosteronism, 214
Idiopathic hypercalcemia of infancy, 131
Idiopathic hypopituitarism, 172–173
Idiopathic hypopituitary dwarfism,
  23–24
Idiopathic precocious puberty, 186
IGF, 58, 72
IGF-1, 6, 6*f*, 17, 59, 110
  laboratory values, 338–339
IGFBP
  laboratory values, 339
Incomplete precocious puberty, 189–190
  boys, 189–190
  girls, 189
Incomplete syndrome of androgen
    insensitivity, 152–153
Infant
  hypocalcemia, 113–114
  measuring length, 45, 47
Infantometer, 47
Insulin, 60, 308, 308*t*
  actions, 232*t*
  adjustments, 241–242
  administration, 232–233
  diabetic ketoacidosis, 297
  laboratory values
    free, 340
    serum, 340
  multiple dose injections (MDI), 233–234
    time of action, 238–243
  short term correction, 237*t*
  subcutaneous
    administration, 231*f*
Insulin antibodies
  highly sensitive
    laboratory values, 340
  laboratory values, 339
Insulin-dependent diabetes mellitus,
    243. *See also* Type 1 diabetes
    mellitus (insulin-dependent dia-
    betes mellitus)

Insulin growth factor (IGF), 58, 72
Insulin growth factor binding protein
    (IGFBP)
  laboratory values, 339
Insulin-like growth factor 1 (IGF-1), 6,
    6*f*, 17, 59, 110
  laboratory values, 338–339
Insulin pump, 234
Insulin receptors, 6, 6*f*
Insulin-receptor substrates (IRS), 9
Insulin therapy
  diabetic ketoacidosis, 223*t*, 228–229
  type 1 diabetes mellitus (insulin-
    dependent diabetes mellitus),
    230–236
Internal sexual ducts
  development, 139*f*
Intrauterine growth charts, 46*f*
Intrauterine hyperglycemia, 272
Iodine
  hyperthyroidism, 104
IRS, 9
Islet cell adenomas, 290
Islet cell antibody
  laboratory values, 340–341
Isolated gonadotropin deficiency, 170

J

Jak kinases, 5
Jakob-Creutzfeldt disease, 72–73
Jamaican vomiting disease, 277
Juvenile pause, 165
Juvenile rheumatoid arthritis
  stature, 62

K

Kallmann syndrome, 170–171
Ketone bodies, 279
17-ketosteroids
  24-hour urine
    laboratory values, 341
Ketotic hypoglycemia, 275
Klinefelter syndrome, 15, 49, 80, 99,
    136, 149, 176, 178, 191
Knock knees, 119–120
Kwalatmala, 152

L

Laboratory values, 314–356
Langerhans cell histiocytosis, 22, 288
Late onset 21-hydroxylase deficiency
  skin pigmentation, 145
Lateral tibial prominence, 113
Laurence-Moon syndrome, 173
L-Dopa, 71
Length-for-age
  boys, 50*f*
  girls, 51*f*
Leptin, 252
  serum
    laboratory values, 341
Letterer-Siwe disease, 22
LH
  beta gene mutations, 171

serum
   laboratory values, 341–342
Lipoid congenital adrenal hyperplasia,
   150
Liver hemangioma, 100
Luteinizing hormone (LH), 5, 140, 165
   beta gene mutations, 171
   serum
      laboratory values, 341–342
Luteomas
   ovaries, 291
Lymphocytic thyroiditis
   chronic, 99
Lyon hypothesis, 134
Lypressin
   central diabetes insipidus, 38
Lysine vasopressin
   central diabetes insipidus, 38

M

Magnesium, 112
   deficiency, 118
Magnesium sulfate, 308–309
Males
   blood pressure, 256t–257t
   body mass index, 251f
   genetic virilization, 150
   genital development, 161, 162f–163f
   growth-velocity charts, 52f
   incomplete precocious puberty,
      189–190
   length-for-age, 50f
   pseudohermaphroditism, 142, 150,
      157
   pubertal age at onset, 164
   pubic hair, 162f–163f
   secondary sexual development,
      179f–180f
   sexual differentiation, 141f
      genes and hormones, 137f
   weight-for-age, 50f
Malnutrition, 68, 277
Mannitol, 309
Maple syrup urine disease, 274
Marfan syndrome, 79
Master gland, 1
Maternal deprivation, 74
Maternal smoking, 66
Maternal substance abuse, 66
Maturity onset diabetes of the young
   (MODY), 245, 246t
MCAD
   mutations, 274
McCune-Albright syndrome, 6, 188–189
MCT, 107, 289
MDI
   insulin, 233–234
      time of action, 238–243
Medications, 306–313
   history, 11
Medium-chain acyl-CoA dehydrogenase
   (MCAD)
   mutations, 274
Medroxyprogesterone acetate, 309

Medullary carcinoma of the thyroid
   (MCT), 107, 289
Melanocyte-stimulating hormone
   (MSH), 253
MEN, 217, 291–294, 292t–293t
Menarche, 164
Menses
   childhood obesity, 255
Mental retardation, 80
Metanephrine
   laboratory values
      24-hour urine, 342–343, 343–344
      random urine, 343
Metformin, 309
Methimazole, 309
   hyperthyroidism, 103–104
Metric system, 49
Metyrapone
   Cushing disease, 213
Mexican Americans
   obesity, 248
Microphallus, 69, 173
Microprolactinomas, 22
MIF, 136
Mineralocorticoids, 207
   21-hydroxylase deficiency, 147–148
MIT, 85
MODY, 245, 246t
Monoiodotyrosine (MIT), 85
MSH, 253
Mullerian duct inhibitory factor (MIF),
   136
Multiple dose injections (MDI)
   insulin, 233–234
      time of action, 238–243
Multiple endocrine neoplasia (MEN),
   217, 291–294, 292t–293t
Munchausen by proxy, 278
Myxedema
   pretibial, 101

N

National Center for Health Statistics
   charts of stature for age, 49
Nelson syndrome, 210
Neonates
   diabetes mellitus, 243–244
   Graves disease, 105
   hyperthyroidism, 299
   hypoglycemia, 269–275
   hypothyroidism, 89–98
      screening, 93–94
   transient hyperparathyroidism, 129
Nephrogenic diabetes insipidus, 32–33
   treatment, 39
Nesidioblastosis, 273
Neuroblastoma, 217–218
Neurofibromatosis type 1, 288
Neurologic examination, 16
Neuropeptide Y (NPY), 253
Neurophysin II, 26
Neutral protamine Hagedorn (NPH),
   232, 233, 238
Newborn. See Neonates

New Guinea, 152
Nitroprusside, 309
Noninsulin-dependent diabetes mellitus.
    See Type 2 diabetes mellitus
    (noninsulin-dependent diabetes
    mellitus)
Noonan syndrome, 67, 175
Norepinephrine, 253
    laboratory values
        24-hour urine, 319
        plasma, 320, 344
        random urine, 320
Normal sexual differentiation, 134–142
NPH, 232, 233, 238
NPY, 253
Nuclear medicine
    hyperthyroidism, 104–105
Nutrition, 62
Nutritional pattern, 11
Nutritional rickets, 121

O

Obesity, 248–263
    comorbidities, 253–263, 254–255
    laboratory evaluation, 255–261
    pathophysiology, 249–253
    prevention, 262–263
    psychological toll, 254
    treatment, 260–262
    type 2 diabetes mellitus (noninsulin-
        dependent diabetes mellitus), 244
Obstructive sleep apnea
    childhood obesity, 254–255
Octreotide
    hypoglycemia, 285
Online Mendelian Inheritance in Man
    web site, 10
Optic astrocytomas, 21
Optic dysplasia, 172
Optic gliomas, 21
Optic nerve hypoplasia, 24
Oral calcium carbonate
    renal osteodystrophy, 119
Orbital hypotelorism, 23–24
Osmolality
    laboratory values
        random urine, 344
        serum, 344
Osmolality disturbances
    causes, 30*t*–31*t*
Osteocalcin
    serum
        laboratory values, 345
Osteopenia, 131
Osteoporosis, 131–132
    bisphosphonates, 132
Ovaries
    arrhenoblastomas, 291
    luteomas, 291
    thecoma, 291

P

Painful thyroid gland, 108
Pamidronate, 309–310

Pancreatectomy
    hypoglycemia, 285
Panhypopituitarism, 172–173
Papillary carcinoma, 107
Paracrine effects, 2*f*
Parathyroid adenomas, 129, 290
Parathyroid hormone (PTH), 110,
        111–112, 117
    laboratory values
        C-terminal, 345
        serum, 345–346
    resistance, 4
Parathyroid hormone (PTH) antibody
    serum
        laboratory values, 345
Parathyroid hormone releasing protein
        (PTHrP), 110, 112
    laboratory values, 346
Parents, 13
    modeling obesity, 262–263
Partial androgen insensitivity
    sex of rearing, 157
Pathological hypoparathyroidism,
        116–117
Pendred syndrome, 94
Penis, 140
Peptide hormones, 5
    binding, 7*f*
Persistent hyperinsulinemic hypo-
        glycemia of infancy, 273
Phenotypic sex, 136–140
Phenoxybenzamine
    pheochromocytoma, 215–216
Phenylalanine
    plasma
        laboratory values, 346
Phenytoin (Dilantin), 101
Pheochromocytoma, 215–216, 290
    hypertension, 305
    phenoxybenzamine, 215–216
Phosphate
    hypercalcemia, 131, 298
Phosphorus supplements, 310
Physical examination, 11–12, 13–14,
        14*f*–15*f*
    abnormal growth, 44
    hypocalcemia, 113
    short stature, 76
Pituitary adenomas, 4–5
Pituitary dwarfism, 70
Pituitary gigantism, 80
    treatment, 81
Pituitary gland, 1
    anatomy, 18*f*
    tumors, 21–22
Pituitary-hypothalamic axis, 1
Pituitary/hypothalamic hormone
        deficiencies
    genetic forms, 24*f*
Pituitary stalk transection, 24, 32*f*
Plasma osmolality, 28
Plasma renin activity (PRA), 207
Polydipsia, 34
    diagnosis, 35*f*

psychogenic
diagnosis, 37
Polyuria, 34
diagnosis, 35*f*
POMC, 196, 252
Postnatal growth
endocrine factors, 58–62
Potassium
deficit
diabetic ketoacidosis, 228
supplements, 310–311
Potassium iodide, 310
PRA, 207
Prader orchidometer, 161
Prader-Willi syndrome, 67, 73, 173
Precocious puberty, 22, 23, 80
central (complete or true), 186–189
central nervous system (CNS), 188
constitutional, 186
diagnosis, 182*f*–184*f*
differential diagnosis, 192
idiopathic, 186
incomplete, 189–190
boys, 189–190
girls, 189
psychological support, 193
treatment, 192–193
Prednisone, 204
Pregnancy, 11
Pregnenolone
serum
laboratory values, 346
Premature adrenarche, 191
Premature sexual development
hypothyroidism, 99
Premature thelarche, 190–191
Pretibial myxedema, 101
Primary hyperparathyroidism, 128–132
Progesterone, 165
serum
laboratory values, 347
Proinsulin
serum
laboratory values, 347
Prolactin, 17, 110
serum
laboratory values, 347–348
Prolactinomas, 289
Pro-opiomelanocortin (POMC), 196, 252
Propranolol, 311
adverse effects, 277
hyperthyroidism, 104, 105–106
neonatal hyperthyroidism, 299
thyroid storm, 299
Propylthiouracil (PTU), 89, 103, 106,
311–312
neonatal hyperthyroidism, 299
thyroid storm, 300
Protein-sparing modified fast (PSMF),
262
Pseudohermaphroditism
female, 142–147
congenital adrenal hyperplasia, 149
male, 142, 150, 157

Pseudohypoparathyroidism, 67, 74,
117–118
Pseudotumor cerebri
childhood obesity, 255
Pseudovitamin D deficiency rickets,
124–125
PSMF, 262
Psychogenic polydipsia
diagnosis, 37
Psychological support
precocious puberty, 193
Psychosocial dwarfism, 62, 73–74
PTH. *See* Parathyroid hormone (PTH)
PTHrP, 110, 112
laboratory values, 346
PTU. *See* Propylthiouracil (PTU)
Puberty, 59
age at onset, 163–164
African Americans females, 164
childhood obesity, 255
delayed. *See* Delayed puberty
disorders, 159–193
early
variations of, 190–191
endocrine changes of, 164–167
growth spurt, 163
physical, 159–163
stage, 16
temporary delayed, 167–170
Pubic hair
development, 161*f*
female, 159–160
male, 161–163, 162*f*–163*f*
Pure gonadal dysgenesis, 149–150
Pygmies, 70

R
Rachitic rosary, 121
Radioactive iodine
Graves disease
pregnancy, 95
hyperthyroidism, 104–105
Rathke-cleft cyst, 20–21
Rathke pouch
tumors, 171–172
REE, 252
Reifenstein syndrome, 191
Renal disease
chronic, 34
Renal osteodystrophy, 119
Renin activity
plasma
laboratory values, 348
Resting energy expenditure (REE), 252
Retinal cerebellar hemangioblastomato-
sis, 294
Retinoid-X receptor (RXR), 9
Rickets, 119–120
1 alpha-hydroxylation deficiency,
124–125, 130
hepatocellular, 121–124
hydroxylation deficiency, 124–125,
130
inherited causes of, 124–125

Rickets (*contd.*)
  nutritional, 121
  pseudovitamin D deficiency, 124–125
  types, 122*t*–123*t*
  vitamin D-dependency, 124–125
  vitamin D-resistant, 124–125
Rickets of prematurity, 124
Roche Wainer Thissen (RWT) method, 57
Russell-Silver dwarfism syndrome, 66
RWT method, 57
RXR, 9

S
Salts
  vasopressin, 28
Schmidt syndrome, 99
Secretagogues, 71
Sedentary time
  obesity, 263
Sella turcica, 20
Septooptic dysplasia, 24, 69, 172
Septum pellucidum
  absent, 24
Serotonin, 253
Serum glucose
  regulation, 268
Serum osmolality, 3
17 alpha-hydroxylase deficiency, 151
17 beta-hydroxysteroid dehydrogenase type 3, 151
17-hydroxycorticosteroids
  24-hours urine
    laboratory values, 335
17-hydroxypregnenolone
  serum
    laboratory values, 336–337
17-hydroxyprogesterone
  serum
    laboratory values, 337
17-ketosteroids
  24-hour urine
    laboratory values, 341
Sex
  phenotypic, 136–140
Sex hormone-binding globulin (SHBG)
  laboratory values, 348–349
Sex Maturity Rating (SMR), 159
Sex steroids, 17, 60
  delayed puberty, 181
Sexual development
  premature
    hypothyroidism, 99
Sexual differentiation
  disorders, 134–157, 142–157
    males, 141*f*
  normal, 134–142
Sexual infantilism
  permanent conditions of, 170–171
Sexual precocity, 186–193
  causes and classification, 187*t*–188*t*
SGA, 66
SHBG
  laboratory values, 348–349

Short stature, 62–73
  acquired hypothyroidism, 98
  diagnosis, 74–77, 75*f*, 76*t*
  endocrine causes, 68–69
  etiology, 63*f*–64*f*
  genetic, 66
  nonendocrine causes, 62–68
  physical examination, 76
  psychological effects, 73
SHOX gene, 174
SIAHD. *See* Syndrome of inappropriate secretion of ADH (SIADH)
Sick day management
  type 1 diabetes mellitus (insulin-dependent diabetes mellitus), 236–237
Signal transducer and activator of transcription (STAT), 5
Skeleton
  development, 49
Skin
  examination, 16
Slipped capital femoral epiphysis
  childhood obesity, 255
Small for gestational age (SGA), 66
Smith's Recognizable Patterns of Human Malformation, 66
Smoking
  maternal, 66
SMR, 159
Social gender, 140–142
Soda
  obesity, 263
Sodium, 3
  regulation, 27*f*
Sodium bicarbonate, 312
  hyponatremia/hyperkalemia, 302–303
Sodium chloride
  hypercalcemia, 131
Sodium phosphate
  hypercalcemia, 298
Sodium sulfate
  hypercalcemia, 298
Somatomedins. *See* Insulin growth factor (IGF)
Somatostatin
  laboratory values, 349
Somatotropin-releasing inhibiting factor (SRIF), 5, 17
Somogyi phenomenon, 237
Soto syndrome, 78
Spironolactone, 312
SRIF, 5, 17
SRY gene, 134
Stadiometer, 45, 48*f*
StAR, 150
STAT, 5
Stature
  charts for age, 49
  juvenile rheumatoid arthritis, 62
  short. *See* Short stature
  tall. *See* Tall stature
Stature-for-age
  girls, 61*f*

Steroid acute regulatory protein (StAR), 150
Steroid hormone, 8f, 9
Steroids
  biosynthetic pathways, 138f
  withdrawal, 208
Stimulatory tests, 72
Stretch receptors, 26
Subacute thyroiditis, 108
Subarachnoid cysts, 22
Subcutaneous insulin
  administration, 231f
Substance abuse
  maternal, 66
Subtotal thyroidectomy
  hyperthyroidism, 104
Summer camps
  type 1 diabetes mellitus (insulin-dependent diabetes mellitus), 242
Suppurative thyroiditis, 108
Sweet urine, 29
Syndrome of inappropriate secretion of ADH (SIADH), 27, 39–42
  diagnosis, 40–41
  hyponatremia, 303–304
  treatment, 41–42
Synthetic thyroxine
  congenital hypothyroidism, 96–97

T

T3 (triiodothyronine), 85
  laboratory values
    free, 349
    radioimmunoassay, 350
    reverse, 349
    serum, 350
T4 (thyroxine), 85, 92, 93, 96
  acquired hypothyroidism, 100–101
  doses by age, 97t
  laboratory values
    binding proteins, 350–351
    direct dialysis serum, 351–352
    electrophoresis, 351
    nondialysis serum, 352
    total serum, 352
  synthetic
    congenital hypothyroidism, 96–97
Tall stature, 77–81
  cause, 78t
  childhood obesity, 255
  diagnosis, 81
  endocrine causes, 80–81
  nonendocrine causes, 77–80
  treatment, 81
Target height
  calculation, 61f
TBG, 85
TBPA, 85
TEE, 252
Television watching
  obesity, 263
Temporary delayed puberty, 167–170
Testes
  fetus, 140

Testicular enzyme defects, 150–153
Testicular feminization, 152
Testicular Leydig cell tumors, 290
Testolactone, 193
Testosterone, 136
  delayed puberty, 181
  fetus, 140
  laboratory values
    serum, 353–354
    total serum, 352–353
TH. *See* Thyroid hormone (TH)
Thecoma
  ovaries, 291
Thelarche
  premature, 190–191
Thiazide
  inducing hypercalcemia, 129–130
  nephrogenic diabetes insipidus, 39
Thirst, 28
Thyroglobulin antibody
  serum
    laboratory values, 354
Thyroglossal duct cyst
  familial, 100
Thyroid-binding globulin (TBG), 85
Thyroidectomy, 108
Thyroid gland
  adenomas, 106
  anatomy and physiology, 83–87
  autoimmune disease, 99
  carcinoma, 89
    follicular, 107
  disorders, 83–108
  dysgenesis, 83, 94
  enlargement
    etiology, 88t
  function
    type 1 diabetes mellitus, 242
  laboratory evaluation, 85–87
  neoplasms, 106–107
  painful, 108
  radioiodine scanning, 86
  ultrasonographic scanning, 86
Thyroid hormone (TH), 59
  composition, 85
  fetal serum concentration, 92–93
  production, 83
  receptors, 9
  resistance, 95
Thyroid hormonogenesis, 94
Thyroiditis
  subacute, 108
  suppurative, 108
Thyroid peroxidase antibody
  serum
    laboratory values, 354
Thyroid releasing factor (TRF), 5
Thyroid stimulating hormone (TSH), 5, 83, 92, 94, 96, 100, 118
  assay, 85–87
  hyperthyroidism, 101
  serum
    laboratory values, 354–355

AAO-9050

Thyroid stimulating immunoglobulins (TSI)
  laboratory values, 355
Thyroid storm, 104, 105, 299–300
Thyroid uptake, 87
Thyrotoxicosis, 80
Thyrotropin releasing factor, 83
Thyrotropin-releasing hormone (TRH), 83
  deficiency, 95
  laboratory values, 354–355
Thyroxin, 17
Thyroxine. *See* T4 (thyroxine)
Thyroxine-binding globulin, 95
  serum
    laboratory values, 355
Thyroxine-binding prealbumin (TBPA), 85
Total energy expenditure (TEE), 252
Transient hyperparathyroidism
  neonates, 129
Transient hyperthyrotropinemia, 96
Transsphenoidal microsurgery, 20
  Cushing disease, 213
TRF, 5
TRH, 83
  deficiency, 95
  laboratory values, 354–355
Triiodothyronine. *See* T3 (triiodothyronine)
Trousseau sign, 113
TSH. *See* Thyroid stimulating hormone (TSH)
TSI
  laboratory values, 355
Turner syndrome, 67, 72, 99, 136, 149, 174–175, 178, 185
Type 1 diabetes mellitus (insulin-dependent diabetes mellitus), 218–246
  clinical presentation, 221–222, 221*f*
  diabetic ketoacidosis, 222–229
  dietary management, 235–236
  environmental factors, 220
  honeymoon period, 240
  hypoglycemia, 240
  insulin therapy, 230–236
  long-term management, 229–238
  sick day management, 236–237
  summer camps, 242
  thyroid function, 242
  without diabetic ketoacidosis, 229
Type 2 diabetes mellitus (noninsulin-dependent diabetes mellitus), 244–246
  African Americans, 244
  childhood obesity, 254
  obesity, 244

Type 1 polyglandular syndrome, 202
Type 2 polyglandular syndrome, 202

U
Uniparental disomy (UPD), 67
UPD, 67
Upper-to-lower-segment ratio, 57*f*
Urinary tract infection, 34

V
Vanillylmandelic acid (VMA), 290
  laboratory values
    24-hour urine, 356
    random urine, 355–356
Vasopressin, 5, 312–313
  biologic effects, 27–28
  metabolic disorders, 29–43
  normal physiology, 29–30
  salts, 28
  secretion, 43
Velocardiofacial syndrome, 116–117
Virilization, 140, 290
  genetic females, 142–147
  genetic male, 150
Vitamin D, 110
  serum
    laboratory values, 356
Vitamin D2, 307
Vitamin D3 (cholecalciferol), 110
Vitamin D-dependency rickets, 124–125
Vitamin D-resistant rickets, 124–125
VMA. *See* Vanillylmandelic acid (VMA)
Voided urine sample, 3
Von Hippel-Lindau disease, 294

W
Water
  regulation, 27*f*
Water-deprivation test, 34*t*
Weaver syndrome, 79
Weight
  gestational age, 15
Weight-for-age
  boys, 50*f*
  girls, 51*f*
Weight loss, 173–174
Weight management, 260–262, 261*f*
Werner syndrome, 217, 291
Williams syndrome, 130
Wolman disease, 202

X
X chromosome, 135*f*
X-linked hypophosphatemia, 125

Y
Y chromosome, 134, 135*f*